AF449430

Diseases of the Esophagus

Volume II
Benign Diseases

Editors:

Alex G. Little, M.D.
Chairman, Department of Surgery
University of Nevada School of Medicine
Las Vegas, Nevada

Mark K. Ferguson, M.D.
Chief, Section of Thoracic Surgery
Department of Surgery
The University of Chicago
Chicago, Illinois

David B. Skinner, M.D.
President, New York Hospital
Cornell Medical Center
New York, New York

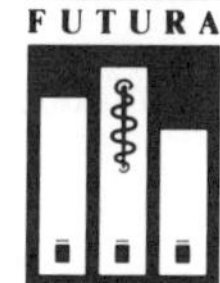

**Futura Publishing
Company, Inc.**
Mount Kisco, NY
1990

Library of Congress Cataloging-in-Publication Data

Diseases of the esophagus / editors, Mark K. Ferguson, Alex G. Little,
   David B. Skinner.
        p.   cm.
     Based on the Fourth World Congress of the International Society
   for Diseases of the Esophagus, held Sept. 6–8, 1989 in Chicago, Ill.
     Includes bibliographical references.
     Contents: Vol. 1 Malignant diseases — v. 2. Benign diseases /
   editors, Alex G. Little, Mark K. Ferguson, David B. Skinner.
     ISBN 0-87993-367-4 (v.   1). — ISBN 0-87993-368-2 (v.   2)
     1. Esophagus—Diseases—Congresses.   2. Esophagus—Cancer—
   —Congresses.   I. Ferguson, Mark K. II. Little, Alex G.
   III. Skinner, David B., 1935-   .   IV. International Society for
   Diseases of the Esophagus. Congress (4th : 1989 : Chicago, Ill.)
     [DNLM: 1. Esophageal Diseases—congresses.   WI 250 D61105 1989]
   RC815.7.D574   1990
   616.3'2—dc20
   DNLM/DLC
   for Library of Congress   90-2918
                                                                      CPI

Copyright   1990

Futura Publishing Company, Inc.

Published by:
   Futura Publishing Company, Inc.
   2 Bedford Ridge Road, P.O. Box 330
   Mount Kisco, New York 10549

LC #: 90-2918
ISBN #: 0-87993-368-2

Every effort has been made to ensure that the information in this book is as up to
date and as accurate as possible at the time of publication. However, due to the
constant developments in medicine, neither the author, nor the editor, nor the
publisher can accept any legal or any other responsibility for any errors or omissions
that may occur.

All rights reserved.

No part of this book may be translated or reproduced in any form without the written
permission of the publisher.

Printed in the United States of America.

To Louise, Ashley, and Jody,
  without whose support this book
  would not have been possible.

Alex G. Little

To Phyllis,
  for her patient support and understanding.

Mark K. Ferguson

To the many Residents and Fellows
  who have contributed so much to our work
  on esophageal diseases over the past 20 years.

David B. Skinner

Contributors

Ian Adams, B.Sc.
Regional Department of Thoracic Surgery, East Birmingham Hospital, Birmingham, England

R. Peter Altman, M.D.
Department of Surgery, The Babies Hospital, Columbia-Presbyterian Medical Center, New York, New York

P. Alziar, M.D.
Department of Thoracic Surgery, Hopital Salvator, Marseilles, France

Antonino Appignani, M.D.
Department of Pediatric Surgery, Bologna University, Bologna, Italy

R. Arca
Department of Surgery, University of Rome-Tor Vergata, Rome, Italy

Massimo Asolati, M.D.
The First Department of Surgery, University of Padua Medical School, Padua, Italy

Stephen E. A. Attwood, M.D.
Creighton University School of Medicine, Department of Surgery, Omaha, Nebraska

L. Backman, M.D., Ph.D.
Department of Surgery, Danderyd's Hospital, Danderyd, Sweden

Marco Baessato, M.D.
The First Department of Surgery, University of Padua Medical School, Padua, Italy

B. Bake, M.D., Ph.D.
Department of Clinical Physiology, Sahlgrens Hospital, Gothenburg, Sweden

Christopher S. Ball, M.D.
Royal Lancaster Infirmary, Lancaster, England

John Bancewicz, Ch.M.
University of Manchester, Department of Surgery, Hope Hospital, Salford, England

Romeo Bardini, M.D.
The First Department of Surgery, University of Padua Medical School, Padua, Italy

Antony P. Barlow, M.D.
Creighton University School of Medicine, Department of Surgery, Omaha, Nebraska

C. Thomas Bombeck, M.D.
Professor, Department of Surgery, University of Illinois, Chicago, Illinois

Luigi Bonavina, M.D.
The First Department of Surgery, University of Padua Medical School, Padua, Italy

Rudolf Bumm, M.D.
Department of Surgery, Klinikum rechts der Isar, Muenchen, Federal Republic of Germany

P. J. Byrne, M.Sc.
Department of Surgery, St. James Hospital, Dublin, Ireland

A. Caamano, M.D.
Department of Thoracic Surgery, Hôpital Salvator, Marseilles, France

Alan J. Cameron, M.D.
Mayo Clinic, Rochester, Minnesota

P. Campan, M.D.
Department of Thoracic Surgery, Hôpital Salvator, Marseilles, France

David N. Campbell, M.D.
Department of Surgery, University of Colorado Health Sciences Center, Denver, Colorado

M. Caporossi, M.D.
Policlinico Umberto I, I Istituto di Clinica Chirugica, Rome, Italy

N. J. H. Carroll, Ph.D.
Astra Clinical Research Unit, Edinburgh, Scotland

P. Carvalho, M.D.
University of Illinois Hospital, Chicago, Illinois

Ivan Cecconello, M.D.
Digestive Surgery Department, Sao Paulo University School of Medicine, Sao Paulo, Brazil

Suriya Chakkaphak, M.D.
Ramathibodi Hospital, Bankok, Thailand

P. Addario Chieco
Department of Surgery, University of Rome-Tor Vergata, Rome, Italy

R. Christiaens, M.D.
Department of Surgery, Catholic University, Leuven, Belgium

D. Colin-Jones, M.D.
Department of Medicine, Queen Alexandra Hospital, Portsmouth, United Kingdom

P. J. Collins, M.D.
Department of Surgery, Royal Adelaide Hospital, Adelaide, Australia

W. Coosemans, M.D.
Department of Surgery, Catholic University, Leuven, Belgium

F. Cuan-Orozco
Department of Surgery and Medicine, Heinz-Kalk Hospital, Bad Kissingen, West Germany

Antonio Cusumano, M.D.
The First Department of Surgery, University of Padua Medical School, Padua, Italy

Isi Dab, M.D.
Department of Pediatrics, Respiratory and Cystic Fibrosis Clinic, University Hospital VUB, Brussels, Belgium

Thomas C. B. Dehn, M.S.
Department of Surgery, John Radcliffe Hospital, Oxford, England

Tom R. DeMeester, M.D.
Professor and Chairman, Department of Surgery, Creighton University School of Medicine, Omaha, Nebraska

C. Deschamps
Department of Surgery, University of Montreal, Montreal, Canada

R. Dom, M.D.
Laboratory of Neuropathology, Catholic University, Leuven, Belgium

Remigio Dòmini, M.D.
Department of Pediatric Surgery, Bologna University, Bologna, Italy

Philip E. Donahue, M.D.
Professor of Surgery, University of Illinois, Chicago, Illinois

B. Dupin, M.D.
Department of Thoracic Surgery, Hopital Salvator, Marseilles, France

André Duranceau, M.D.
Department of Thoracic Surgery, Hotel-Dieu de Montreal, University of Montreal, Montreal, Quebec, Canada

L. Durif, M.D.
Department of Thoracic Surgery, Hopital Salvator, Marseilles, France

F. Henry Ellis, Jr., M.D., Ph.D.
Senior Surgical Consultant, Department of Thoracic and Cardiovascular Surgery, Lahey Clinic Medical Center, Burlington, Massachusetts; Chief, Division of Thoracic and Cardiovascular Surgery, New England Deaconess Hospital; Clinical Professor of Surgery, Harvard Medical School, Boston, Massachusetts

viii / CONTRIBUTORS

Carsten Emde, M.D.
Department of Surgery, Klinikum rechts der Isar, Muenchen, Federal Republic of Germany

L.-C. Enander, M.D.
Department of Surgery, Central Hospital, Karlstad, Sweden

G. Etienne, M.D.
Department of Digestive Surgery, Hôpital Beaujon, Paris, France

Ernst P. Eypasch, M.D.
Department of Surgery, Creighton University School of Medicine, Omaha, Nebraska

W. H. Falor, M.D.
Akron City Hospital, Akron, Ohio

S. W. Fannin, M.D.
Akron City Hospital, Akron, Ohio

O. Farges, M.D.
Department of Digestive Surgery, Hôpital Beaujon, Paris, France

O. Fausa, M.D., Ph.D.
Department of Medicine, Rikshospitalet, Oslo, Norway

Françoise Fékété, M.D.
Department of Digestive Surgery, Hôpital Beaujon, Paris, France

Mark K. Ferguson, M.D.
Associate Professor of Surgery, Chief, Section of Thoracic Surgery, The University of Chicago, Chicago, Illinois

Hubertus Feussner, M.D.
Department of Surgery, Technical University of Munich, Munich, Federal Republic of Germany

Valentino Fontebasso, B.S.
The First Department of Surgery, University of Padua Medical School, Padua, Italy

William O. Frank, M.D.
Clinical Development–North America, Smith Kline and French Laboratories, Philadelphia, Pennsylvania

Brice Gayet, M.D.
Department of Digestive Surgery, Hôpital Beaujon, Paris, France

K. Geboes, M.D.
Laboratory of Histochemistry and Cytochemistry, Catholic University, Leuven, Belgium

Zoran Gerzic, M.D., Ph.D.
Professor of Surgery, Director, Center for Esophageal Surgery, Institute for Digestive Diseases, University Clinical Center–Belgrade, Center for Esophageal Surgery, Belgrade, Yugoslavia

S. Peter Gibb, M.D.
Chairman, Department of Gastroenterology, Lahey Clinic Medical Center, Burlington, Massachusetts

P. Gillen, M.Ch.
Department of Surgery, St. James Hospital, Dublin, Ireland

P. Ginevri
Department of Surgery, University of Rome-Tor Vergata, Rome, Italy

Margherita Giocoli, M.D.
Clinical Pediatrica II, University of Bari, Bari, Italy

H. G. Gooszen, M.D.
Department of Surgery, University Hospital Leiden, Leiden, The Netherlands

T. F. Gorey, M.Ch.
Department of Surgery, St. James Hospital, Dublin, Ireland

V. Greczanik, B.S.
Akron, Ohio

Giovanni Grillone, M.D.
Department of Anesthesia and Intensive Care, Bologna University, Bologna, Italy

Jacques Aime Gruwez, M.D.
Department of Surgery, Catholic University, Leuven, Belgium

P. Guelinckx, M.D.
Department of Surgery, Catholic University, Leuven, Belgium

Roberta J. Hall, M.D.
Department of Surgery, University of Colorado Health Sciences Center, Denver, Colorado

Jean Marie Hay, M.D.
French University Association for Surgical Research, Bois-Colombes, France

T. P. J. Hennessy, M.Ch.
Department of Surgery, St. James Hospital, Dublin, Ireland

Arnulf H. Hölscher, M.D.
Department of Surgery, Klinikum rechts der Isar, Muenchen, Federal Republic of Germany

Arnulf H. Hölscher, M.D.
Department of Surgery, Technical University of Munich, Munich, Federal Republic of Germany

Wolfgang Holzgreve, M.D.
Zentrum fur Frauenheilkunde, Westf. Wilhelms-Universitat Munster, Munster, Austria

Joost M. L. M. Horbach, M.D.
Department of Surgery, University Hospital Leiden, Leiden, The Netherlands

M. Horowitz, M.D.
Department of Surgery, Royal Adelaide Hospital, Adelaide, Australia

Clemente Iascone, M.D.
Associate Professor of Surgery, I Department of Surgery, University of Rome-La Sapienza, Rome, Italy

Jouko Isolauri, M.D.
Department of Surgery, Technical University of Munich, Munich, Federal Republic of Germany

Mannon Jadliwalla, M.D.
Department of Thoracic Surgery, Hotel-Dieu de Montreal, University of Montreal, Montreal, Quebec, Canada

Glyn Garfield Jamieson, M.D.
Department of Surgery, Royal Adelaide Hospital, Adelaide, Australia

E. H. Jansen, M.D.
Department of Gastroenterology, University Hospital Leiden, Leiden, The Netherlands

J. B. M. J. Jansen, M.D.
Department of Gastroenterology, University Hospital Leiden, Leiden, The Netherlands

Harry Jenkins, M.D.
Department of Surgery, Creighton University School of Medicine, Omaha, Nebraska

Lloyd R. Jenkinson, M.D.
Royal Lancaster Infirmary, Lancaster, England

E. Jones, M.D.
Department of Pathology, St. James Hospital, Dublin, Ireland

J.-Fr. Kalk, M.D.
Department of Surgery and Medicine, Heinz-Kalk Hospital, Bad Kissingen, West Germany

Mardi R. Karin, M.D.
Department of Surgery, University of Iowa Hospitals and Clinics, Iowa City, Iowa

M. G. W. Kettlewell, M. Chir.
Department of Surgery, John Radcliffe Hospital, Oxford, England

Jelena Knezevic, M.D.
Attending Surgeon, Institute for Digestive Diseases, University Clinical Center–Belgrade, Center for Esophageal Surgery, Belgrade, Yugoslavia

P. Koussouris, M.D.
Department of Surgery and Medicine, Heinz-Kalk Hospital, Bad Kissingen, West Germany

J. M. Kraus, M.D.
Akron City Hospital, Akron, Ohio

Edwin Lafontaine, M.D.
Department of Thoracic Surgery, Hotel-Dieu de Montreal, University of Montreal, Montreal, Quebec, Canada

C. B. H. W. Lamers, M.D.
Department of Gastroenterology, University Hospital Leiden, Leiden, The Netherlands

Toni Lerut, M.D.
Department of Surgery, Catholic University, Leuven, Belgium

John R. Lilly, M.D.
Department of Surgery, University of Colorado Health Sciences Center, Denver, Colorado

Mario Lima, M.D.
Department of Pediatric Surgery, Bologna University, Bologna, Italy

T. Lind, M.D., Ph.D.
Department of Medicine, Rikshospitalet, Oslo, Norway

Alex G. Little, M.D.
Chairman, Department of Surgery, University of Nevada School of Medicine, Las Vegas, Nevada

H. Lönroth, M.D.
Department of Medicine, Rikshospitalet, Oslo, Norway

Lars Lundell, M.D., Ph.D.
Department of Surgery, Sahlgren's Hospital, University of Gothenburg, Gothenburg, Sweden

G. L. Maddern, M.D.
Department of Surgery, Royal Adelaide Hospital, Adelaide, Australia

C. Maffi, M.D.
Policlinico Umberto I, I Istituto di Clinica Chirurgica, Rome, Italy

James W. Maher, M.D.
Department of Surgery, University of Iowa Hospitals and Clinics, Iowa City, Iowa

Alfonso M. Maiorana, M.D.
Hospital Policlinico, Clinica Chirurgica, Palermo, Italy

Anne Malfroot, M.D.
Department of Pediatrics, Respiratory and Cystic Fibrosis Clinic, University Hospital VUB, Brussels, Belgium

M. Maragakis, M.D.
Klinik und Poliklinik fur Kinderund, Neugeborenenchirurgie, Westf. Wilhelms-Universitat, Munster, West Germany

Luis A. Martinez, M.D.
Department of Surgery, University of Colorado Health Sciences Center, Denver, Colorado

Hugoe R. Matthews, M.D.
Regional Department of Thoracic Surgery, East Birmingham Hospital, Bordesley Green East, Birmingham, England

J. A. McGuigan, M.D.
Regional Department of Thoracic Surgery, East Birmingham Hospital, Bordesley Green East, Birmingham, England

James E. McGuigan, M.D.
Department of Medicine, University of Florida, Gainesville, Florida

J. Mebis, M.D.
Laboratory of Histochemistry and Cytochemistry, Catholic University, Leuven, Belgium

M. A. Mercado, M.D.
Department of Surgery and Medicine, Heinz-Kalk Hospital, Bad Kissingen, West Germany

Stefano Merigliano, M.D.
The First Department of Surgery, University of Padua Medical School, Padua, Italy

I. Miidla, M.D.
University of Illinois Hospital, Chicago, Illinois

Miroslav Milicevic, M.D., Ph.D.
Associate Professor of Surgery, Institute for Digestive Diseases, University Clinical Center–Belgrade, Center for Esophageal Surgery, Belgrade, Yugoslavia

J. M. Miller, M.D.
Akron City Hospital, Akron, Ohio

I. M. Mitchell, M.D.
Regional Department of Thoracic Surgery, East Birmingham Hospital, Bordesley Green East, Birmingham, England

Aldo Moraldi, M.D.
Associate Professor of Surgery, Department of Surgery, University of Rome-Tor Vergata, Rome, Italy

J. C. Myers, M.D.
Department of Surgery, Royal Adelaide Hospital, Adelaide, Australia

Ary Nasi, M.D.
Digestive Surgery Department, Sao Paulo University School of Medicine, Sao Paulo, Brazil

Michel J. Noirclerc, M.D.
Department of Thoracic Surgery, Hôpital Salvator, Marseilles, France

N. Nolan, M.R.C. Path.
Department of Pathology, St. James Hospital, Dublin, Ireland

Lorenzo Norberto, M.D.
The First Department of Surgery, University of Padua Medical School, Padua, Italy

Tracey L. Norris, B.Sc.
Royal Lancaster Infirmary, Lancaster, England

Lloyd M. Nyhus, M.D.
Professor and Chairman, Department of Surgery, Chicago, Illinois

Tim O'Hanrahan, M.D.
University of Manchester, Department of Surgery, Hope Hospital, Salford, England

L. Olbe, M.D., Ph.D.
Department of Surgery, Sahlgrens Hospital, Gothenburg, Sweden

Mark B. Orringer, M.D.
Professor and Head, Section of Thoracic Surgery, University of Michigan Medical Center, Ann Arbor, Michigan

Robert H. Palmer, M.D.
Clinical Development–North America, Smith Kline and French Laboratories, Philadelphia, Pennsylvania

Giovanni I. Pappagallo, M.D.
Clinical Trials Unit, University of Padua Medical School, Padua, Italy

K.-J. Paquet, M.D.
Department of Surgery and Medicine, Heinz-Kalk Hospital, Bad Kissingen, West Germany

Maurizio Pavanello, M.D.
The First Department of Surgery, University of Padua Medical School, Padua, Italy

E. Pellerin, M.D.
Department of Thoracic Surgery, Hotel-Dieu de Montreal, University of Montreal, Montreal, Quebec, Canada

Alberto Peracchia, M.D.
The First Department of Surgery, University of Padua Medical School, Padua, Italy

M. Piccio
Department of Surgery, University of Rome-Tor Vergata, Rome, Italy

Henrique Walter Pinotti, M.D.
Digestive Surgery Department, Sao Paulo University School of Medicine, Sao Paulo, Brazil

Didier Pottier, M.D.
French University Association for Surgical Research, Bois-Colombes, France

W. Rambach, M.D.
Department of Surgery and Medicine, Heinz-Kalk Hospital, Bad Kissingen, West Germany

Giovanni Ruggeri, M.D.
Department of Pediatric Surgery, Bologna University, Bologna, Italy

Alberto Ruol, M.D.
The First Department of Surgery, University of Padua Medical School, Padua, Italy

M. Ruth, M.D.
Department of Otorhinolaryngology, Sahlgrens Hospital, Gothenburg, Sweden

N. Sandberg, M.D., Ph.D.
Department of Otorhinolaryngology, Sahlgrens Hospital, Gothenburg, Sweden

Anthony D. Sandler, M.D.
Department of Surgery, University of Iowa Hospitals and Clinics, Iowa City, Iowa

S. Sandmark, M.D., Ph.D.
Department of Otorhinolaryngology, Regionsjukhuset, Orebro, Sweden

B. Sandzén, M.D.
Department of Surgery, University Hospital, Umea, Sweden

Jerry F. Schlegel, B.S.
Department of Surgery, University of Iowa Hospitals and Clinics, Iowa City, Iowa

Philippe Segol
French University Association for Surgical Research, Bois-Colombes, France

U. Seligsson, M.D.
Department of Surgery, Sodersjukhuset, Stockholm, Sweden

Y.-S. Shen, M.D.
University of Chicago Hospital, Chicago, Illinois

H. A. Shepherd, M.D.
Department of Medicine, Royal Hampshire County Hospital, Winchester, England

F. Siemens, M.D.
Department of Surgery and Medicine, Heinz-Kalk Hospital, Bad Kissingen, West Germany

Jörg Ruediger Siewert, M.D.
Department of Surgery, Technical University of Munich, Munich, Federal Republic of Germany

David B. Skinner, M.D.
President, New York Hospital, Cornell Medical Center, New York, New York

C. Söderlund, M.D.
Department of Surgery, Sodersjukhuset, Stockholm, Sweden

Thomas C. Smyrk, M.D.
Departments of Surgery and Pathology, Creighton University School of Medicine, Omaha, Nebraska

Hubert J. Stein, M.D.
Department of Surgery, Creighton University School of Medicine, Omaha, Nebraska

Sergio Stipa, M.D.
Chief of Surgery, I Department of Surgery, University of Rome-La Sapienza, Rome, Italy

R. C. Stuart, M.D.
Department of Surgery, St. James Hospital, Dublin, Ireland

Raymond Taillefer, M.D.
Department of Nuclear Medicine, Hotel-Dieu de Montreal, University of Montreal, Montreal, Quebec, Canada

B. C. Taylor, Ph.D.
Bio-Engineering Research Center, University of Akron, Akron, Ohio

Ermanno Tiso, M.D.
The First Department of Surgery, University of Padua Medical School, Padua, Italy

S. Törngren, M.D.
Department of Surgery, Sodersjukhuset, Stockholm, Sweden

P. Unge, M.D.
Department of Medicine, Sanvikens Hospital, Sandvileen, Sweden

P. Van Clooster, M.D.
Department of Surgery, Catholic University, Leuven, Belgium

J. N. Van Leeuwen, M.D.
Department of Surgery, Catholic University, Leuven, Belgium

D. Van Raemdonck, M.D.
Department of Surgery, Catholic University, Leuven, Belgium

K. H. Vestweber, M.D.
University of Cologne, II Department of Surgery, Cologne, West Germany

Steven J. Walker, M.D.
East Birmingham Hospital, Birmingham, England

Anthony Watson, M.D.
Consultant Surgeon, Royal Lancaster Infirmary, Lancaster, England

I. H. Westin, B.Sc.
Clinical Pharmacology and Medicine, Ab Hassle, Molndal, Sweden

Jeffrey D. Wetherington, Ph.D.
Regulatory Affairs, Smith Kline and French Laboratories, Philadelphia, Pennsylvania

G. Heinrich Willital, M.D.
Klinik und Poliklinik fur Kinderund Neugeborenenchirurgie, Westf. Wilhelms-Universitat Munster, Munster, Austria

Michael D. Young, M.D., Ph.D.
Regulatory Affairs, Smith Kline and French Laboratories, Philadelphia, Pennsylvania

Guy Zeitoun, M.D.
French University Association for Surgical Research, Bois-Colombes, France

Bruno Zilberstein, M.D.
Digestive Surgery Department, Sao Paulo University School of Medicine, Sao Paulo, Brazil

Foreword

The fourth triennial congress of the International Society for Diseases of the Esophagus (ISDE) was successfully held in Chicago, Illinois, under the presidency of David B. Skinner, M.D. It included unforgettable events that particularly featured a well-organized and high-quality scientific program from which contributions were solicited for a publication representing the state-of-the-art of our understanding of esophageal physiology and pathology. I hope that the publication will make these efforts available to wider scientific readership in this field. I am also pleased that the ISDE is now firmly established and I am sure that we can look forward to even more development with the fifth congress.

Finally, I would like to express my heartfelt appreciation to Professor Skinner and his staff for their great contribution toward the huge success of the congress.

Kiyoshi Inokuchi, M.D.
The Immediate-past President of
International Society for
Diseases of the Esophagus

Preface

This book is made up of chapters based on presentations that were made at the Fourth World Congress of the International Society for Diseases of the Esophagus. From the 350 oral and poster presentations, the chapters in this book were specifically written for this publication. The goal of the editors was to focus on benign diseases of the esophagus, emphasizing primarily original and innovative material which addresses controversial and unsettled subjects in pathophysiology, diagnosis, and treatment of esophageal disease.

Selection from the material presented at the Congress has resulted in a book which reflects the viewpoints of international leaders from the several disciplines interested in the esophagus. On occasion, this has resulted in chapters which present differing opinions or disparate conclusions from similar material. This is the state of the art regarding esophageal diseases today and best provides the reader with a realistic understanding of current concepts. The editors have provided overviews of the different sections, providing some guidelines for interpretation and resolution of new and/or conflicting reports.

One clear implication of the design of this book is that it will be more useful to the clinician with some experience than to the novice. It will be of greater utility for someone interested in delving into specific and "cutting edge" information than for the student who wishes to acquire general information about settled areas.

Preparation of this book was possible only through the contributions of a large group of people. The leadership, identified on the following page, and members of the International Society of Diseases of the Esophagus both provided the chapters and orchestrated the world congress which facilitated interaction of international specialists. It is such an open exchange of ideas which actually permits development of a book such as this. In addition, the book would not have been possible without the continuing and unflagging dedication of Ms. Darlene Buczak who collected the manuscripts and kept the editors organized and Ms. Linda Shaw, our editor, who never lacked patience and whose editorial skills managed to remedy most of the failings of the editors.

Alex G. Little, M.D.
Mark K. Ferguson, M.D.
David B. Skinner, M.D.

Members of the Scientific Program Committee Fourth World Congress of the International Society for Diseases of the Esophagus

President: David B. Skinner, New York, New York

Steering:

Hiroshi Akiyama
Tokyo, Japan

Tom R. DeMeester
Omaha, Nebraska

André Duranceau
Montreal, Quebec, Canada

Mark K. Ferguson
Chicago, Illinois

E. Moreno Gonzalez
Madrid, Spain

Glyn G. Jamieson
Adelaide, Australia

Bernard Launois
Rennes, France

Toni Lerut
Leuven, Belgium

Alex G. Little
Las Vegas, Nevada

Hugoe R. Matthews
Birmingham, England

Alberto Peracchia
Padova, Italy

Charles S. Winans
Chicago, Illinois

John Wong
Hong Kong

Bruno Zilberstein
Sao Paulo, Brazil

Ex-Officio:

G. Castrini
Rome, Italy

M. Endo
Tokyo, Japan

Advisory:

C. Thomas Bombeck
Chicago, Illinois

Attila Csendes
Santiago, Chile

Henry F. Ellis
Boston, Massachusetts

François Fékété
Paris, France

Robert Giuli
Paris, France

Vincente Guarner
Mexico City, Mexico

Min-Hsiung Huang
Taipei, Taiwan, R.O.C.

Jean-Min Sheh
Taipei, Taiwan, R.O.C.

Mark B. Orringer
Ann Arbor, Michigan

Henrique Walter Pinotti
Sao Paulo, Brazil

Sergio Stipa
Rome, Italy

Anthony Watson
Lancaster, England

J. Rudiger Siewert
Munich, West Germany

K. Inokuchi
Saga-shi, Japan

K. Nabeya
Tokyo, Japan

Contents

I.

Congenital Disease:
Editors' Overview

The first two papers in this section deal with two important aspects of esophageal atresia. Chapter 1 discusses utilization of an amniotic fluid assay for acetylcholinesterase as a marker for esophageal atresia. Although there is not enough experience to accept this test as the definitive one which should become routine in the evaluation of polyhydramnios, it seems to be an assay with high specificity for esophageal atresia and its role should continue to be evaluated.

Chapter 2 deals with the pulmonary disorders that are seen in infants with esophageal atresia. This experience documents the frequency of severe pulmonary complications in the pre- and postoperative time periods in these infants. This study also emphasizes the importance of early diagnosis which serves to highlight the value of establishing the acetylcholinesterase assay as helpful in prenatal diagnosis.

Chapters 3 and 4 deal with congenital esophageal disorders that require surgical intervention. Trifurcation tracheoesophageal fistula is an unusual variant of esophageal atresia which is important to both pediatricians and pediatric surgeons. In particular, surgeons need to be aware of this possible anatomy and take the precautions outlined to be sure that surgical complications are avoided.

The final chapter in this section deals with indications, technique, and results of colon interposition in children. The most frequent diagnosis in this series is that of esophageal atresia. One important aspect of the surgical technique is the author's recommendation of flexibility of selection of the part of the colon which should be used. The decision should be based upon the vascularization pattern of the colon which is identified intraoperatively. Most frequently this results

1

in utilization of a segment of colon based upon the ascending branch of the left colic artery but on other occasions transverse or even right colon is more appropriate. It is clear from the results that this procedure can be performed with very low mortality and acceptable long-term function.

Improved Method for Prenatal Diagnosis of Esophageal Atresia

Wolfgang Holzgreve, M. Maragakis,
G. Heinrich Willital

Introduction

Many congenital anomalies can now be detected prenatally early in pregnancy by sonography. In some of the fetal anatomic malformations, the diagnosis in utero influences the perinatal management, including the timing of delivery and preparation for an early correction after birth in a specialized pediatric surgery center.[1,2]

In esophageal atresia, prenatal diagnosis is important for two reasons. (1) Because of the known association between esophageal atresia and other anomalies,[3] for example, Vater association[4] or trisomies 18 and 13, an ultrasound examination suggesting esophageal atresia should alert the obstetrician to perform detailed sonographic evaluation and prenatal chromosome analysis. (2) By suspecting an esophageal atresia prenatally, the risk of accidental postpartum aspiration pneumonia due to improper feeding of the affected baby and metabolic disturbances caused by repeated vomiting can be decreased, and all necessary preparations for postnatal correction by an experienced surgical team can be performed.

Because the prenatal diagnosis of esophageal atresias by ultra-

Little AG, Ferguson MK, Skinner DB: Diseases of the Esophagus, Vol. II: Benign Diseases. Futura Publishing Company, Inc., Mount Kisco, NY, © 1990.

sound alone is still difficult and in some cases of tracheoesophageal fistula may be impossible, there is a need for additional tests such as the one described here.

Sonographic Findings

Hydramnios, sometimes also called "polyhydramnios," can be defined either semiquantitavely by invasive dilutional techniques or clinically by the estimation of amniotic fluid volume. Sonographically, formulae for estimating amniotic fluid volume (taking the pockets of fluid in four quadrants into account) have been developed, but a simple clinical definition is that polyhydramnios can be diagnosed if there is enough space for an additional fetus within the amniotic cavity. The incidence of polyhydramnios is reported to vary between at least 0.4 and 1.5%[5,6] and can be suspected on clinical grounds if the uterus is bigger than expected at the calculated duration of pregnancy and if identification of the small parts of the fetus is difficult.

In about 40% of cases with polyhydramnios, fetal-placental abnormalities or maternal diabetes can be found.[7] In one series,[5] an even higher rate of developmental defects (83%) was detected in the presence of hydramnios.

About 40% of the total amount of water leaving the amniotic cavity goes through the fetus, and in esophageal atresia, accumulation of fluid in the stomach and proximal duodenum can be recognized easily from the classic finding of the "double bubble" phenomenon (Fig. 1).

Rare anomalies that may cause polyhydramnios, such as congenital neck teratoma and fetal diaphragmatic hernia, can be differentiated antenatally by ultrasound examination. The association between polyhydramnios and upper intestinal or esophageal obstruction was first recognized by Ehrlich from Tel Aviv.[8] Jeffcoate and Scott[9] found polyhydramnios in 12 out of 13 cases of esophageal atresia except for one case with an indirect communication of the upper and lower parts of the esophagus via the trachea. Lloyd and Clatworthy,[10] however, reported only seven cases of polyhydramnios in a series of 53 infants with esophageal atresia. Summarizing different series, it can be concluded that between 2% and 10% of infants without overt other anomalies, delivered from mothers with polyhydramnios, have a congenital esophageal obstruction.

Esophageal atresia is reported to occur once in every 1500 live

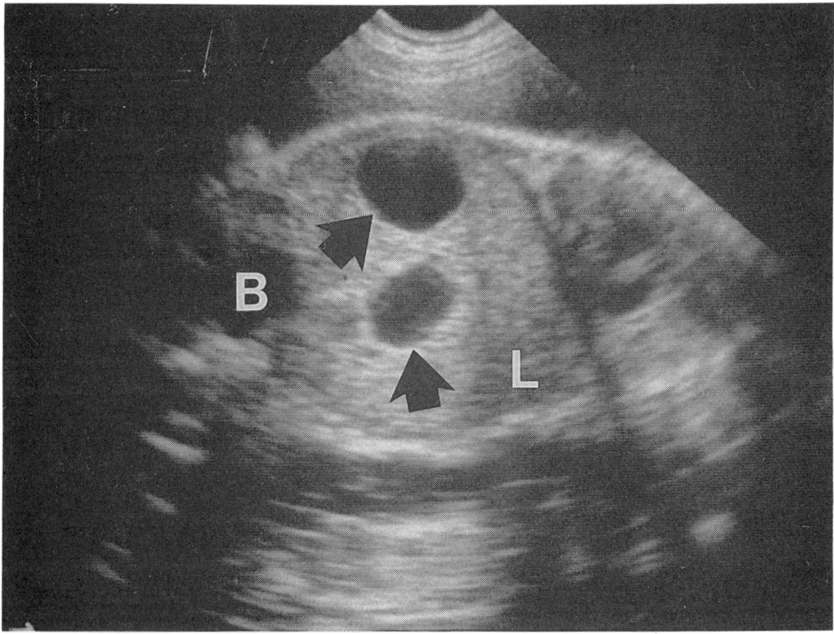

Figure 1: Longitudinal ultrasonogram of "double bubble" phenomenon (arrows) caused by dilated stomach and proximal duodenum in duodenal atresia (L = liver, B = bladder).

births, and only 1 in 15,000 has esophageal atresia with no fistula to the trachea.[11] In these cases, the correct prenatal diagnosis is easier because of the sonographically detectable lack of stomach fluid and a frequently found discrepancy in the ratio of abdominal diameter to head diameter[12] in addition to the polyhydramnios. In the remaining 90% of cases with tracheoesophageal fistulae, fluid can enter the stomach, thus making the sonographic diagnosis much more difficult or even impossible without additional techniques.

Prenatal diagnoses of esophageal atresias by ultrasound were first reported in 1981[13] and 1982.[14] In 1983 it was pointed out[15] that an additional ultrasound finding in esophageal atresia is the alternating filling and emptying of the esophagus proximal to the site of atresia. It is now easily possible to visualize the fetal mouth and it is well documented that fetal swallowing is a normal in utero activity (Fig. 2) that occurs intermittently with one or two movements per minute of different speed, and that in cases of esophageal atresia even "fetal vomiting" may be observed sonographically.[16,17]

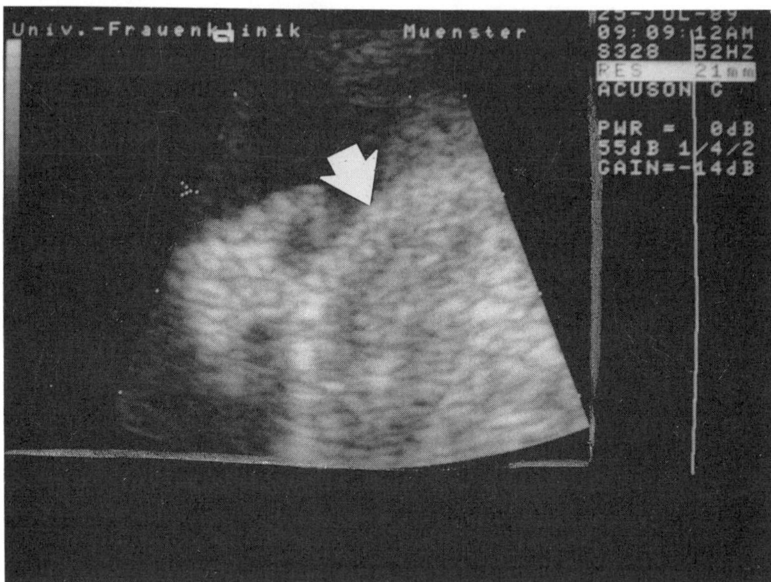

Figure 2: Ultrasonogram of closed fetal mouth (arrow). Note the fetal nose with nares on the left side of the picture.

Gestational Age at Time of Sonographic Diagnosis

From embryologic investigations it is known[18] that the primitive foregut is formed during the fourth fetal week, giving rise to the pharynx, larynx, trachea, lower respiratory system, and esophagus. The tracheoesophageal septum originally divides the traches from the esophagus and by the end of the embryonic period the trachea, hypopharynx, larynx, and esophagus have differentiated into their final form. Already by the middle of the second trimester the fetal hypopharynx, larynx, and trachea have attained adequate size so that they can be visualized on prenatal ultrasound examination.[18] The fetal esophagus may also be visualized before the 24th week of pregnancy and is readily apparent posterior to the trachea if it is distended.

In neonates with atresia of the midesophagus, which is the most common form of esophageal atresia, the distended proximal esophageal pouch displaces the upper trachea anteriorly so that a dilated fluid-filled esophagus can be visualized on lateral X-ray films.

Also prenatally, an intra-amniotic injection of a radiopaque dye sometimes shows the distended proximal esophageal pouch,[19] but in cases of esophageal atresia with tracheoesophageal fistula, the partial passage of the contrast medium into the fetal intestine may obscure the diagnosis.

Acetylcholinesterase Test for Detection of Esophageal Atresia

Because of the difficulties of reliably diagnosing esophageal atresia by ultrasonography and amniofetography, a simple and readily available biochemical marker present in amniotic fluid would be of great practical importance.

In 1983 we suggested amniotic fluid acetylcholinesterase as a possible marker for the prenatal diagnosis of esophageal atresia based on a case with a positive acetylcholinesterase test in the presence of polyhydramnios and fetal esophageal atresia.[20] The amniotic fluid alpha-fetoprotein (AFP) concentration was within the double median range by radioimmunoassay, and we suggested that this may have been an "artifact" caused by dilutional effect. This is supported by the observation that the AFP concentration in cases of esophageal atresia may either be increased[21] or found within the normal range depending on the degree of polyhydramnios.

In a subsequent study,[22] we retrospectively examined further samples of clear amniotic fluid obtained at second trimester amniocenteses of three pregnancies, each of which proved to be complicated by upper gastrointestinal atresia. Two of these cases had a positive fast-running acetylcholinesterase band on polyacrylamide gel electrophoresis and normal AFP concentrations. We have now evaluated a total of 14 pregnancies with esophageal atresia, and only three with tracheoesophageal fistula did not have an acetylcholinesterase band on electrophoresis (Table I). We therefore conclude that in cases of polyhydramnios without another explanation for its origin, amniocentesis is indicated not only to search for a possible chromosomal etiology but also to determine the presence of acetylcholinesterase.

In neural tube defects, the demonstration of AChE is associated with AFP increases whereas this is characteristically not true for obstructions of the upper intestinal tract (Table I).

It is of interest that in opposition to suspected neural tube defects and other disorders, fetal esophageal atresia is the only situation where AChE testing offers significantly more information than the quick, accurate, and economic AFP testing.

Table I
Polyhydramnios and Obstructions of the Upper Intestinal Tract

Diagnosis	n	AFP		AChE	
		Incr.	*Normal*	+	−
Esophageal atresia	14	3	11	11	3
Duodenal stenosis	7	1	6	4	2
Stenosis of the ileum/ jejunum	3	1	2	1	2
Total	24			16	

As with other congenital anomalies, the incidence of esophageal atresia detected in prenatal diagnosis programs is probably higher than the figures quoted in the pediatric or surgical literature because some children with esophageal atresias and associated anomalies, e.g., chromosomal aneuploidies, may never enter any pediatric surgery series.

References

1. Harrison MR, Golbus MS, Filly RA: The unborn patient: Prenatal Diagnosis and Treatment. Orlando/San Diego/San Francisco, Grune & Stratton, 1984.
2. Golbus MS, Holzgreve W, Harrison MR: Intrauterine Direktbehandlung des Feten. Gynäkologe 17:62, 1984.
3. Szendrey T, Danyi G, Czeizel A: Etiological study on isolated esophageal atresia. Hum Genet 70:51, 1985.
4. Knudtzon J, Jordheim O, Smedsrud B: Twins discordant for Vater association: Obstructed labor of second twin due to ascites and persistent cloaca without communication to the exterior. Acta Obstet Gynecol Scand 65:185, 1986.
5. Quinlan RW, Cruz AC, Martin M: Hydramnios: Ultrasound diagnosis and its impact on perinatal management and pregnan-outcome. Am J Obstet Gynecol 145:306, 1983.
6. Zamah NM, Gillieson MS, Walters JH, Hall PF: Sonographic detection of polyhydramnios: A five-year experience. Am J Obstet Gynecol 143:523, 1982.
7. Wallenburg HCS, Wladimiroff JW: The amniotic fluid. II. Polyhydramnios and oligohydramnios. J Perinat Med 6:233, 1977.

8. Ehrlich AW: Der diagnostische Wert des Hydramnion für die Erkenntnis hochsitzender, kongenitaler Verschlüsse des Verdauungstrakts. Ann Pediatr 199:596, 1962.

9. Jeffcoate TNA, Scott JS: Polyhydramnios and oligohydramnios. Can Med Assoc J 80:77, 1959.

10. Lloyd JR, Clatworthy HW: Hydramnios as an aid to the early diagnosis of congenital obstruction of the alimentary tract. Pediatrics 21:903, 1958.

11. Farrant P: The antenatal diagnosis of esophageal atresia by ultrasound. Br J Radiol 52:1202, 1980.

12. Pretorius DH, Meier PR, Johnson ML: Diagnosis of esophageal atresia in utero. J Ultrasound Med 2:475, 1983.

13. Zemlyn S: Prenatal detection of esophageal atresia. Clin Ultrasound 9:453, 1981.

14. Jassani MN, Gauderer MWL, Fanaroff AA, Fletcher B, Markatz IR: A perinatal approach to the diagnosis and management of gastrointestinal malformations. Obstet Gynecol 59:33, 1982.

15. Eyheremendy E, Phister M: Antenatal real-time diagnosis of esophageal atresias. J Clin Ultrasound II:395:1983.

16. Bowie JP, Clair MR: Fetal swallowing and regurgitation: Observation of normal and abnormal activity. Radiology 144:877, 1982.

17. Utsu M, Sahahibara S, Ishida T, Chiba Y, Hasegawa T: Dynamics of tracheal fluid flow in the human fetus, studied with pulsed Doppler ultrasound. Acta Obstet Gynecol Jpn 35:2017, 1983.

18. Moore KL: The Developing Human. Philadelphia, W.B. Saunders, 1974.

19. Cooper C, Mahoney BS, Bowie JP, Albright RT, Callen PW: Ultrasound evaluation of the normal fetal upper airway and esophagus. J Ultrasound Med 4:343, 1985.

20. Holzgreve W, Beller FK, Pawlowitzki IH: Amniotic fluid acetylcholinesterase as a marker in prenatal diagnosis of esophageal atresia. Am J Obstet Gynecol 145:641, 1983.

21. Seppälä M: Increased alpha-fetoprotein in amniotic fluid associated with a congenital esophageal atresia of the fetus. Obstet Gynecol 42:613, 1973.

22. Holzgreve W, Golbus MS: Amniotic fluid acetylcholinesterase as a prenatal diagnostic marker for upper gastrointestinal atresias. Am J Obstet Gynecol 147:837, 1983.

2

Pulmonary Aspects in Esophageal Atresia

Toni Lerut, P. Van Clooster, J. N. Van Leeuwen,
Jacques A. Gruwez

Introduction

Over the last decades, surgical correction of esophageal atresia (EA) has been characterized by a steady improvement in survival. Today a baby born with esophageal atresia has a virtual 100% chance of survival provided there are no associated congenital anomalies or pulmonary pathology. Consequently more attention has been paid to the quality of survival especially related to esophageal and/or pulmonary symptoms.[1] In view of this perspective, our patient material has been analyzed more specifically in relation to its pulmonary aspects. From 1967 until 1987, 136 patients have been treated for one of the classic forms of esophageal atresia (Fig. 1). This series is divided into two equal groups: group I (1967–1980) 69 patients; group II (1981–1987) 67 patients, allowing comparison of progress over the years. According to birthweight, seriousness of associated congenital anomalies and pulmonary condition patients are classified in Waterston's classification (Table I).[2]

Results

An early diagnosis is of paramount importance as patients with EA quickly will develop aspiration of saliva into their lungs as long

Little AG, Ferguson MK, Skinner DB: Diseases of the Esophagus, Vol. II: Benign Diseases. Futura Publishing Company, Inc., Mount Kisco, NY, © 1990.

ESOPHAGEAL ATRESIA
1967-1987

136 PATIENTS

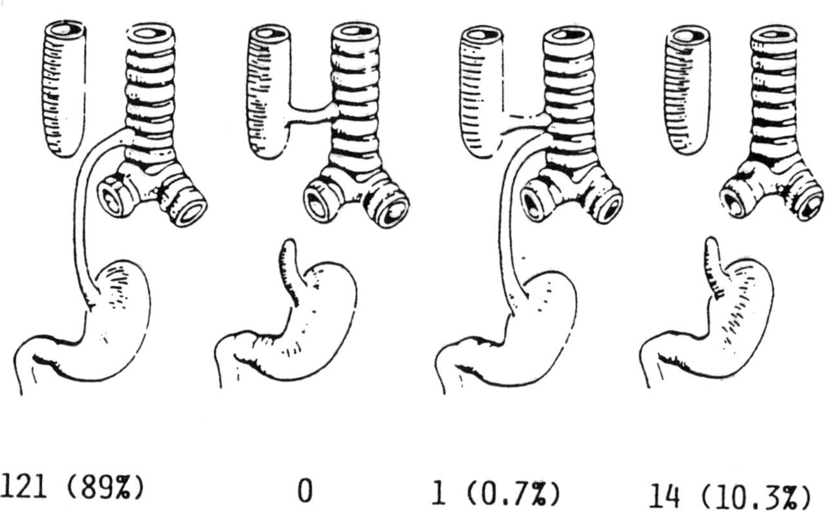

121 (89%)   0   1 (0.7%)   14 (10.3%)

Figure 1

Table I
Waterston Classification

	Group I	Group II	Group III
Class A	17/69 24.6%	25/67 37%	42/136 30.9%
Class B	31/69 45%	21/67 31.5%	52/136 37.8%
Class C	21/69 30%	21/67 31.5%	42/136 30.9%

as continuity has not been restored. In the presence of a tracheoe-sophageal fistula (TEF) with the distal segment, 80% in our experience, gastric juice regurgitates into the lungs causing a chemical pneumonitis. Those patients will develop an incidence of pneumonia which is three times as high as compared to an atresia without fistula.[3] Therefore, early feeding attempts should be avoided in order to prevent aspiration and consequent pneumonia.

In our series, feeding attempt before diagnosis was done in 25 out of 136 patients (18%). Four out of these died: two as a consequence of pneumonia, one of cardiac pathology, and one of serratia meningitis. Only four patients were referred more than 4 days after birth, and although none of them died, three developed major pulmonary problems. Perhaps further diagnostic improvement can still be expected by prenatal echography.

There is no doubt that the higher the degree of prematurity, the higher the degree of pulmonary immaturity will be. In our series, 43 out of 136 patients (31.6%) showed some degree of prematurity, 16 of them having a birth weight of less than 2,000 g. Half of those were categorized in Waterston's class C because of their bad pulmonary status. Moreover, this group of patients had a much higher number of associated congenital anomalies compared to the overall incidence. Seven of the 16 had life-threatening anomalies, five of them being cardiopathies. Five of the 16 died, two of them because of anomalies incompatible with life.

Before deciding any treatment, diagnosis should be as exact as possible. This can be obtained by means of a plain X-ray of the baby. Air in the abdomen indicates a TEF with the distal segment and a stiff radiopaque nasogastric tube allows the surgeon to appreciate the depth of the upper pouch.[4]

Nevertheless many published papers recommend the use of contrast material to opacify the upper pouch allowing the visualization of a possible TEF between the upper pouch and the trachea.[5] Such an examination, however, if not performed under optimal conditions, initially leads to aspiration of contrast material into the lungs resulting in an important narrowing of bronchial lumen whatever the contrast material may be.[6] Increased risk of pneumonia will be the penalty. In our series, radiologic opacification attempts were common, usually before referral to our institute. Eighty-four patients had a documented opacification study, 41 had no opacification study (Table II). An iatrogenic X-ray documented bronchography was noticed in 19 out of 84 patients (22.5%).

Table II
Comparison of Opacification and Non-Opacification Groups

	Overall Classification		*Pulmonary Anastomosis*	
	Non-Opacification N = 41	*Opacifcation N = 84*	*Non-Opacification*	*Opacifcation*
Class A	21 (51%)	23 (27.5%)		
Class B	13 (31%)	48 (57%)	3/13 (23%)	17/48 (35.5%)
Class C	7 (17%)	13 (15%)	1/7 (14%)	5/13 (38.5%)
		Total	4/41 (10%)	22/84 (26%)

Opacification = Radiologic Contrast Examination

In the nonopacification group, twice as many of the patients belong to Waterston class A (51%). On the contrary, in the opacification group, twice as many of the patients belong to class B (57%). Although the numbers are about equal for class C, five patients of the opacification group were classified as such only because of their pulmonary condition whereas only one of the nonopacification group fell in class C only because of his pulmonary condition. In other words, a downstaging of the pulmonary condition was seen in 26% (22/84) of the patients in the opacification group versus only 10% (4/41) in the nonopacification group.

It is clear that associated congenital malformations can compromise the pulmonary status: they appeared in 46% of our patients (19/30), 21.5% of them being life-threatening. In particular, the cyanotic cardiopathies influence pulmonary function. Sixteen babies had important associated cardiopathies of which six belonged to Waterston class C because of their serious pulmonary condition. This combination of severe cardiopathy and unhealthy lungs resulted in four postoperative deaths while two (monoventricle) were not even considered for further treatment.

The surgical treatment in an uncomplicated situation consists of ligation of TEF and primary anastomosis as soon as possible. More difficult is the operative strategy in case of life-threatening associated anomalies and/or prematurity and poor pulmonary condition. Some authors recommend a decompressive gastrostomy as a first step followed by a delayed anastomosis when the general condition has improved.[4] This approach, however, results in a sharp decrease in in-

Table III
Waterson Classification and Postoperative Mortality

	Group I	Group II		
	1967–1980	*1981–1987*	*Total*	*%*
Class A	2/17 11.7%	0/25 0%	2/42	4.7%
Class B	4/31 12.9%	1/21 4.7%	5/52	9.6%
Class C	8/21 3.8%	4/19 21%	12/40	30%
Total	14/69 20.8%	5/65 7.7%	19/134	14%

N = 134 number of operated patients.

trapulmonary pressure through the TEF, leading to an acute loss of effective ventilatory pressure making resuscitation impossible in case of poor lung compliance.[7] We used this method in seven patients with a fatal outcome in six. Therefore, it is our conviction to ligate the TEF as soon as possible in order to prevent further air leak and reflux of gastric juice in the lungs.[8]

Special care is required for the group with immature respiratory distress syndrome for which ventilatory pressure may indeed result in severe abdominal distention, eventually even gastric rupture. Eight patients in our series required ventilatory support preoperatively, twice followed by gastric rupture with fatal outcome in two patients (one with gastric laceration). Nevertheless, it appears that the improved support facilities may offer a chance to a small group of patients who 10–15 years ago never would have had any chance to survive.

The overall postoperative mortality in our series was 14%, decreasing from 20% in group I to 7% in group II (Table III). Out of the 19 deaths, four were a direct consequence of combined severe cardiopathy and pulmonary complications. Thus, more than half of the postoperative mortality was due to poor pulmonary status whether or not associated with life-threatening cardiopathies. If radiologic contrast opacification had been used, postoperative mortality was 20% versus 5%. Two patients (10%) died as a direct consequence of an iatrogenic bronchography and consequent pneumonia.

In addition to the postoperative mortality, nine other patients (6.7%) died in the late follow-up. Here tracheopulmonary problems played a major role as two died of a documented tracheomalacia and two as a consequence of apnea, probably an unrecognized tracheo-

Table IV
Long-Term Follow-Up

	<3 Yrs *N = 84*	*≥3 Yrs* *N = 63*
Symptom-Free	18 (21%)	36 (57%)
Symptomatic	66	27
Pulmonary + Esophageal	43* (65%)	20 (74%)
Esophageal	18	1
Pulmonary	5 (7%)	6 (22%)

* 15 with gastroesophageal reflux.

malacia. Tracheomalacia clearly remains a major threat for patients born with an esophageal atresia[9] and perhaps earlier treatment with a tracheo- or aortopexy could have prevented a fatal outcome.[10]

Postoperative morbidity caused by pulmonary complications is frequent. Forty-two percent were free of postoperative pulmonary problems, with an increase from 35% in group I to 49% in group II. In group II, only 13% had major pulmonary problems mostly belonging to Waterston class C or again having had a constrast study prior to operation. Eighty-four patients have been followed for more than 1 year (Table IV). On an arbitrary basis, results before the age of 3 years are compared to results after 3 years (63 patients). Initially only 21% are totally asymptomatic gradually increasing to 57% at the age of 3 years (36/63).

It is striking that in the group of symptomatic patients, the vast majority—43/66 (65%) and 20/27 (74%)—had both pulmonary and gastrointestinal (GI) problems. Only 7% (5/66) and 22% (6/27) had pulmonary problems without any associated problems, suggesting that as long as GI problems persist, the patient will be more vulnerable to pulmonary problems.[11,12]

If pulmonary symptoms persist, there was in 75% a combination of pulmonary and GI problems. In this perspective the possible role of gastroesophageal reflux (GER) as a cause of chronic pulmonary infections is striking. Fifteen patients had a problem of GER and all of them had associated pulmonary symptoms. After intensive medical treatment (11 patients) or an antireflux procedure (four patients) a marked improvement of the pulmonary condition was noticed in seven. In two medically treated patients, an antireflux procedure was eventually required. Besides GER, a large variety of problems may cause pulmonary problems. Therefore, a careful investigation of this often complex pathology before starting any treatment[9,13] is essential. Despite the fact that many patients become clinically asymptomatic, recent studies indicate a persistent decreased pulmonary function of a restrictive or obstructive pattern even to adult age.[1,14]

Finally, a separate group is formed by infants with long gap atresia in which a primary anastomosis is impossible, 26 patients in our series. They have more problems as prematurity and congenital anomalies are more frequent. Sixty percent belonged to Waterston class C (26% had a Vater syndrome). It is logical therefore to expect that in this group pulmonary problems will determine in a substantial way morbidity and mortality. To restore continuity we have been using mainly two methods: Howard elongation[15] (11 patients) to bridge moderare gaps and coloplasty according to Belsey (13 patients)[16,17] to bridge large gaps. Rehbein's guide fistulization was used twice.[18] Our experience demonstrates a much higher incidence of pulmonary problems for Howard elongation; in one patient the treatment had to be interrupted because of severe apneic spells. Severe bronchitis was seen in three patients and four patients developed severe GER with important repercussions on the pulmonary condition. In contrast there were only three patients with important pulmonary problems after coloplasty.

Conclusion

Pulmonary complications are common in the pre-, peri-, and postoperative periods of a baby born with esophageal atresia. Early diagnosis is of paramount importance, avoiding lung damage by aspiration of saliva and food or refluxing gastric juice if TEF is present. Adequate further investigation requires a perfect understanding of the physiopathology, especially the deleterious consequences of contrast material. As early as possible ligation of TEF allowing adequate ventilation of the lung and preventing further acid reflux is the cardinal step in the treatment. Meticulous anastomotic techniques avoiding traction and early removal of the nasogastric tube are the best guarantees of preventing anastomotic strictures and GER. Esophageal problems such as GER and persistent anastomotic strictures are to be detected and treated as soon as possible in order to minimize their negative repercussions on pulmonary function.

References

1. Biller AJ, Allen JL, Schuster SR, Treves ST, Winter HS: Long-term evaluation of esophageal and pulmonary function in patients with repaired esophageal atresia and tracheoesophageal fistula. Dig Dis Sci 32:985, 1987.
2. Waterston DJ, Bonham-Carter RE, Aberdeen C: Oesophageal atresia-tracheo-oesophageal fistula. Lancet 2:819, 1962.
3. Meeker IA: In Hays DM, Woolley MM, Snyder WH: Changing techniques in the management of esophageal atresia. Arch Surg 92:611, 1966.
4. Holder TM, Ashcraft KW, Sharp RJ, Amoury RA: Care of infants with esophageal atresia, tracheoesophageal fistula and associated anomalies. J Thorac Cardiovasc Surg 94:828, 1987.
5. Myers NA: Oesophageal atresia: The epitome of modern surgery. Ann R Coll Surg Engl 54:276, 1973.
6. Koop CE: Recent advances in the surgery of oesophageal atresia. In: Progress in Pediatric Surgery, Vol. 2, Rickmann PP, Hecker WC, Prévot J (eds), Paris, Masson, 1971.
7. Templeton JM, Templeton JJ, Schnaufer L, et al: Management of esophageal atresia and tracheoesophageal fistula in the neonate with severe respiratory distress syndrome. J Pediatr Surg 20:394, 1985.
8. Belsey RHR, Dennison CP: Congential atresia of the oesophagus. Br Med J 3:324, 1950.
9. Benjamin B, Cohen D, Glasson M: Tracheomalacia in association with tracheo-oesophageal fistula. Surgery 79:504, 1976.
10. Conroy PT, Bennett NR: Management of tracheomalacia in association with congenital tracheo-oesophageal fistula. Br J Anaesthesiol 59:1313, 1987.
11. Orringer MB, Kirsch MM, Sloan H: Long-term esophageal function following repair of esophageal atresia. Ann Surg 186:436, 1977.
12. Shermeta DW, Whitington PF, Seto DS, Haller JA: Lower esophageal sphincter dysfunction in esophageal atresia: Nocturnal regurgitation and aspiration pneumonia. J Pediatr Surg 12:871, 1977.
13. Bargy F, Manachy Y, Helardot P, Bienayne J: Le risque récurrentiel dans la chirurgie de l'atrésie de l'oesophage. Chir Pédiatr 24:130, 1983.
14. Milligan DWA, Levison H: Lung function in children following repair of tracheooesophageal fistula. J Pediatr 95:24, 1979.
15. Howard R, Meyers NA: Esophageal atresia: A technique for elongating the upper pouch. Surgery 58:725, 1965.
16. Belsey RHR: Reconstruction of the esophagus with left colon. J Thorac Cardiovasc Surg 49:33, 1965.
17. Lerut T, Otte JB, Rahardjo T, Focquet M, Fraga J, Decannière L, Gruwez JA: De behandeling van slokdarmatresie en de congenitale tracheo-oesophageale fistel. Acta Chir Belg 82:321, 1982.
18. Rehbein F, Schweder N: Neue Wege in der Rekonstruktion der kinderlichen Spieseröhre. Med Woch 97:757, 1972.

3

Trifurcation Tracheoesophageal Fistula

Roberta J. Hall, David N. Campbell, John R. Lilly,
Luis A. Martinez, R. Peter Altman

Introduction

Trifurcation tracheoesophageal fistula (TEF) is an unusual variant of standard esophageal atresia with fistula in which the distal esophageal fistula is attached to the caudal rim of the carina rather than to the posterior trachea. Surgical implications are: first, the esophageal fistula appears identical to the mainstem bronchi. Second, because of its caudal dislocation, approximately 1.5 cm of distal esophagus, normally present for anastomosis, is not available. Third, the tethering effect of the distal esophageal blood supply is absent so that the esophagus retracts into the mediastinum after fistula division. As a consequence of the latter two factors, esophageal repair is complex despite an otherwise acceptable location of the proximal esophageal pouch.

All but one of five consecutive infants with trifurcation TEF operated upon during the past 13 years developed surgical complications. Two patients died, one from mediastinitis secondary to an intractable anastomotic leak, the other from division of the left mainstem bronchus along with the esophageal fistula. Similarly, a third patient had division of the right intermediate bronchus when

Little AG, Ferguson MK, Skinner DB: Diseases of the Esophagus, Vol. II: Benign Diseases. Futura Publishing Company, Inc., Mount Kisco, NY, © 1990.

it was mistaken for the esophageal fistula but survived. Despite a single upper esophageal myotomy, one other patient developed a rigid esophageal stricture which necessitated prolonged dilatations and finally excision with reanastomosis. The exceptional patient had two adjunctive myotomies which satisfactorily reduced anastomotic tension and has done well.

Trifurcation TEF is encountered unexpectedly at thoracotomy. Secure identification of both bronchi must be done as a first step before fistula division. Since anatomically the malformation is more closely akin to esophageal atresia *without* fistula, primary esophageal repair should be abandoned unless sufficient esophageal myotomy is feasible.

Trifurcation tracheal esophageal fistula is an unusual variant of esophageal atresia in which the fistula arises from the caudal rim of the carina instead of from the posterior trachea (Fig. 1). We have chosen the term "trifurcation" for this anomaly because at operation the esophageal fistula has the peculiar appearance of a third mainstem bronchus. Ladd described this malformation in 1944, calling it a type IV[1] but its inclusion in subsequent publications has been rare or absent.

During the past 13 years, approximately 195 infants have undergone operation for esophageal atresia with TEF at our combined institutions, but only five (3%) had the trifurcation variant. The purpose of this communication is to review the embryologic basis of the malformation, to briefly describe the clinical course of these five patients, and to make specific recommendations for surgical treatment for this anomaly.

Embryology

Embryologically, the trachea and esophagus originate in common from a diverticulum of the primitive foregut which develops between day 22 and day 23 of gestation. Division of this anlage into separate respiratory and digestive portions is accomplished as paired lateral ridges of endoderm grow toward the midline, creating the tracheo-esophageal grooves. These grooves advance in a rostral-caudal direction, fusing at the midline to make the separation of the two tubes complete by 34–36 days of gestation.[2–4] A rich capillary network that forms the splanchnic bed surrounds both tubes, formed primarily from branches from the dorsal 5th and 6th arches. Well-defined

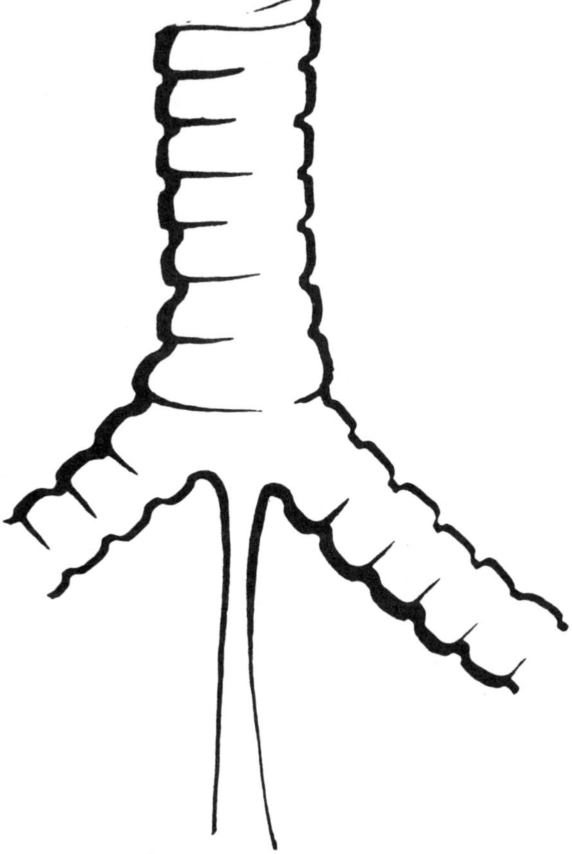

Figure 1: In trifurcation TEF, the distal esophageal segment arises from the carina instead of the posterior trachea.

esophageal branches from the aorta are normally present by the 7th week. Imperfect fusion of the tracheoesophageal grooves,[5] probably in response to an interruption of blood supply occurring in the 4th or 5th week of growth, the so-called "fetal vascular accident,"[6] may result in a persistent connection between esophagus and trachea at any point along their length creating a tracheoesophageal fistula. At the same time, the rich vascular plexus is interrupted at different points along the esophagus. If the insult occurs later, after complete separation of the trachea and esophagus, the result will be esophageal atresia without tracheoesophageal fistula. If it occurs just prior to

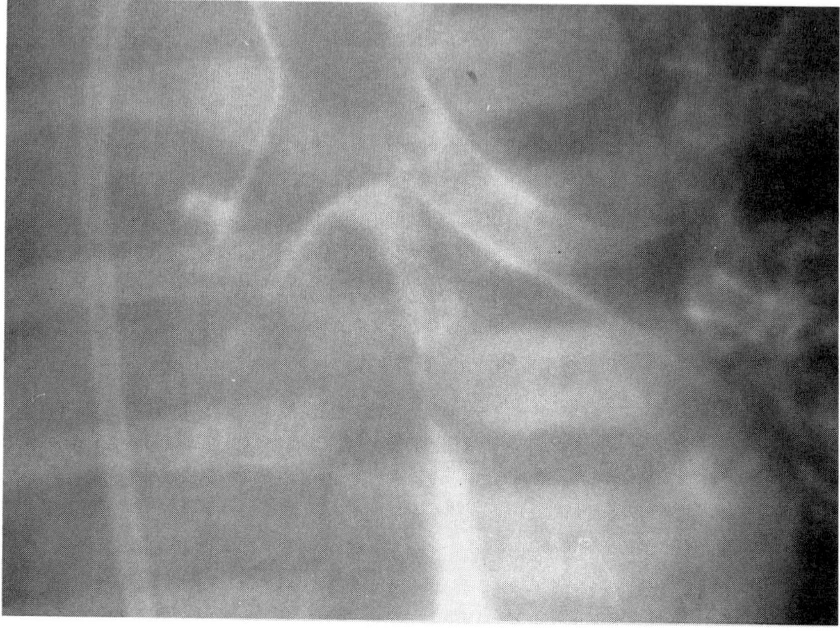

Figure 2: Posteroanterior view following esophagram. Barium showing anatomy of trifurcation TEF.

complete separation, we hypothesize the result would be a trifurcation TEF. Disruption of the esophageal blood supply at this point would not allow sufficient collateral to the lower esophageal segment to develop from the superior plexus (5th arch). Support for this contention is that the lower esophageal segment is not tethered in the middle mediastinum, and in fact, it appears to be supplied mainly from abdominal branches, placing inferior traction on the segment. Thus, trifurcation TEF may be the link between esophageal atresia without fistula and the standard TEF.

Patients

Infant #1. A 6-day-old male was transferred to our hospital after having undergone a right thoracotomy for TEF during the first 24 hours of life. The esophageal fistula was not found, the chest was closed, and a gastrostomy was performed. Following a barium study

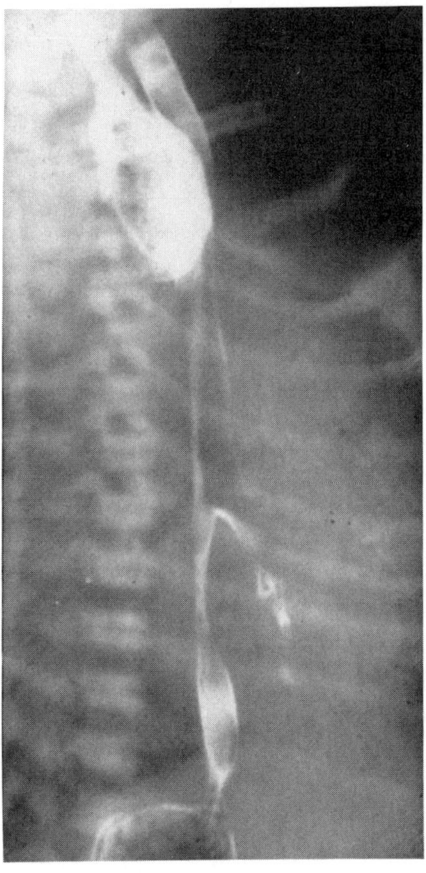

Figure 3: Lateral chest film showing takeoff of trifurcation TEF at carina.

(Figs. 2, 3), bronchoscopy was done and the TEF was identified arising from the distal carina between the right and left mainstem bronchi. A #3 Fogarty catheter was introduced through the bronchoscope into the fistula and secured (Fig. 4). The thoracotomy wound was re-opened, and a structure was identified in the mediastinum which appeared to enter the carina posterior to the right mainstem bronchus and was thought to be the trifurcation TEF. The structure was divided but unfortunately it turned out to be the bronchus intermedius. A structure of similar size was identified coursing directly from the carina which contained the Fogarty catheter. The fistula was divided, and the distal end oversewn. The transsected bronchus intermedius

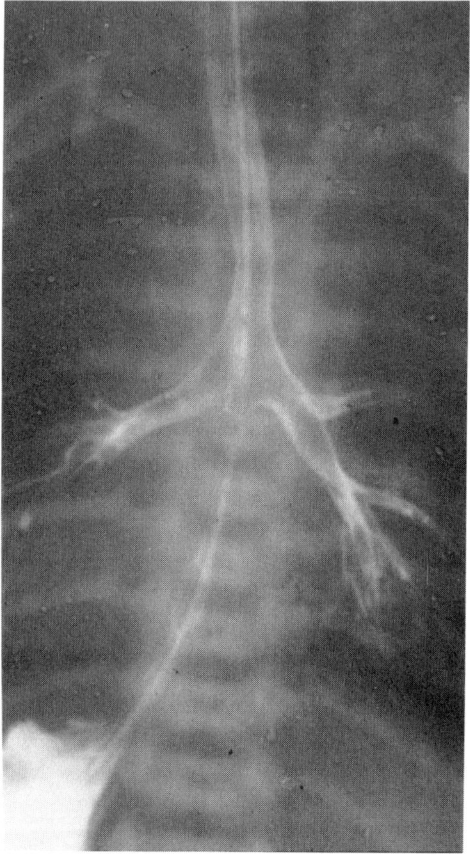

Figure 4: #3 Fogarty catheter is passed through the trifurcation TEF to identify the fistula.

was reattached to the trachea at the origin of the fistula. The proximal end of the bronchus intermedius was closed with sutures and a cervical esophagostomy was done. Subsequently the child has had a gastric tube interposition procedure and is doing well.

Infant #2. A 2390-gram newborn male was determined to have esophageal atresia by barium study of the proximal pouch. Because of a short proximal esophageal pouch (thoracic vertebra 2), repair was delayed and only a gastrostomy was done. At 7 days of age, the proximal pouch had descended to thoracic vertebra 4, indicating an adequate length for primary repair. At thoracotomy, a trifurcation

TEF was identified. The upper esophageal pouch permitted only a single Livaditis myotomy and the esophageal anastomosis was done under moderate tension. Six days postoperatively the patient developed an anastomotic leak. The leak healed 10 days after chest tube drainage, and the patient was started on oral feedings. He was discharged from the hospital and was doing well shortly thereafter.

He was readmitted at 5 months of age, weighing only 3.16 kg and was found to have a recurrent esophageal anastomotic leak and mediastinal abscess cavity. Chest tube drainage was reinstituted in conjunction with total parenteral nutrition, and 3 weeks later he underwent Nissen fundoplication. Postoperatively, the patient developed right upper lobe pneumonitis which resolved with difficulty. After 4 months of hospitalization, he was finally discharged, but at 10 months of age, he died suddenly at home. Autopsy revealed a 1-mm anastomotic leak.

Infant #3. A 2430-gm newborn male with esophageal atresia and TEF was treated by gastrostomy and parenteral nutrition because of a short proximal esophageal pouch (thoracic vertebra 1). After 22 days, the upper esophageal pouch had descended to vertebral body 3 and he underwent exploratory thoractomy. A trifurcation TEF was found, and despite extensive mobilization of the proximal esophageal segment, a primary anastomosis was not attempted because of the distance between the two segments. Therefore, the fistula was divided, both ends oversewn, and the closed end of the distal fistula attached to a vertebral body under some tension.

At reoperation 2 months later, an esophageal anastomosis was possible but with moderate tension. The child developed a marked stricture at the anastomotic site requiring frequent esophageal dilatations. A Nissen fundoplication was performed at 7 months of age because of gastroesophageal reflux. At 2 years of age, the tightly stenotic anastomosis was excised and the anastomosis redone. He has done well following this procedure.

Infant #4. A 2100-gm male infant was diagnosed at birth as having esophageal atresia without fistula because of a blind ending upper esophageal pouch and a gasless abdomen on the abdominal roentgenogram. A gastrostomy was performed. A barium study through the gastrostomy demonstrated a distal tracheoesophageal fistula, and at subsequent thoracotomy, a trifurcation TEF was found. After extensive mobilization of the upper pouch and two serial esophageal myotomies, primary esophageal anastomosis was achieved under modest tension. Recovery was uneventful and he remains well several years later.

Infant #5. A male newborn of 36 weeks' gestational age with oligohydramnios rapidly developed severe respiratory distress. The diagnosis of TEF was confirmed. However, preoperative chest X-ray was distinctly abnormal and was interpreted as complete collapse of the left lung. At operation, a gastrostomy was performed. Because of the continuous escape of air from the stomach, ventilation was inadequate. Emergency right thoracotomy and ligation of presumed large tracheoesophageal fistula were carried out. The patient expired within 24 hours of respiratory failure. At autopsy the fistula and left mainstem bronchus had been ligated together with a single tie and transsected. The TEF was of the trifurcation type.

Discussion

Variations of fistula location are not infrequent in patients with tracheoesophageal fistula. For example, fistulas to the upper pouch, multiple fistulas, and fistula to the right mainstem bronchus have been reported.[7-9] Although requiring precise identification, the operative management is altered little by these variants. Such is not the case for trifurcation TEF. In fact, surgical management is closer to that of esophageal atresia without fistula than to a standard TEF. To our knowledge, the specific surgical technique for repair of trifurcation TEF has not been described. The surgical approach should include the following maneuvers which may avoid some of the pitfalls associated with this difficult anomaly.

First, recognition of the trifurcation variant is crucial. If the fistula is not found in its usual location on the posterior trachea, meticulous identification of all structures arising from the carina is required, i.e., right and left mainstem bronchi and the tracheoesophageal fistula. As illustrated in patients #1 and #5, failure to make positive identification of all three structures can be disastrous. If a trifurcation fistula is suspected before operation, we strongly advocate the passage of a catheter across the fistula (Fig. 5) to help identify the true trifurcation fistula.

Second, because of an absolute absence of 1.5–2.0 cm of distal esophagus ordinarily present for anastomosis, mobilization of the upper pouch is always necessary. After full mobilization, a determination must be made as to the feasibility of a primary anastomosis.

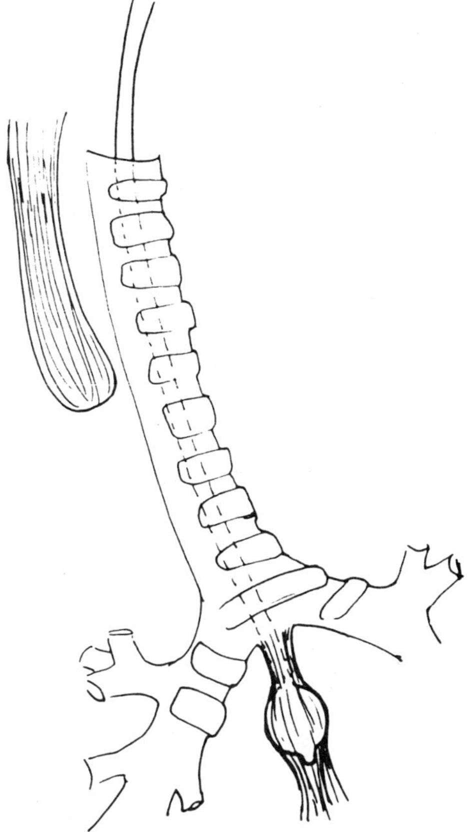

Figure 5: The passage of a Fogarty catheter through the fistula to help identify the distal fistula should be routinely carried out by bronchoscopy if a trifurcation TEF is suspected.

If a myotomy as described by Livaditis[10] will provide adequate length of the upper esophagus to achieve primary anastomosis, it should be carried out, but the upper esophageal segment should not be opened until this determination is made. If adequate length cannot be obtained with one or two upper esophageal myotomies, then the fistula should be transsected and closed, and primary anastomosis should be abandoned, at least initially. In this respect, management of this anomaly closely resembles esophageal atresia without fistula. A later attempt at primary repair may be feasible (as in patient #3) if sufficient downward growth of the upper pouch and elongation of the lower segment subsequently occurs.

Third, because the esophageal fistula is suspended from the trachea without benefit of the usual tethering produced by a direct esophageal blood supply, it retracts into the mediastinum like a severed stretched rubber band when divided. Consequently, if primary anastomosis is elected, division of the fistula should be done in stepwise fashion. Stay sutures are placed in the fistula as it is divided.

Fourth, the delicate, thin-walled distal esophageal segment usually seen with trifurcation TEF will only accommodate a single rather than two-layer closure.

In conclusion, trifurcation tracheoesophageal fistula is an uncommon variant of esophageal atresia with a very high complication rate because of its inherent anatomy. Extreme care should be exercised when confronted with this type of anomaly. The two mainstem bronchi as well as the fistula should be completely defined prior to any definitive procedure, and since anatomically, the malformation is more closely akin to esophageal atresia *without* fistula, primary esophageal repair should be abandoned unless extensive myotomy is feasible.

Finally, one caveat is worth mentioning concerning diagnosis of TEF. Many textbooks suggest that passage of a catheter into the stomach with return of gastric contents rules out TEF. This is not always true. In fact, as we have seen at least once in our experience, the catheter can be passed across the trachea through the fistula and into the stomach.

References

1. Ladd W: The surgical treatment of esophageal atresia and tracheoesophageal fistulas. N Engl J Med 230:625, 1944.
2. Smith EI: The early development of the trachea and the esophagus in relation to atresia of the esophagus and tracheoesophageal fistula. Contr Embryol Carnegie Inst Wash 245:35:41, 1957.
3. O'Rahilly R, Muller F: Chevalier Jackson Lecture. Respiratory and alimentary relations in staged human embryos. New embryological data and congenital anomalies. Ann Otol Rhino Laryngol 93:421, 1984.
4. Judson GR: Esophageal atresia and congenital stenosis. In: Pediatric Surgery, 4th ed., Welch, Randolph-Ravitch, O'Neill Jr, Rove (eds), Chicago, Year Book Medical Publishers, Inc, 1986, p 682.
5. Snell RS (ed): The respiratory system. In: Clinical Embryology for Medical Students, 2nd ed., Boston, Little Brown and Company, 1975, p 177.

6. Barnard CW: The genesis of intestinal atresia. Surg Forum 7:393, 1956.
7. Goodwin CD, Ashcraft KW, Holder TM, et al: Esophageal atresia with double tracheoesophageal fistula. J Pediatr Surg 13:269, 1987.
8. Babbitt DP: Double tracheoesophageal fistula without atresia: Report of a case. N Engl J Med 257:713, 1957.
9. Holder TM, Cloud DT, Lewis JE Jr, et al: Esophageal atresia and tracheoesophageal fistula: A survey of its members by the surgical section of the AAP. Pediatrics 34:542, 1961.
10. Livaditis A: Esophageal atresia, a method of overbridging large segmental gaps. Z Kinderchir 13:298, 1973.

4

The Retrosternal Procedure for Esophagus Replacement with Colon in Children:
Indications, Surgical Technique and Results

Remigio Dòmini, Antonino Appignani, Mario Lima, Giovanni Grillone, Giovanni Ruggeri

Introduction

Surgical techniques for esophagus substitution in pediatric patients include intrathoracic or retrosternal placement.[1-5] Our experience with the latter approach has led us to consider it the elective technique of choice. We present here our indications, our cases, and results.[1-4]

In the Department of Pediatric Surgery of the University of Bologna, from 1974 to 1988, 70 operations were performed according to the indications[1-4,6,7] described in Table I.

In esophageal atresia, retrosternal colon conduit (RCC) was the final solution for cases in which primary repair was not indicated or possible, for those in which dehiscence of a primary repair occurred and for those previously treated elsewhere unsuccessfully. There are 16 out of 57 cases presented in Table I.

Little AG, Ferguson MK, Skinner DB: Diseases of the Esophagus, Vol. II: Benign Diseases. Futura Publishing Company, Inc., Mount Kisco, NY, © 1990.

Table I
Indications for Retrosternal Colon Conduit (RCC)

	No. of Cases	No. of RCC	%
Esophageal Atresia	165	41	24.8
Esophageal Atresia in patients unsuccessfully operated on elsewhere	16	16	100
Peptic Stenosis	29*	8	27.8
Burn Stenosis	25	2	8
Portal Hypertension	99	2	2
Epidermolysis Bullosa	1	1	100

* 7 cases were operated on with intrathoracic technique, the remaining 14 cases were treated with dilations and Nissen fundoplication.

In peptic and burn stenosis,[5,6,8] the operation was reserved for the cases in which either esophageal dilatations weren't indicated or were ineffective. Although portal hypertension is rarely one of the indications for this kind of operation, there are two cases in our experience in which the management of varices caused esophageal perforation, and in these, the ultimate and definitive solution was the substitution of the organ.

Finally, the only case of epidermolysis bullosa,[9,10] carrying a long, tight stenosis of the esophagus, was also treated successfully with this technique.

Surgical Technique

We consider the first year as the ideal age for the patient to undergo the operation, when the body weight is at least 10 kg. In most of the cases we used the left colon (55 times, 78%) fed by the left colic pedicle. When its vascularization was uncertain, we alternatively chose the transverse colon (11 times, 15%) vascularized by midcolic vessels or seldom the last ileal loop and the first part of the colon with the ileo-colic blood supply (4 times, 5%, two of which were first operations and the other two were reoperations) (Table II).

While the vascularization of the colon is easily tested in a few minutes once the vessels are isolated and clamped, a lot of attention must also be paid to evaluating the venous drainage that can turn

Table II
Colic Segment Employed

	No. of Cases	%
Left	55	78.5
Transverse	11	15.7
Ileo-colon	4	5.8

out to be insufficient. The time between the preparation of the chosen loop and its resection is used to perform a wide retrosternal tunnel according to the classic technique,[1,2,4] which is a combined maneuver using fingers and dilators together, trying not to open the parietal pleura.

A particular technique to avoid compression of the interposed loop is to fix the anterior hepatic edge to the rib arch with a few stitches of gross catgut. Then the loop is resected and passed through the retrosternal tunnel, following a big rubber tube that envelops completely its upper stump to avoid mediastinal contamination. The loop is placed following its peristaltic orientation. After the end-to-end colo-colic anastomosis (extra-mucosal layer), the colo-gastric end-to-side anastomosis on the posterior wall of the stomach is made in triple layer, to act as an antireflux mechanism. Afterwards, the abdominal wall is closed, but previously a Penrose drain is placed in the mediastinum; gastrostomy, if previously performed as in esophageal atresia or in very strict stenosis, is maintained. In other cases, if possible, we prefer to leave a nasogastric tube, correctly placed before the closure of the abdomen. The last step of operation is the esophago-colic end-to-end anastomosis, performed with full-thickness stitches in one layer, over a transanastomotic tube, previously placed in the nose, if there is not already a nasogastric tube in situ.

A technical remark must be added for patients affected by esophageal stenosis, where the damaged esophagus isn't removed at the same operation but is delayed a few months to avoid further serious stress, due to thoracotomy and the prolonged time necessary for operation. The postoperative period in these patients lasts 15 days and is generally good; the merits of these results are due to two very important therapeutic managements: antibiotic prophylaxis and total parenteral nutrition executed through a central venous catheter, usually the Broviak type.

Table III
Complications Treated Conservatively: 10 Cases

Leak of esophago-colic anastomosis	8 cases
Surgical wound infection	2 cases

At discharge, children are regularly fed per os and gastrostomy is maintained for another month as a safety caution.

Results

In our experience, retrosternal colon interposition resulted in no intraoperative mortality and there was only one case of postoperative death, due to septicemia 5 days after the operation, 9 years ago. Complications can be divided into two groups: those treated conservatively (Table III) and those submitted to surgical operation (Tables IV and V).

In the first group (10 cases, 14%) are included eight cases of leak of the esophago-colic anastomosis and two cases of infection of the wound. The second group (10 cases, 14%) can be further divided into two groups: one group including serious but non-life-threatening complications and one group of very serious complications that can be life-threatening for the patient. Three cases of stricture of the esophago-colic anastomosis belong to the first subgroup. They were treated with resection of the stenosis and remaking of the anastomosis. Included in this same subgroup were two cases of intestinal obstruction due to adhesions, treated with laparotomy and lysis.

In the second group, including very serious complications, there were five cases (7%): three cases of peptic disease of the interposed loop caused by gastrocolic reflux, treated and solved with a personal technique,[11] and two cases of necrosis of the loop promptly removed

Table IV
Complications Requiring Reoperation: 5 Cases

Stricture of the esophago-colic anastomosis	3 cases
Intestinal obstruction due to adhesions	2 cases

Table V
Serious Complications Requiring Reoperation:
5 Cases

Peptic disease of the colon conduit	3 cases
Necrosis of the colon conduit	2 cases

with construction of esophagostomy and gastrostomy. The operation was repeated successfully 1 year later using ileo-colon.

Conclusions

From the data above, we can say that the colon conduit performed with retrosternal technique is the safest method for substituting the esophagus in children. Its characteristics as far as reliability is concerned are: no intraoperative mortality; exceptional postoperative mortality: only 1 case out of 70 patients (1.4% mortality); few complications needing surgical correction, and among them, the most serious are rare (7%); very high percentage of complete and definitive success (98%); good functioning of the neo-esophagus[12] shown by the regular growth of height and weight of operated patients; the possibility of reintervening using a different colic segment with a good prospect of success.

References

1. Peracchia A: Chirurgia dell'esofago. In: Trattato di Tecnica Chirurgica. Vol. 4, Utet, Torino, 1982, p 159.
2. Randolph JG, Enderson KD: Replacement of the esophagus. In: Pediatric Surgery, Ravitch MM, et al (eds), Chicago, Year Book Medical Publishers, 1979, pp 482–488.
3. Domini R, Appignani A, Lima M: Retrosternal esophagocoloplasty in esophageal atresia. Congress of esophageal surgery, Munich, 1986.
4. Neville W, Najem A: Colon replacement of the esophagus for congenital and benign disease. Ann Thorac Surg 36:626–633, 1983.
5. Domini R: Chirurgia delle ernie diaframmatiche e del reflusso gastroesofageo. Padua Piccin Ed, 1972.
6. Domini R, Appignani A, Lima M: Esophagocoloplasty procedure in children suffering from peptic stenosis: Our experience in 14 cases. O.E.S.O. Second international polydisciplinary congress, Paris, 1987.
7. Domini R, Appignani A, Lima M: Esophagocoloplasty procedure in pe-

II.

Gastroesophageal Reflux Disease:
Editors' Overview

A. Diagnosis

The diagnosis of gastroesophageal reflux disease must begin with the ability to differentiate normal from abnormal. Chapter 5 definitively identifies the pH patterns which are found in normal volunteers, in both the esophagus and the stomach over a 24-hour period. It is increasingly clear, as this chapter emphasizes, that the stomach and the esophagus, along with the duodenum, function as an interrelated, upper gastrointestinal, functional complex and investigations of one organ frequently require studies of its neighbor. Along these lines, Chapter 6 reports an experience using simultaneous esophageal and gastric pH monitoring in the investigation of 100 consecutive patients. This report documents the usefulness and importance of this dual investigation in selected patients.

Chapter 7 shows that patients with pathological gastroesophageal reflux may have acid reflux within the proximal esophagus. This ability to detect the cephalad extent of acid reflux documents the possibility of occult aspiration and secondary pulmonary disease in this population of patients.

The final chapter reports the specificity and the sensitivity of various histologic parameters, utilizing endoscopic biopsy material, in the identification of pathological gastroesophageal reflux, using the results of esophageal pH monitoring as the comparison. A combination of parameters is more accurate than any single parameter

37

alone. The important point, as stressed by the authors, is that abnormal histology in the presence of a normal esophageal pH study should prompt a search for an alternative diagnosis.

B. Pathophysiology

Chapter 9 addresses the well-known and unequivocal fact that the pressure and length characteristics of the manometric lower esophageal sphincter are not sufficient to explain the barrier against gastroesophageal reflux that exists at the gastroesophageal junction. Specifically, the authors provide evidence to support the concept of a gastric component to the reflux barrier. Further defining the relationship between the stomach and the esophagus, the authors also show that gastric distention can provoke relaxation of the lower esophageal sphincter which may be an important factor in postprandial gastroesophageal reflux.

Chapter 10 provides data derived from dogs that peptone infusion into the duodenum decreases the pressure within the lower esophageal sphincter through a centrally mediated action which is dependent upon the vagal nerves and cholinergic neurotransmission. Understanding as we do that lower esophageal muscle tone is an important component of the reflux barrier and that this pressure varies over time, this study helps to identify one of the causes of this fluctuation in pressure.

Chapter 11 analyzes the interaction of gastroesophageal reflux and esophageal motility in normal volunteers with physiological gastroesophageal reflux in an attempt to define a perhaps regulatory interplay between esophageal motor activity and reflux. Both the frequency and the nature of esophageal contractions vary before, during, and following reflux episodes. This does suggest a motor response to reflux which can easily be supposed important in the protective response which serves to clear acid and other reflux material from the esophagus. The following chapter continues on the theme of the reflux/motor function relationship in reflux patients with increasing degrees of mucosal changes. This analysis shows that the contraction amplitude in the esophageal body decreases with worsening of esophagitis. Contraction duration is increased and contraction velocity is diminished. Patients with a Barrett's esophagus have esophageal body motility abnormalities similar to patients with advanced esophagitis. It is clear from these two chapters that alterations of esophageal motor function are seen in correlation with reflux episodes and that motor function in patients with reflux esophagitis is impaired.

Chapter 13 shows that the delay in gastric emptying which is seen in some patients with gastroesophageal reflux is caused by retention within the proximal stomach. Emptying from the distal stomach is normal. Understanding, as shown in Chapter 1, that proximal gastric distention may decrease lower esophageal sphincter pressure, it is clear that this may be an important factor in patients with reflux disease.

The final chapter focuses on nonesophageal pathophysiologic sequelae of reflux by documenting the frequency of gastroesophageal reflux in children with asthmatic symptoms. The authors provide data to support a pathophysiologic sequence, whereby exposure of the esophageal mucosa to acid causes a reflex, neurally mediated, bronchoconstriction, rather than microaspiration, as the explanation for this connection.

C. Medical Therapy

Chapters 15 and 16 report the results of prospective randomized studies comparing H_2 blockers to a proton pump inhibitor in the treatment of patients with reflux esophagitis. Both studies demonstrate that omeprazole is superior for the acute healing of reflux esophagitis. Both studies are careful to point out that many patients also respond to H_2 blockers even though dose escalation may be necessary and to emphasize that the studies report only short-term results. Utilization of omeprazole as a long-term treatment has not yet been reported so its role is unclear. In contrast, Chapter 17 specifically focuses on patients with documented gastroesophageal reflux without endoscopic esophagitis. These patients were entered into a prospective randomized study which documented that cimetidine was superior to placebo in alleviating daytime heartburn. In fact, approximately 75% of treated patients had relief of symptoms during the course of the study. Further evaluation showed that patients with esophagitis had a similar symptomatic response. The use of H_2 blockers can be effective in treating the symptom of heartburn in patients with gastroesophageal reflux disease.

These chapters all document that there are some patients who will not respond, either symptomatically or with healing of esophagitis, to pharmacologic treatment of their gastroesophageal reflux.

Chapters 18 and 19 utilize pH monitoring, esophageal manometry, and endoscopy to identify characteristics of patients who are likely to fail medical therapy. These characteristics are the presence of severe, that is grade 2 or 3, esophagitis, increased acid exposure, a very low pressure in the LES, and/or the presence of abnormal esophageal body motor function. This information suggests that patients with these characteristics should be followed closely when medical management is begun and considered for early operative therapy if there is not a prompt response.

D. Surgical Therapy

Chapter 20 addresses the dilemma of variable results of surgical treatment of gastroesophageal reflux disease among institutions. Not surprisingly, at least part of the difference is due to differences in patient selection and therefore variations in the severity of disease in the patient populations. This is an important point to be emphasized and explains the need for careful definition of entry criteria for either medical or surgical treatment in any report that addresses therapeutic results.

Chapters 21 and 22 provide results regarding the efficacy of several standard operations for gastroesophageal reflux disease. The first report addresses results when a Belsey Mark IV operation is the exclusive one employed and documents the excellent outcome that can be obtained when the operating team is experienced in the utilization of this operation. The following chapter, in contrast, is a randomized, prospective study in which several different operations were used. Their results show that in this setting, with multiple surgeons involved performing several operations, that the Nissen fundoplication provides the best outcome.

The final three chapters in this section discuss important issues in surgical treatment. Chapter 23 addresses the relationship between gastroesophageal reflux and pulmonary disease. The results seem contradictory as there was actually a decrease in spirometry values following antireflux surgery even though respiratory symptoms such as cough and dyspnea were improved by surgery in the group of symptomatic patients. The penultimate chapter makes an interesting identification of postfundoplication vagal nerve damage in 21% of patients. This is almost certainly a functional rather than an anatomic disruption; nonetheless, this is a surprisingly high number. Despite this observation, results of the operative treatment of reflux are good, suggesting to the authors that vagotomy may be helpful through suppression of acid production. This has been suggested previously by others but results of primary antireflux surgery at present do not justify routine performance of either truncal or selective vagotomy in patients with primary gastroesophageal reflux.

The final chapter reports a surgical approach to patients with very complicated and/or recurrent gastroesophageal reflux disease following prior antireflux surgery. This study suggests that when total duodenal bypass is required that vagotomy be delayed and not performed unless clinically required.

5

Twenty-Four-Hour Esophageal pH Monitoring:
An In-Depth Study of 50 Normal Subjects

Stephen E. A. Attwood, Antony P. Barlow,
Tom R. DeMeester

Introduction

The definition of gastroesophageal reflux disease is an increased exposure of the esophagus to gastric juice. The controversies that surround the use of 24-hour esophageal pH monitoring to discriminate the disease state from normal centers around variations in the technique of pH monitoring and the lack of normal values. The former problem has been resolved to a large degree by the introduction of computer programs to process and analyze pH monitoring data.

It is important to emphasize that 24-hour esophageal pH monitoring is not a test for reflux, but rather a measurement of esophageal exposure to gastric juice. This exposure can be measured by determining the cumulative time the esophageal pH is outside the normal range during the 24-hour period, and the nature of the exposure can be determined by measuring the time at different pH thresholds. These measurements, although precise, do not reflect how the exposure occurred. To do this, it is necessary to measure the frequency

Little AG, Ferguson MK, Skinner DB: Diseases of the Esophagus, Vol. II: Benign Diseases. Futura Publishing Company, Inc., Mount Kisco, NY, © 1990.

and duration of each exposure below or above the various pH thresholds. To combine cumulative exposure, frequency of exposure, and continuous duration of exposure into a holistic measurement, a score has been devised.[1] By consent, a pH of 4 has been used as a threshold point. With current technology, it is a simple process to calculate the score for each pH threshold and to graphically display the data. This has improved the interpretation of the test.

Measurements of gastric juice exposure in the esophagus are not normally distributed and thus percentile values are required to establish a normal range.[2] To identify with confidence a 95th percentile, 50 normal volunteers were studied and the nature of their esophageal exposure to gastric juice assessed. These normal values are now applied in the routine clinical investigation of patients with foregut symptoms, using esophageal pH monitoring for the diagnosis of gastroesophageal reflux disease.

Methods

Subjects

Fifty normal volunteers were studied after history, physical examination, barium esophogram, and esophageal manometry had ruled out esophageal or gastric pathology. The study was ethically approved by the Creighton University IRB and full informed consent was obtained from each subject.

pH Monitoring

Twenty-four-hour intraluminal pH monitoring was performed using a glass electrode (Ingold Electronics, Switzerland) placed 5 cm above the upper border of the manometrically defined lower esophageal sphincter. The pH monitoring system was standardized at pH values of 1 and 7 at the beginning and at the end of the test period. The diet was standardized only by limiting food and beverages to those with a pH value between 4 and 7. All subjects tested were instructed to record their symptoms, such as heartburn, regurgitation, dysphagia, chest pain, cough, and wheeze, in a diary and mark the time on the recorder. They were asked to remain upright while awake and to lie flat on retiring for the night. The data were stored on Synectics (Sweden) and Proxima (Casalecchio di Reno, Italy) re-

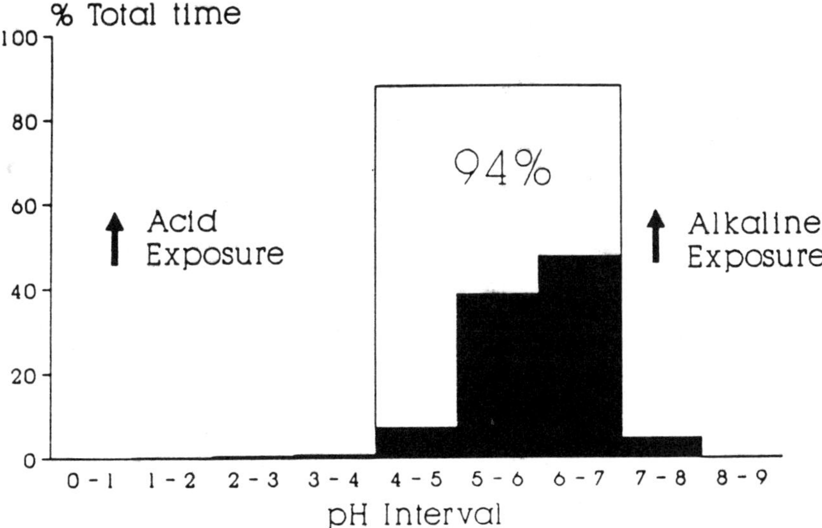

Figure 1: The normal range of esophageal pH, expressed using the median percentage of the total time spent at each pH interval. Ninety-four percent of the time is spent within the pH bands 4–7, underlining the value of using pH 4 and 7 as the limit of normality.

corders. Subsequent analysis was performed with the Gastrosoft program (Gastrosoft, Dallas, TX) using a data conversion program for the Proxima recorders.

Results

To determine the normal esophageal exposure, the time spent at each pH interval, 0–1, 1–2, etc., was determined and plotted graphically. Figure 1 shows the median percent time spent at each pH interval and illustrates that 94% of the time the pH was between 4 and 7. In normal individuals, exposure outside this range is minimal.

To measure the pH exposure outside the pH range 4–7, the time spent below the pH thresholds 4, 3, 2, 1 or above 7 and 8 was calculated and expressed as the percent time the pH was above or below a value for the total time and the time spent in the upright and supine position. To define the nature of this exposure, the total number of episodes, the number of episodes longer than 5 minutes, and the time of the longest episode in minutes was calculated for each pH range. The results were expressed graphically for each component

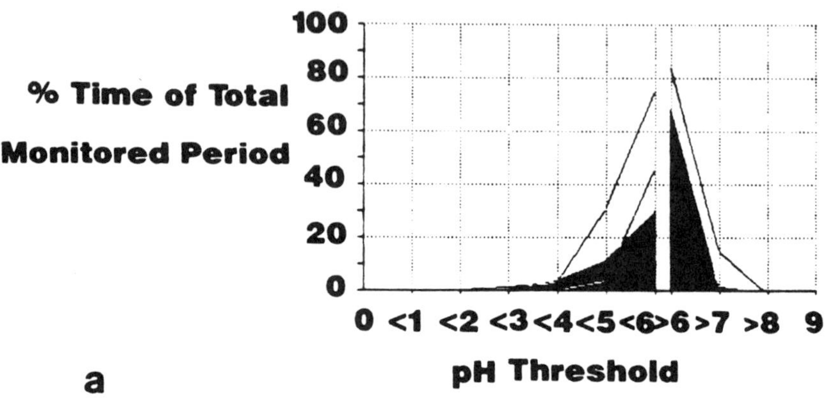

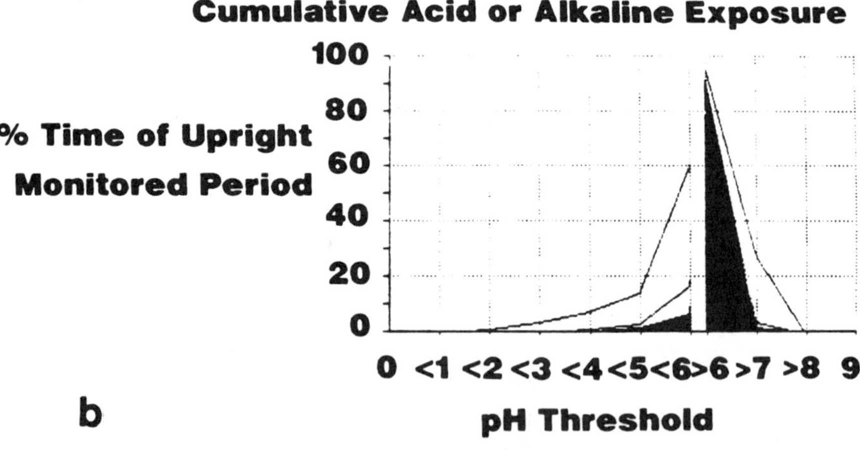

Figure 2a–f: Graphic display showing the median and 95th percentile levels in 50 normal individuals, using whole pH values above and below 6 as thresholds. The black area represents measurements made in the patient. The lower line shows the median and the upper line the 95th percentile value for the 50 normal subjects. When the black area exceeds the 95th percentile line for a given pH threshold, the patient has an abnormal value for the component measured. (a) Percent cumulative exposure for total time. (b) Percent cumulative exposure for upright time. (c) Percent cumulative exposure for supine time. (d) Number of episodes. (e) Number of episodes greater than 5 minutes in length. (f) Length of longest episode.

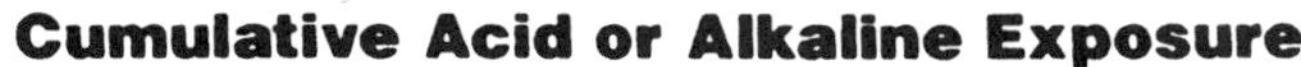

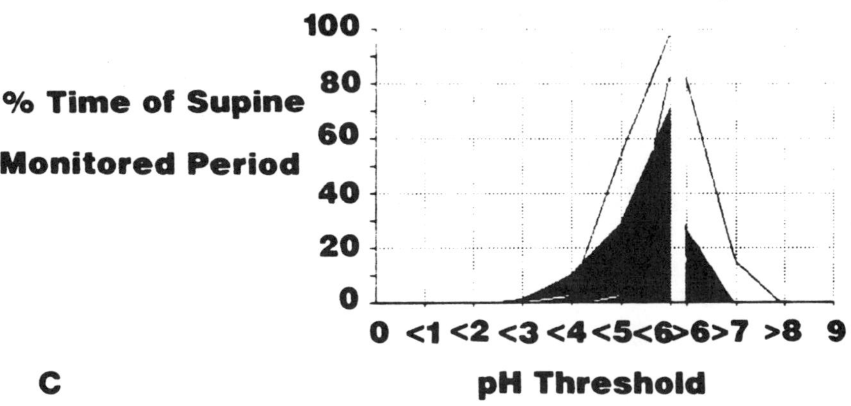

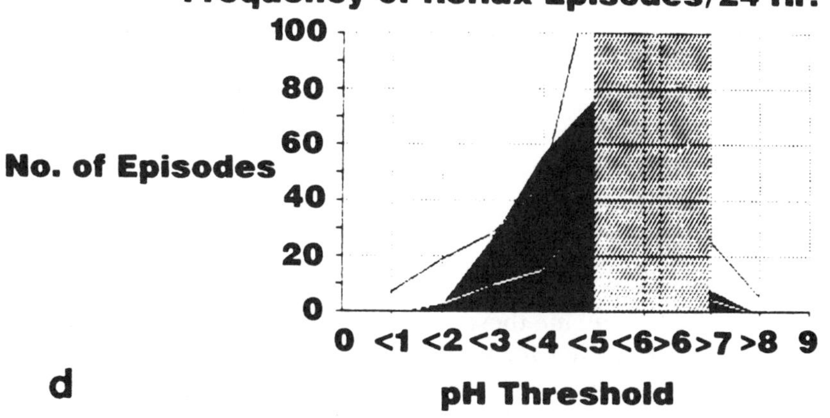

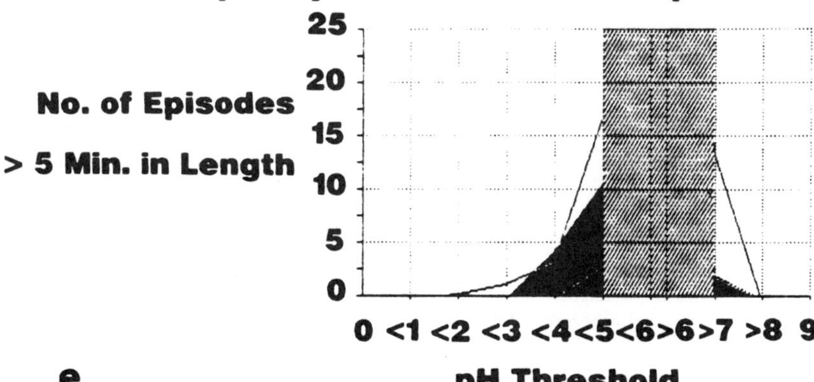

Figure 2c–e: See legend 2

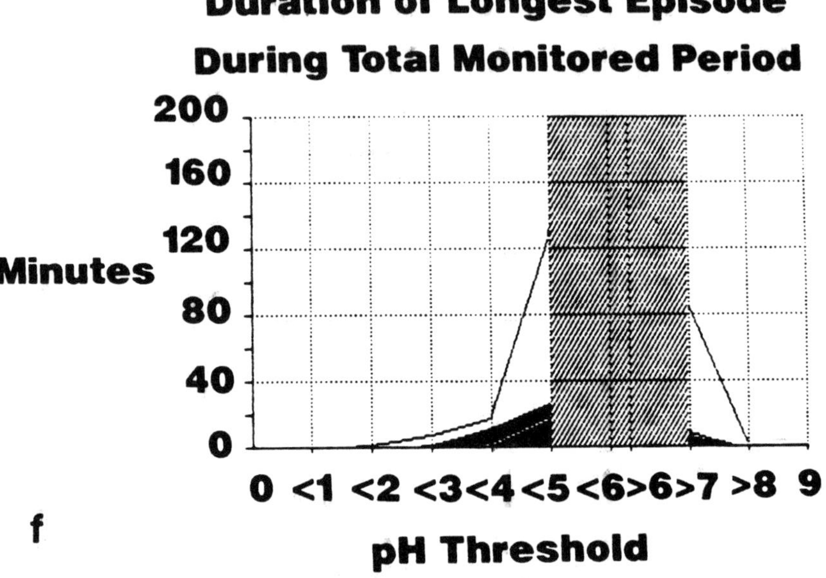

Figure 2f: See legend 2

(Fig. 2a–f) and allowed the patient's results to be compared with the median and the 95th percentile of the normal subjects. Values above the 95th percentile are considered abnormal.

In order to combine these measurements into one holistic value, a score was calculated for each component based on the standard deviation of its mean value and added to make a composite score. In order to use the standard deviation in this manner, it was necessary to deal with the data as though it were parametric. To do so, a zero point was established 2 standard deviations below the mean for each particular component. Thus, any measured value could be referenced to this zero point and awarded points on the basis of how far it varied from the mean using the standard deviation as the weighing unit (Fig. 3).

The formula use for performing the calculation illustrated in Figure 3 is

$$\text{Component Score} = \frac{\text{Patient Value} - \text{Mean}^*}{\text{Standard Deviation}^*} + 1$$

---

* The mean and standard deviation of 50 normal subjects for the component being scored.

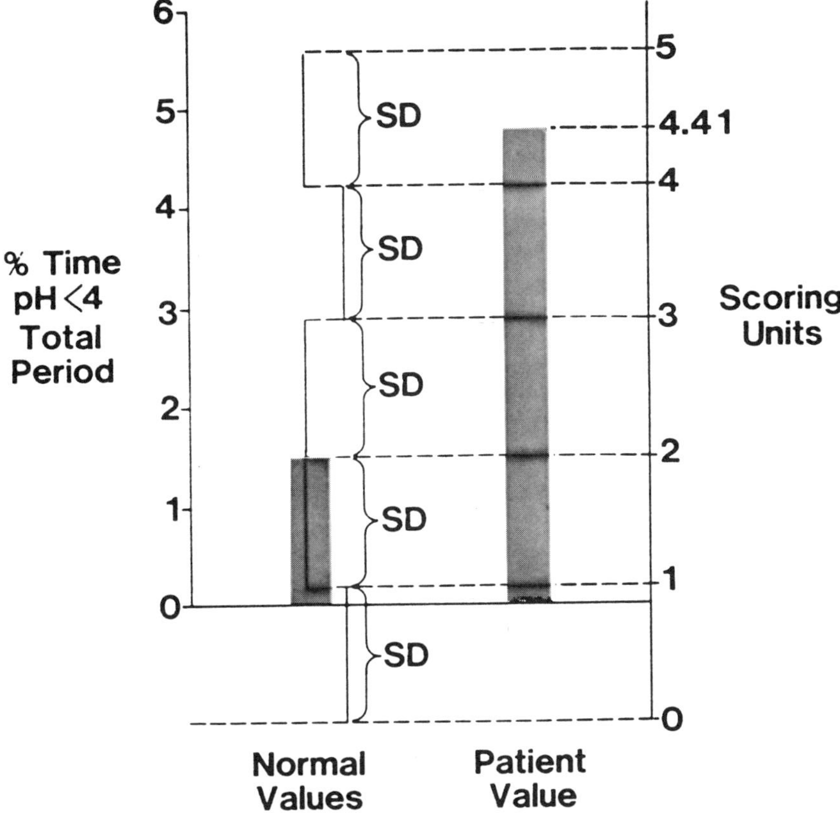

Figure 3: Concept of using the standard deviation as the scoring unit to score the component percent time pH<4 for the total period. Note the establishment of an abstract zero point 2 standard deviations below the mean value for total-period acid exposure measured in normals. Theoretically, this allows scoring the measurement in patients as though the normal values were parametric. By this method, a patient who had a total acid exposure below pH 4 of 4.8% would have a score for this component of 4.41.

Each component score was then added to produce a composite score for each pH range. The upper limits of normal for each of these scores is given in Table I and illustrated in Figure 4. A patient's values may then be superimposed on this graph and his/her esophageal pH exposure evaluated in relation to that measured in the normal subjects.

Table I
The Composite Scores at the Upper Limits of Normal for Each pH Interval

			Upper Limit of Composite Scores					
pH threshold	<1	<2	<3	<4	<5	<6	>7	>8
95th percentile	14.1	17.4	14.1	14.7	15.8	12.8	14.9	8.5
97.5 percentile	20.1	25.0	15.9	17.6	16.5	14.7	22.7	23.5

Discussion

The advantage of computerized analysis of 24-hour pH records is that it allows rapid, detailed evaluation of esophageal acid exposure that would be time-consuming to perform by manual means. It removes observer error and allows gastrointestinal laboratories in different locations to handle the data in a similar fashion. Ideally, each laboratory should perform studies on normal individuals to set its own range of normal, as a quality check. In practice, these normal

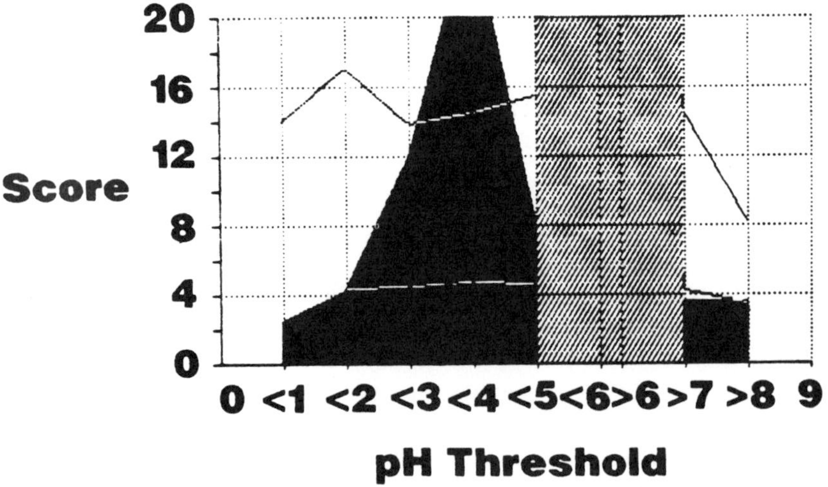

Figure 4: The composite score used to express the overall pH result. The lower line represents the median score and the upper line the 95th percentile of 50 normal subjects. The black area represents the composite score of the patient with increased esophageal acid and alkaline exposure measured at pH of <2, <3, <4, >7, and >8.

values are surprisingly similar throughout the world.[3] Performing studies in normals is both expensive and time-consuming, and in some areas it is not possible to recruit adequate numbers of normal subjects to achieve statistical confidence limits. Careful screening must be done to exclude the presence of foregut disease. In our unit, two out of three volunteers are rejected.

Although the pH of 4 has been shown to be the best single discriminator of normal from gastroesophageal reflux disease, useful information can be gained from the full pH profile. The nature of the gastric juice, i.e., the degree of acidity suggesting the presence of hypersecretion or the presence of an alkalinity suggestive of bile reflux is evident from the pH profile. It can be seen from Figure 1 that exposure to pH values below 4 and above 7 are unusual. Exposure to a pH<4 is a dependable and reliable sign of gastroesophageal reflux. A shift in the patient values towards the left may indicate hyperacidity in the stomach, suggesting that the patient may be a hypersecretor. Exposure to a pH above 7 indicates alkaline gastroesophageal reflux, but is a less dependable sign than acid reflux for the following reasons. First, errors in calibration will have a much greater effect at the border of abnormal alkalinity than at the border of abnormal acidity (Fig. 1). For this reason we use glass probes which are more reliable at the higher pH scales, and each probe is calibrated before and after the study to ensure the absence of drift. Second, the presence of dental infection may increase the pH of saliva. Third, the presence of esophageal obstruction can cause pooling of saliva in the esophagus with bacterial overgrowth and an increase in pH. To avoid the latter, we routinely perform pH monitoring after endoscopy has been carried out and any strictures dilated. When alkaline pH exposure in the esophagus is increased, and dental infection and esophageal obstruction have been excluded, the observation is a reliable indication of alkaline duodenogastric and gastroesophageal reflux. The presence of alkaline exposure has recently been shown to be important in the development of complications of the disease, i.e., erosive esophagitis, stricture, and Barrett's esophagus.[4]

Esophageal pH monitoring is a highly accurate predictor of gastroesophageal reflux disease. In sequential studies performed in 18 subjects in differing environments, we have shown that although the individual components varied, the composite score for each individual remained the same in 17. In addition, the sensitivity and specificity of pH monitoring applied to a group of known refluxers and normal volunteers was 96%.[5]

Although different etiologies for gastroesophageal reflux disease exist, their common effect is to increase the exposure of the esophagus to gastric juice and therefore identification and quantification of that exposure is the most accurate indicator of the disease. We have used pH monitoring in over 2000 patients presenting with symptoms of foregut disease and have found it extremely useful in documenting which patients have increased esophageal acid exposure. Furthermore, it has proven to be safe and free from morbidity or mortality. Its routine application has allowed the detection and description of gastroesophageal reflux disease in many atypical patients. pH monitoring gives objectivity to the diagnosis in patients with atypical symptoms and signs. In our experience, the presence of significant abnormalities on pH monitoring is useful in establishing the diagnosis of gastroesophageal reflux in patients without esophagitis on endoscopy, and in those patients who have complications of reflux such as Barrett's esophagus, but have few or no symptoms.[6]

Although pH monitoring is the most definitive and descriptive diagnostic tool in the armamentarium of the gastroenterologic physician or surgeon, it must still be used in conjunction with investigations to identify the cause of the increased exposure to gastric juice, such as manometric assessment of the lower esophageal sphincter and esophageal body, and with investigations to assess the complications of the disease, such as endoscopy and biopsy. Only the precise definition of the etiology, the nature of the refluxed material, and its effect in the esophagus will provide the necessary data on which to decide the correct course of management of gastroesophageal reflux disease.

ACKNOWLEDGMENT: The authors would like to acknowledge the work of Mike Walker and Jon Bean in the development of computer applications in the Esophageal Laboratory at Creighton University.

References

1. Johnson LF, DeMeester TR: 24-hour pH monitoring of the distal esophagus: A quantitative measure of gastroesophageal reflux. Am J Gastroenterol 62:325–332, 1974.
2. Herrera BS: The precision of percentiles in establishing normal limits in medicine. J Lab Clin Med 52:34–42, 1958.
3. Emde C, Garner A, Blum A: Technical aspects of intraluminal pH-metry in man. Current status and recommendations. Gut 23:1177–1188, 1987.
4. Attwood SEA, DeMeester TR, Bremner CG, et al: Alkaline gastroesopha-

geal reflux: Implications in the development of complications in Barrett's columnar-lined lower esophagus. Surgery 1989 (in press).
5. Fuchs KH, DeMeester TR, Albertucci M: Specificity and sensitivity of diagnosis of gastroesophageal reflux disease. Surgery 102:575–580, 1987.
6. DeMeester TR, Johnson LF: The evaluation of objective measurements of gastroesophageal reflux disease and their contribution to patient management. Surg Clin North Am 56:39–53, 1976.

6

The Value of Simultaneous 24-Hour Ambulatory Esophageal and Gastric pH Monitoring:
An Analysis of 100 Investigations

Christopher S. Ball, Lloyd R. Jenkinson,
Tracey L. Norris, Anthony Watson

Introduction

Since its introduction as a clinical investigation,[1] 24-hour pH monitoring of the distal esophagus has become well established in the investigation of gastroesophageal reflux (GER). Although esophageal monitoring is highly specific and sensitive as an indicator of acid GER, reflux of gastric fluid with a pH above 4 is not considered abnormal. Consequently, some patients with endoscopic esophagitis and reflux symptoms have a negative esophageal pH test. They do not have abnormal esophageal exposure to acid but may be suffering from reflux of gastric contents of low acidity. This situation may result from low gastric acid secretion as a primary disorder or secondary to surgical vagotomy, gastric resection, or H^2-receptor antagonists; from excessive duodenogastric reflux which again may be primary, or secondary to surgical procedures including pyloroplasty, gastroenterostomy and cholecystectomy; or to the buffering of gastric acid by alkaline food, drink or medicines—an effect enhanced by delayed

Little AG, Ferguson MK, Skinner DB: Diseases of the Esophagus, Vol. II: Benign Diseases. Futura Publishing Company, Inc., Mount Kisco, NY, © 1990.

gastric emptying. Simultaneous monitoring of esophageal and gastric pH is a relatively new technique. It has been used to identify patients with duodenogastric reflux (DGR) who are at risk of GER of solely alkaline, or mixed acid and alkaline type.[2,3] This group of patients are at risk of particularly severe forms of esophagitis from the bile acid and pancreatic enzyme content of duodenal juice.[4]

We have evaluated our initial experience with the simultaneous pH monitoring technique in 100 patients with classic symptoms of GER. Fifteen healthy asymptomatic volunteers were also studied and from the data they provided, a range of normal values was established.

All patients had upper gastrointestinal endoscopy to establish the grade and extent of esophagitis. Patients and controls underwent esophageal manometry to define the exact position of the lower esophageal sphincter. A solid-state digital recorder with twin antimony pH electrodes (Synectics Medical, Stockholm, Sweden) was used for the pH monitoring test. The tips of the electrodes were positioned transnasally at 5 cm above the upper limit, and one at 5 cm below the lower limit of the lower esophageal sphincter. All subjects remained ambulatory for 16 hours of recording in the upright position and lay supine for the remaining 8 hours. Diet was rigidly standardized for timing and content of meals.

From the esophageal pH data, the percentage of total time spent at pH<4 was calculated. An esophageal acid exposure greater than 5% was considered pathological. Following this, the percentage of time spent at each whole pH interval (0–1, 1–2, 2–3 and so on to pH>8) was obtained for upright and supine periods of the study. The 5th and the 95th percentiles of control values for this method of analysis were plotted to produce a graph of the normal range of pH distribution in the esophagus. Patient data were then plotted against the background of normal ranges derived from the control group (Fig. 1). Using this method of pH data analysis and presentation, abnormal shifts in the esophageal pH distribution could be readily identified— acid shifts to the left of the graph and alkaline shifts to the right.

Gastric pH data was analyzed after the alkaline shifts produced by meals had been edited by the computer. Gastric baseline pH, defined as the pH value below pH 2 most frequently registered during the 24 hours study, was calculated. There is a close correlation between gastric baseline pH and gastric secretory status.[5]

The number of alkaline shifts in gastric pH to a pH>4 was obtained and an excessive number of alkaline episodes was considered

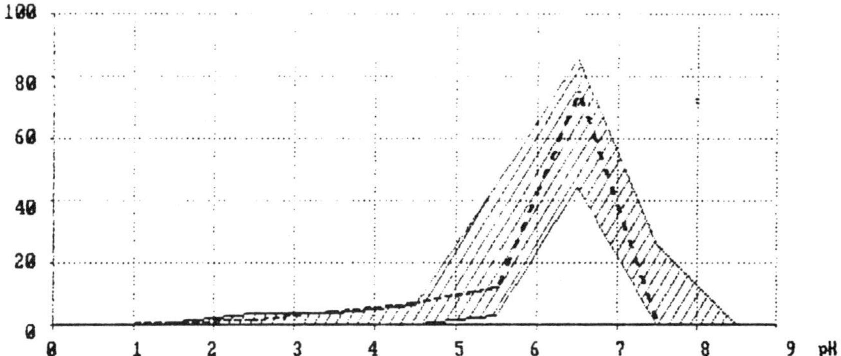

Figure 1: Percent time spent at each pH interval: esophageal data. Normal ranges = shaded area, patient data = broken line.

an indication of DGR. Patient values were compared with controls, and those below the 5th or above the 95th percentile were judged abnormal (Table I).

Gastric data were also presented as percentage time spent at each pH interval so that shifts in the distribution of gastric pH, acid to the left and alkaline to the right, could be identified (Fig. 2).

Abnormal esophageal acid exposure was detected in 74 patients, all of whom had endoscopic esophagitis. The esophageal pH profile was within normal limits in 26 patients, but 20 of these had esophagitis. There were no patients with an abnormal esophageal pH profile and normal endoscopy (Table II). Patients with pathological esophageal acid exposure showed a shift to the left on their pH interval graph but there were no instances of an alkaline shift to the right. Sixty-five patients had gastric pH profiles within normal limits (Table III). Among the 35 abnormal profiles, 21 had acid pH interval shifts to the left and low gastric baseline pH, indicative of gastric

Table I
Gastric pH Data: Control Group Percentiles

	5%	*95%*
gastric baseline pH	1.0	1.8
no. gastric alkaline episodes	0	40

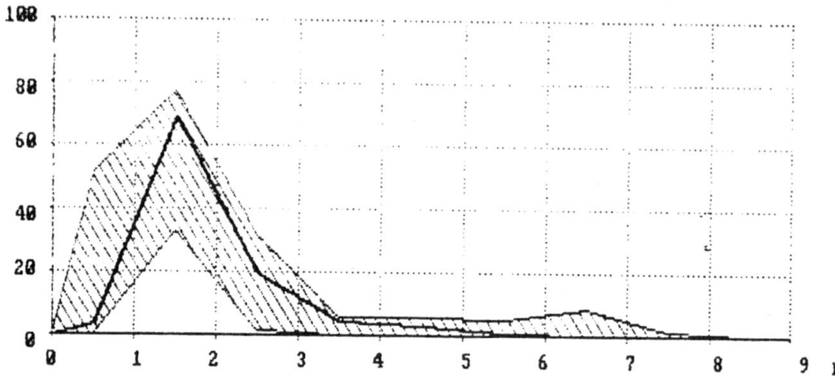

Figure 2: Percent time spent at each pH interval: gastric data. Normal ranges = shaded area, patient data = solid line.

hyperacidity; 14 had alkaline gastric pH interval shifts to the right, consistent with low gastric acidity. The gastric alkaline shift was associated with a high gastric baseline pH and no increase in the number of gastric alkaline episodes in 2 of the 14; these features favor low secretion as the cause of low acidity. The remaining 12 patients had a normal gastric baseline pH but an abnormally large number of alkaline episodes during the upright interprandial and supine periods, strongly suggestive of DGR (Fig. 3).

When the simultaneous pH traces were examined in detail, 4 of the 12 patients with suspected DGR had esophageal reflux episodes coincident with gastric alkaline episodes. These features are a prerequisite for the diagnosis of true alkaline reflux by the simultaneous pH monitoring technique. In the remaining eight patients with suspected DGR, esophageal reflux episodes were not seen at the time of gastric alkaline shifts; this does not exlude the possibility of alkaline GER being undetectable because of the high pH of the refluxate. The

Table II
Endoscopy and Esophageal pH Results in 100 Patients

	Endoscopic Esophagitis	Normal Endoscopy
positive pH test	74	0
negative pH test	20	6

Table III
The Gastric pH Profile in 100
Patients with Symptoms of GER

normal profile	65
hyperacidity	21
low acidity/low secretion	5
low acidity/DGR	9

majority of patients in our study (65%) had a gastric profile with normal limits. Hyperacidity was recorded in 28% of acid refluxers; this is not an unexpected finding considering the high incidence of hypersecretion among refluxers previously described.[6,7] Conventional esophageal pH monitoring in patients with GER and normal

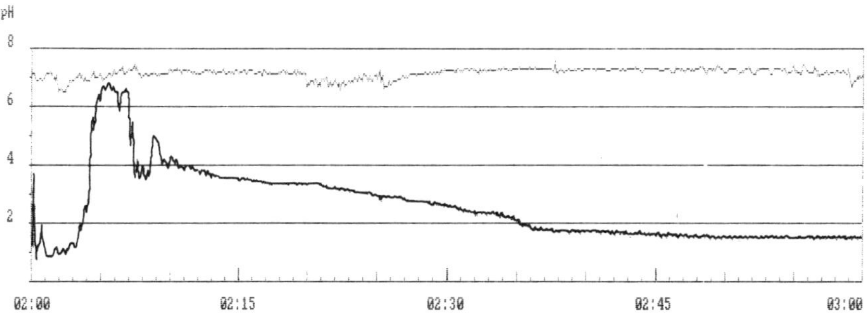

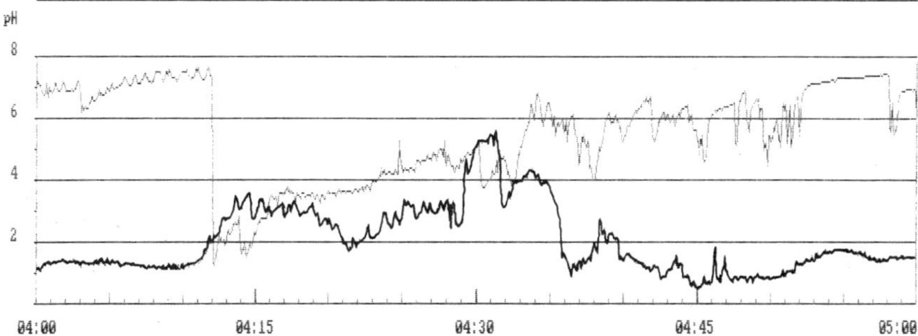

Figure 3: Simultaneous esophageal and gastric pH record showing gastric alkaline episode (top) and mixed esophageal and duodenogastric reflux (bottom).

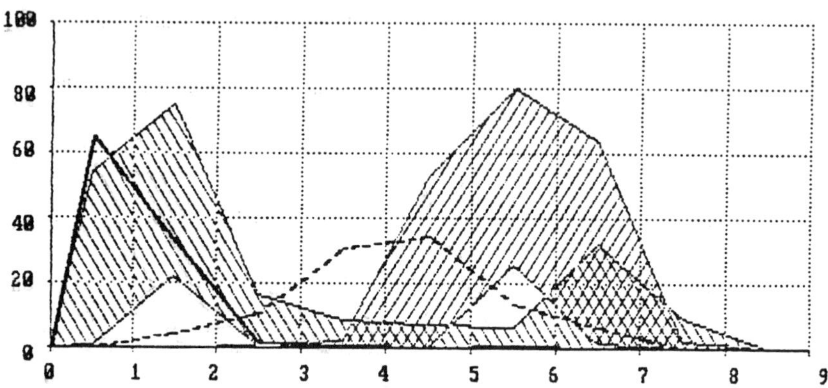

Figure 4: Combined esophageal and gastric pH interval graph. Patient data show combined acid shift of gastric hyperacidity and acid GER.

or high levels of gastric acidity is likely to provide a true estimation of the severity of the disease. Reflux-related esophagitis can occur in low secretion states and, rarely, in achlorhydria.[8] A more common explanation for reduced gastric acidity is DGR. This occurs in the intact stomach,[9] and is probably a physiological event.[10] In these patients, with low acidity but high potency of gastroesophageal refluxate, conventional esophageal pH monitoring may seriously underestimate the severity of reflux. We have found the method of pH interval analysis to be helpful in screening for abnormal esophageal and gastric pH distribution, and pH shifts at both monitoring sites can be displayed by combining the esophageal and gastric data in graphic form on the same axes (Fig. 4).

The routine use of simultaneous esophageal and gastric pH monitoring will help to identify those refluxers whose pathophysiology includes abnormal gastric acidity or DGR. It is of particular value in the evaluation of patients with reflux symptoms and esophagitis but a normal esophageal pH monitoring test.

References

1. Johnson LF, DeMeester TR: 24-hour pH monitoring of the distal esophagus. Am J Gastroenterol 62:325, 1974.
2. Andreoli F, Balloni F, Bigiotti A: Gastroesophageal reflux of mixed type. Minerva Med 75:213 1984.
3. Cortesini C, Pucciani F: Usefulness of combined gastric and esophageal pH monitoring in detecting gastroesophageal alkaline and mixed reflux. Eur Surg Res 16:378, 1984.

4. Gillison EW, Decastro VAM, Nyhus LM, et al: The sigificance of bile in reflux esophagitis. Surg Gynecol Obstet 134:419 1972.
5. Ball CSl Norris TL, Watson A, et al: Clinical applications of simultaneous 24-hour ambulatory gastric and oesophageal pH monitoring. Gut 28:A1377, 1987.
6. Casten DF: Esophageal hiatal hernia and gastric acid secretion. Arch Surg 88:255, 1964.
7. Johansson KE, Tibbling L: Gastric secretion and reflux pattern in reflux oesophagitis before and during ranitidine treatment. Scand J Gastroenterol 21:487, 1986.
8. Palmer ER: Subacute erosive ("peptic") esophagitis associated with achlorhydria. N Engl J Med 262:927, 1960.
9. Tolin RD, Malmud LS: Stelzer F, et al: Enterogastric reflux in normal subjects and patients with Bilroth II gastroenterostomy. Gastroenterology 77:1027, 1979.
10. Muller-Lissner SA, Fimmel CJ, Sonnenberg A, et al: Novel approach to quantify duodenogastric reflux in healthy volunteers and in patients with type I gastric ulcer. Gut 24:510, 1983.

Gastroesophageal Reflux into the Proximal Esophagus: Four-Channel Esophagopharyngeal pH Study in Normal Patients and in Symptomatic Patients

S.W. Fannin, W.H. Falor, J.M. Miller, J.M. Kraus, B.C. Taylor, V. Greczanik

Introduction

Twenty-four-hour esophageal pH monitoring detects and quantifies the amount of gastroesophageal reflux (GER) into the distal esophagus and documents GER's role in the symptoms of heartburn and esophageal injury. Standard recording methods to measure GER use a pH sensitive electrode placed 5 cm above the lower esophageal sphincter (LES).[1]

There has been evidence that GER plays a role in disease processes of the upper esophagus, larynx, and lungs, such as asthma, chronic hoarseness, dysmotility of the upper esophageal sphincter, aspiration pneumonitis, and even sudden infant death syndrome.[2-4] However, standard recording methods fail to detect the extent of cephalad reflux of gastric juices into the proximal portions of the

Little AG, Ferguson MK, Skinner DB: Diseases of the Esophagus, Vol. II: Benign Diseases. Futura Publishing Company, Inc., Mount Kisco, NY, © 1990.

esophagus and pharynx. We have previously described the Esophageal pH Ambulatory Recorder (EpHAR) which measures pH changes simultaneously at four levels in the esophagopharynx.[5,6] The EpHAR, thus, may be used to detect GER into the proximal esophagus and pharynx.

The purpose of this study was to use the EpHAR system to: (1) measure the frequency of GER into the proximal levels of the esophagus in individuals with symptoms of GER and asymptomatic volunteers, (2) determine if any correlation exists between the symptomology of patients and proximal GER, and (3) determine if the lower and upper esophageal sphincter pressure as measured by water perfusion manometry differs in individuals with proximal GER.

Methods

The EpHAR was used to measure ambulatory, out-patient, 24-hour esophagopharyngeal pH at four levels above the LES (5, 11, 17, and 23 cm) in 128 individuals, 83 symptomatic from presumed GER and 45 asymptomatic volunteers. The symptomatic group were patients who were referred for evaluation to Akron City Hospital's Esophageal Laboratory. Sixty-nine individuals from the symptomatic group had esophageal manometry performed with measurement of lower esophageal pressure (LESP) and upper esophageal pressure (UESP). A symptomatic individual was classified in one of three groups: (1) typical symptoms of GER (heartburn, regurgitation, or dysphagia), (2) atypical symptoms of GER (cough, wheezing, hoarseness, atypical chest pain, etc.), or (3) combined symptoms (typical and atypical). Of the 83 symptomatic individuals, 29 had typical symptoms of GER, 13 had atypical symptoms, and 41 had combined symptoms. The asymptomatic group were volunteers with no history suggestive of GER. Esophageal water perfusion manometry was not performed in the asymptomatic group.

Data recorded 5 cm above the LES were analyzed and scored by the Johnson and DeMeester algorithm. Individuals were classified as either a pathological refluxer (PR group) or a normal refluxer (NR group). From the data recorded at 5, 11, 17, and 23 cm above the LES, the percent time pH<4 was calculated for the total, erect, and supine time periods. Individuals were classified as having abnormal acid exposure at each level of the esophagus if the percent time pH<4 was greater than the mean percent time pH<4 plus 2 standard de-

Table I
Mean and Standard Deviation of the Percent Time pH <4 for the Asymptomatic and Symptomatic Groups at Each Level of the Esophagus above the LES for Each Time Period*

Level	Time Period	Asymptomatic % time pH <4 Mean ± SD N = 45	Symptomatic % time pH <4 Mean ± SD N = 83	p
5 cm	Total	3.6 ± 3.3	11.5 ± 17.9	<.05
	Erect	5.4 ± 5.5	12.4 ± 19.1	<.05
	Supine	1.2 ± 2.0	10.2 ± 19.1	<.05
11 cm	Total	1.3 ± 1.9	5.5 ± 10.4	<.05
	Erect	2.1 ± 3.3	5.3 ± 9.1	<.05
	Supine	0.3 ± 0.5	5.8 ± 14.3	<.05
17 cm	Total	0.9 ± 1.4	3.2 ± 7.8	<.05
	Erect	1.4 ± 2.3	3.4 ± 9.2	<.05
	Supine	0.3 ± 0.9	2.8 ± 7.7	<.05
23 cm	Total	0.2 ± 0.6	1.0 ± 2.5	<.05
	Erect	0.3 ± 0.9	1.1 ± 4.0	<.05
	Supine	0.0 ± 0.2	0.5 ± 1.8	<.05

* Statistical significance at the 0.05 level.

viations calculated for the NR group. The percentage of pathological refluxers with normal and abnormal acid exposure were calculated at each level of the esophagus for each test period and symptom classification. The mean LESP and UESP were calculated for each group. Student's *t*-test, goodness of fit analysis, and the Mann-Whitney test were used to compare groups.

Results

The mean percent time pH<4 is shown in Table I for the asymptomatic and symptomatic groups. The symptomatic group had statistically greater acid exposure at all four levels of the esophagus during all test periods (p<0.05).

Based on the Johnson and DeMeester scoring of data recorded 5 cm above the LES, 60.2% of the symptomatic group and 31.1% of the asymptomatic volunteers had abnormal composite scores. Five cm above the LES, 64 (50%) of the 128 individuals (50 symptomatic and 14 asymptomatic) were classified as having pathological reflux

Table II
Mean and Standard Deviation of the Percent Time pH <4 for Normal Refluxers (NR) and Pathological Refluxers (PR) at Each Level of the Esophagus above the LES for Each Time Period*

Level	Time Period	NR Group % time pH <4 Mean ± SD N = 64	PR Group % time pH <4 Mean ± SD N = 64	p
5 cm	Total	1.7 ± 1.5	15.8 ± 18.8	<.05
	Erect	2.5 ± 2.4	17.3 ± 20.0	<.05
	Supine	0.4 ± 0.7	13.6 ± 20.6	<.05
11 cm	Total	0.9 ± 1.2	7.2 ± 11.5	<.05
	Erect	1.2 ± 1.7	7.1 ± 9.9	<.05
	Supine	0.3 ± 0.9	7.3 ± 16.0	<.05
17 cm	Total	0.6 ± 1.0	4.2 ± 8.6	<.05
	Erect	0.8 ± 1.5	4.6 ± 10.2	<.05
	Supine	0.3 ± 1.0	3.5 ± 8.6	<.05
23 cm	Total	0.2 ± 0.3	1.3 ± 2.8	<.05
	Erect	0.2 ± 0.4	1.5 ± 4.6	<.05
	Supine	0.1 ± 0.4	0.7 ± 2.1	<.05

* Statistical significance at the 0.05 level.

(PR group); 64 (50%) (33 symptomatic and 31 asymptomatic volunteers) were classified as having normal reflux (NR group). The mean percent time pH<4 and standard deviation for each group is shown in Table II. The PR group had significantly greater acid exposure at all four levels of the esophagus during all test periods (p<0.05).

Upper limits of normal for acid exposure at 5, 11, 17, and 23 cm during each test period were calculated to be the mean percent time pH<4 of the NR group plus 2 standard deviations. Based on this threshold, the percentage of individuals with abnormal acid exposure at each level of the esophagus in the PR and NR groups is shown in Table III. The PR group had a statistically greater percentage of individuals with abnormal acid exposure at all levels of the esophagus and test periods (p<0.05) except during the supine time period at 23 cm above the LES (p>0.05).

The percentage of individuals with abnormal acid exposure in the PR group were classified according to symptom complex (typical, atypical, combined, or no symptoms) for each test period and level of the esophagus (Fig. 1A-C). Goodness of fit analysis revealed no statistical difference between groups of symptoms (p>0.05).

Table III
The Percentage of Individuals in the Normal Reflux (NR) and Pathological Reflux (PR) Groups with Abnormal Acid Exposure (Mean Percent Time pH <4 Plus 2 Standard Deviations) at Each Level of the Esophagus above the LES for Each Time Period*

Level	Time Period	NR Group % Abnormal N = 64	PR Group % Abnormal N = 64	p
5 cm	Total	3.1	78.1	<.05
	Erect	3.1	70.3	<.05
	Supine	7.8	76.6	<.05
11 cm	Total	6.3	53.1	<.05
	Erect	3.1	42.2	<.05
	Supine	6.2	45.3	<.05
17 cm	Total	4.7	35.9	<.05
	Erect	3.1	29.7	<.05
	Supine	4.7	23.4	<.05
23 cm	Total	6.3	25.0	<.05
	Erect	4.7	21.9	<.05
	Supine	3.1	14.1	NS

* Statistical significance at the 0.05 level. NS = Not significant.

Sixty-nine of the 83 individuals in the symptomatic group had esophageal manometry performed. Differences in LESP and UESP were analyzed between groups of individuals with normal and abnormal acid exposure at each level of the esophagus for each test period. No statistical differences could be detected using the Mann-Whitney U-test. Figure 2A-C shows the mean and standard deviations in normal and abnormal groups at 23 cm above the LES for all time periods.

Discussion

Individuals symptomatic of GER have greater acid exposure at proximal levels of the esophagus compared to asymptomatic individuals for all time periods. Individuals defined to be pathological refluxers (PR) by abnormal Johnson and DeMeester composite scoring of reflux events 5 cm above the LES also have significantly greater acid exposure at proximal levels of the esophagus for all time periods than normal refluxers (NR).

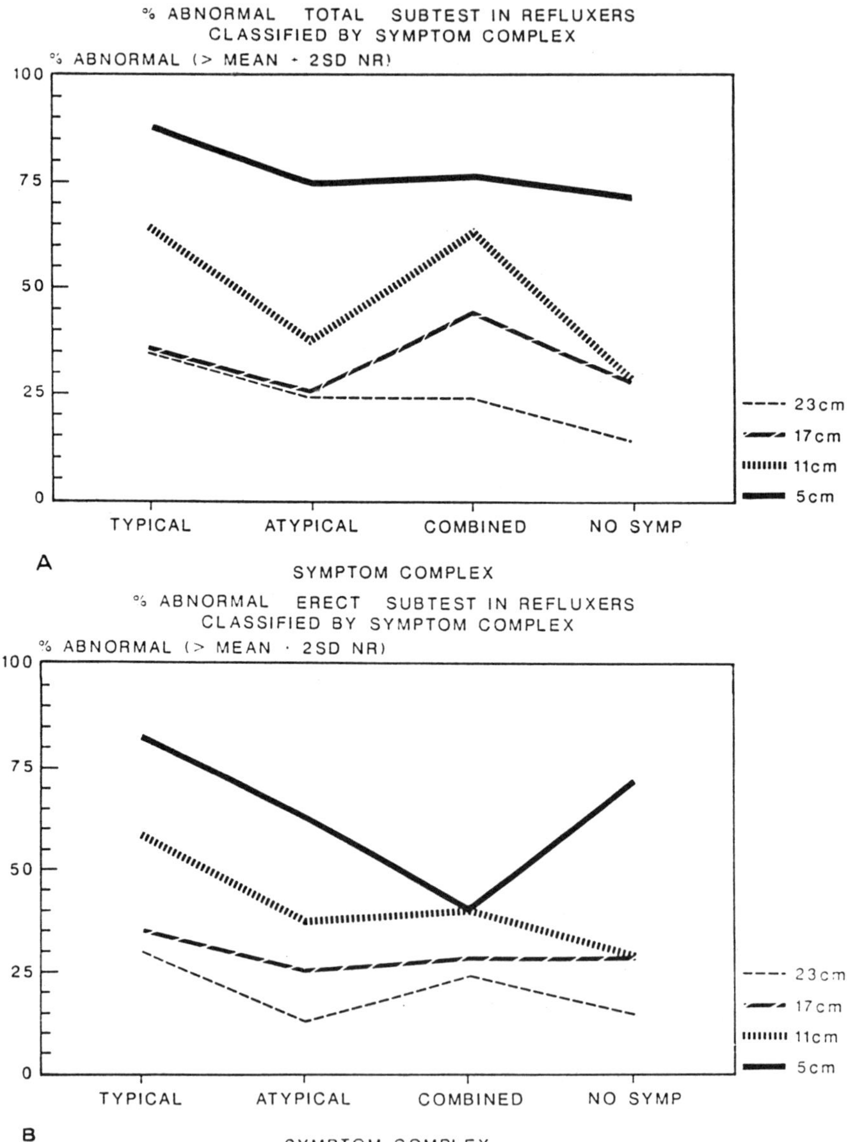

Figure 1: (A-C) The percentage of individuals with abnormal acid exposure in the PR group classified according to symptom group. Figure 1A shows the total test, Figure 1B shows the erect subset, and Figure 1C shows the supine subset. Differences between symptom goups at each level of the esophagus was not significant by goodness of fit analysis (p>0.05).

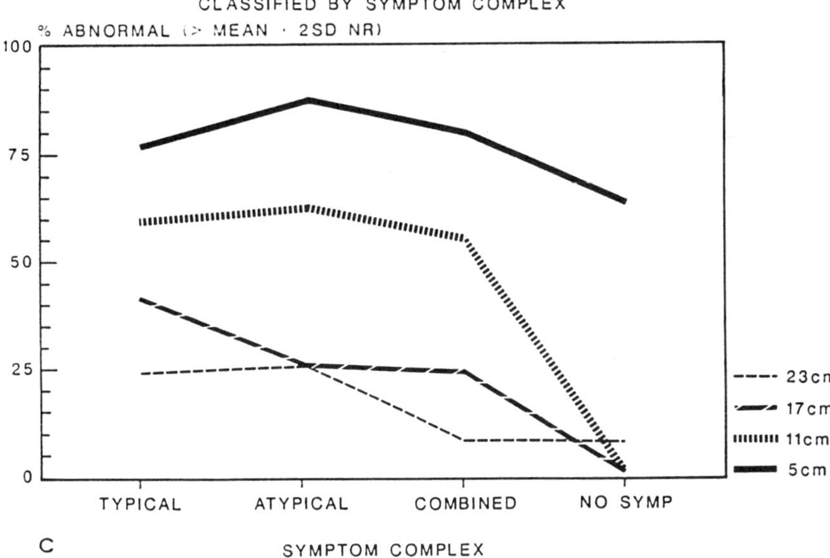

Figure 1: (C)

Upper limits of normal for acid exposure at 5, 11, 17, and 23 cm above the LES were determined from the NR group (mean percent time pH<4 plus 2 standard deviations). In the PR group, 25%, 21.9%, and 14.1% of individuals had abnormal acid exposure documented throughout the esophagus and up to 23 cm above the LES for the total, erect, and supine time periods compared to 6.3%, 4.7%, and 3.1% of individuals in the NR group, respectively.

In the PR group, there were no statistical differences in symptom complex between individuals with abnormal and normal proximal acid exposure nor could differences be detected in the LESP and UESP between groups.

In conclusion, the EpHAR has been shown to be useful in documenting the cephalad extent of GER. A significant percentage of individuals with pathologic reflux determined by Johnson and DeMeester composite scoring have abnormal reflux into the proximal esophagus. Since no specific symptom complex or sphincter pressure measurement could identify individuals with proximal GER, multilevel monitoring of esophageal pH is essential for proximal GER detection.

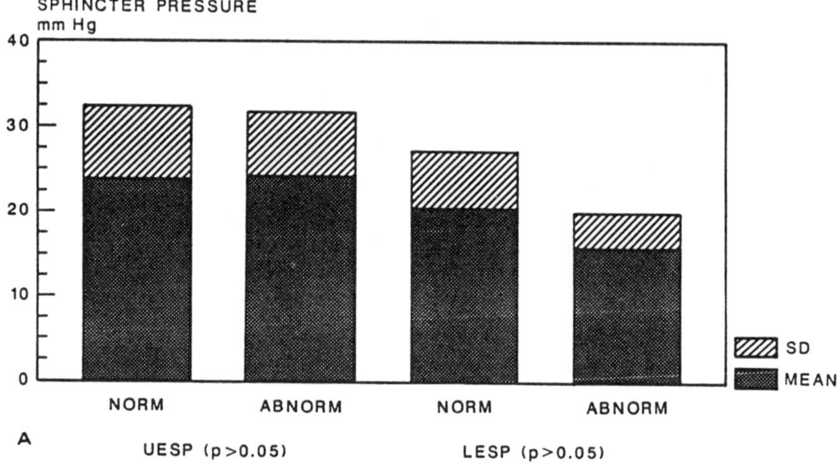

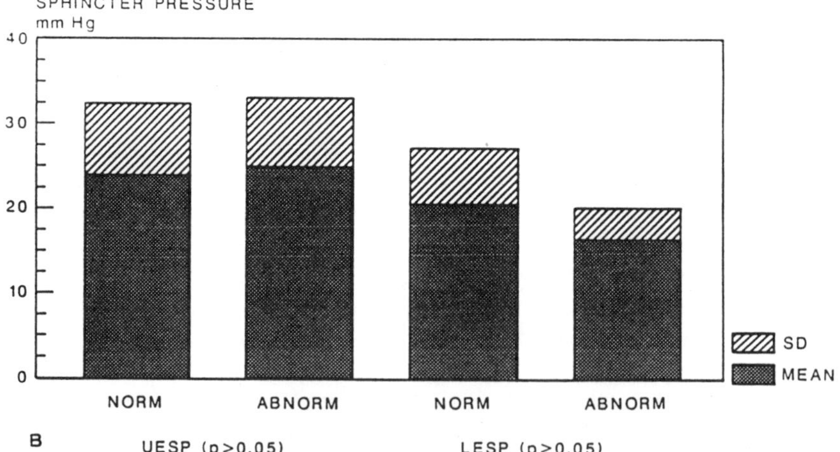

Figure 2: (A-C) The mean UESP and LESP (mmHg) between individuals classified as having normal acid exposure and abnormal acid exposure at 23 cm above the LES. Figure 1A shows the total test, Figure 1B shows the erect subset, and Figure 1C shows the supine subset. Differences in UESP and LESP between normal and abnormal groups at each level of the esophagus were not statistically significant by the Mann-Whitney U-test (p>0.05).

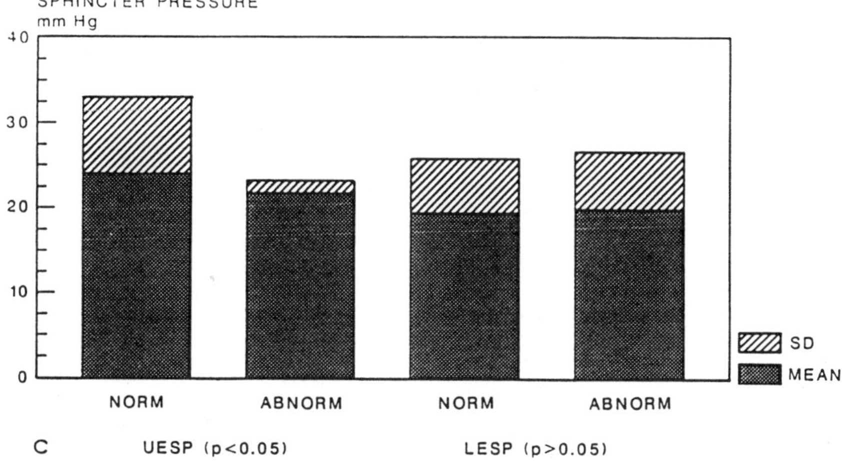

Figure 2: (C)

ACKNOWLEDGMENTS: This work was supported in part by grants from The Akron City Hospital Foundation, The Sisler-McFawn Foundation, and The Musson Charitable Trust.

References

1. DeMeester TR, Johnson LF, Joseph GJ: Patterns of gastroesophageal reflux in health and disease. Ann Surg 184:459, 1976.
2. Allen C, Newhouse M: Gastroesophageal reflux and chronic respiratory disease. Am Rev Respir Dis 129:645, 1984.
3. Boyle JT, Tuchman DN, Altschuler SM, et al: Mechanisms for the association of gastroesophageal reflux and bronchospasm. Am Rev Respir Dis 131:S16, 1985.
4. Ducolone A, Vandevenne A, et al: Gastroesophageal reflux in patients with asthma and chronic bronchitis. Am Rev Respir Dis 135:327, 1987.
5. Falor WH, Miller JM, Kraus J, et al: Outpatient computer- based 32-hour esophageal pH studies teletransmitted to a central esophageal laboratory. Arch Intern Med 145:1617, 1985.
6. Miller JM, Fannin SW, Falor WH, et al: Instrumentation for the automatic recording and analysis of esophageal pH. In: Esophageal Disorders: Pathophysiology and Therapy, New York, Raven Press, 1985, p 133.

8

The Sensitivity and Specificity of Histologic Parameters in the Diagnosis of Gastroesophageal Reflux Disease

Stephen E. A. Attwood, Thomas C. Smyrk,
Antony P. Barlow, Tom R. DeMeester

Introduction

The histologic markers of reflux esophagitis include squamous hyperplasia (increased papillary height and basal zone thickness) and intraepithelial inflammation (polymorphs and eosinophils within the squamous epithelium).[1-4] To this list has recently been added the balloon cell, said to be a marker of cellular damage.[5] While each of these histologic parameters may be present in gastroesophageal reflux disease, it is often difficult in practice to choose a cutoff point that distinguishes the upper limit of normal from disease. In addition, markers of esophageal injury are not necessarily specific for damage by gastroesophageal reflux; histologic esophagitis may result from pill-induced injury and infections such as candida, herpes, and cytomegalovirus.

In order to identify the sensitivity and specificity of histologic abnormalities in the diagnosis of gastroesophageal reflux disease, we

Little AG, Ferguson MK, Skinner DB: Diseases of the Esophagus, Vol. II: Benign Diseases. Futura Publishing Company, Inc., Mount Kisco, NY, © 1990.

evaluated each parameter in patients whose esophageal acid exposure had been assessed by 24-hour pH monitoring.

Methods

Patients

The study group consisted of 100 consecutive patients who had 24-hour pH monitoring and endoscopy with biopsy. All patients had presented with complaints of heartburn or dysphagia. Their mean age was 50 ± 14 years.

Studies Performed

Pinch biopsies were taken in each patient using a grasp forceps. In those patients in whom no macroscopic esophagitis was seen, biopsies were taken at random from the lower esophagus. The number of biopsies per patient ranged from 1 to 18, with a mean of 4.6. Without knowledge of the clinical findings, hematoxylin and eosin stained slides were examined as follows.

All levels were scanned for well-oriented areas, defined as areas in which a subepithelial papilla was visible for its entire length. Epithelial thickness and papillary height were measured using an eyepiece micrometer. The one papilla occupying the greatest proportion of the epithelium was taken to represent papillary height. Basal zone thickness was measured between two well-oriented papillae. The largest value for the basal zone thickness, expressed as a percentage of epithelial thickness, was used. The tissue section with the greatest number of neutrophils was used to count intraepithelial polymorphs (IEP) per section, and IEP per high power field (HPF). Intraepithelial eosinophils (IEE) were counted in the same way. Balloon cells, defined as pale, swollen cells in the stratum spinosum, were graded semiquantitatively on a scale of 1 through 4.

Twenty-four-hour pH monitoring was performed in all patients using a pH probe placed 5 cm above the manometrically defined lower esophageal sphincter.[6] The patients remained ambulatory and recorded their daily events and the time and duration of sleep. Data were accumulated on a portable recorder (Synectics digitrapper) and analyzed by computer using the Gastrosoft program. Pathological acid gastroesophageal reflux was diagnosed by a composite score for the exposure of the esophagus to a pH below 4 of > 14.8, using the scoring system of Johnson and DeMeester.[7]

Statistics

For each parameter, the proportion of true-positive and false-positive diagnoses at specific cutoff points was calculated using the composite score from pH monitoring as the definitive test. For example, 34 of 45 acid refluxers had papillary heights greater than 65% of epithelial thickness compared to 4 of 16 nonrefluxers. Therefore, the point on the curve that represents 65% is plotted at 0.75:0.25. Receiver Operator Characteristic (ROC) curves[8] were constructed for each histologic parameter using a computer program (Rocfast, Robert Centor, Medical College of Virginia, Richmond) which also calculated the area under the curve and the standard error for each curve. The area under each curve was compared to the area under the line of chance (which equaled 0.5) to determine whether a significant difference existed between the two.

The point of maximum likelihood, that is, the point that gives the best combination of sensitivity and specificity, was calculated by computer although it could easily be identified visually from the plotted curve. Using the point of maximum likelihood as the chosen cutoff, a simple scoring system was devised based on the number of histologic abnormalities present, and a sixth curve constructed.

Results

Figures 1a–e show the ROC curves derived for each parameter. The curves for papillary height and basal zone thickness were significantly different from the line of chance. The point of maximum likelihood was 10% for basal zone thickness and 65% for papillary height.

Intraepithelial polymorphs and eosinophils gave curves that were closer to the line of chance, largely because approximately half of the acid refluxers had no intraepithelial inflammation. When more than one inflammatory cell was present in a tissue section, the finding was highly specific.

Balloon cells were frequently seen in refluxers (82%), but the ROC

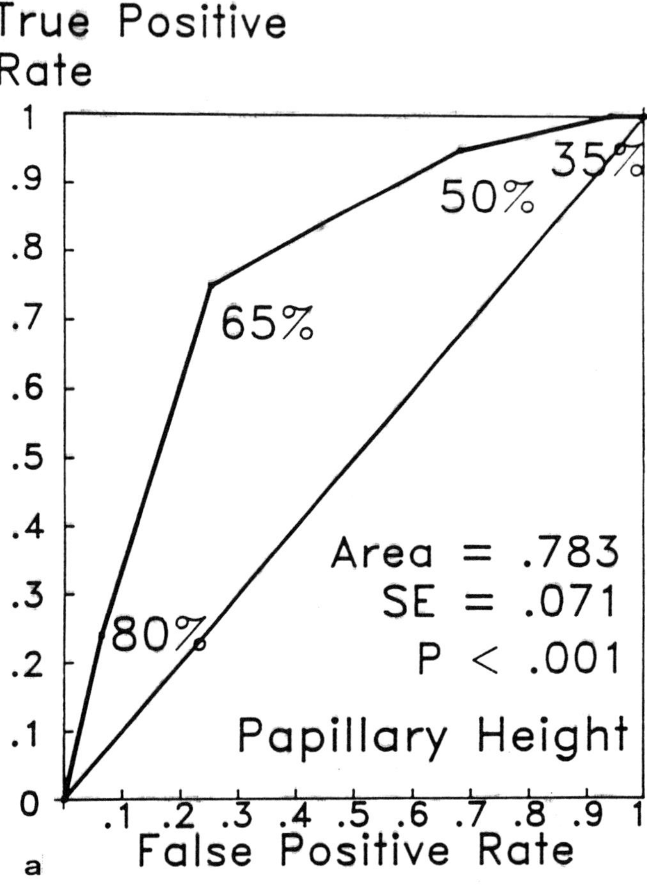

Figure 1: Receive Operator Characteristic curves for histological abnormalities that indicate acid gastroesophageal reflux: (a) papillary height expressed as a percentage of epithelial thickness; (b) basal zone hyperplasia expressed as a percentage of epithelial thickness; (c) intraepithelial polymorphs (IEP) expressed as the number of IEP per section; (d) intraepithelial eosinophils (IEE) expressed as the number of IEE per section; and (e) balloon cells expressed as a semiquantitative estimate of the extent of balloon cell change.

curve showed only a small deviation from the line of chance, resulting in an area under the curve that was not statistically greater than pure chance ($p > 0.05$).

The curve for the combined histologic score (Fig. 2) revealed that with one abnormal histologic parameter there was a sensitivity of 98%

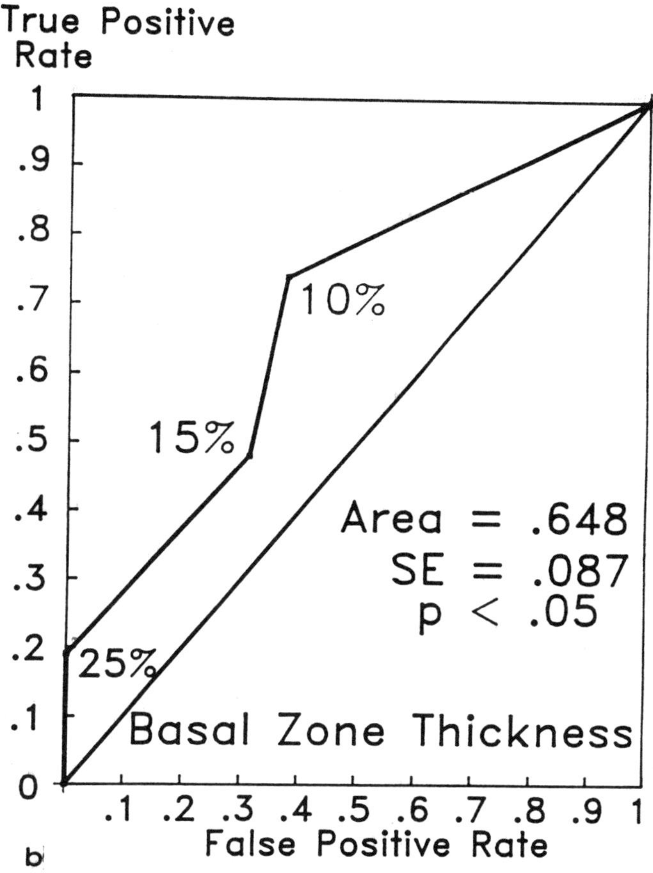

Figure 1B: *Continued*

and with four the specificity was 100%. The point of maximum like-lihood was 2 with a sensitivity at this point of 85% and a specificity of 65%.

Discussion

ROC curves give a visual representation of the performance of a test. By showing the relationship between sensitivity and specificity over a range of cutoff values, they enable the observer to choose a cutoff point of high specificity or sensitivity depending on the role

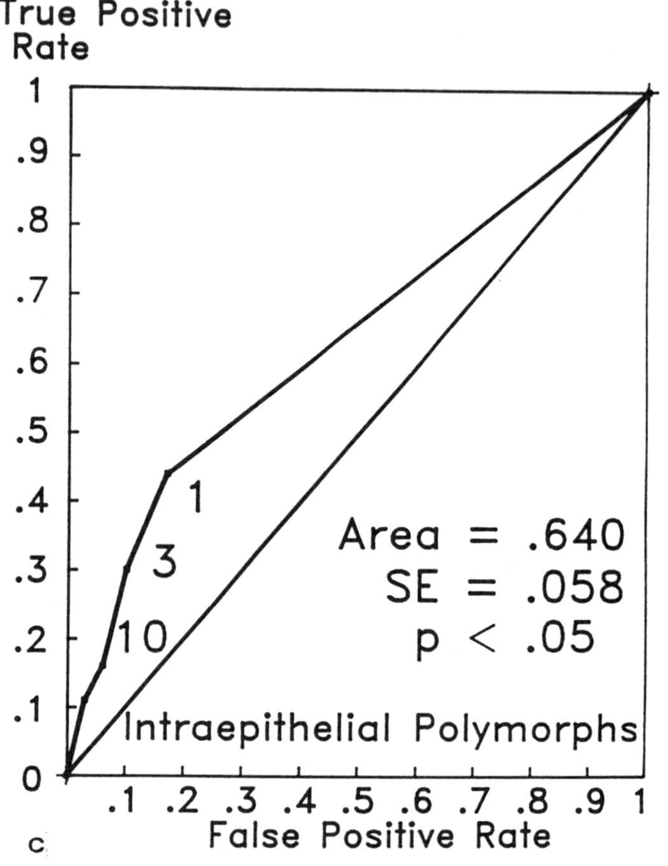

Figure 1C: *Continued*

of the test in the clinical decision-making process. In addition, ROC curves allow statistical analysis and comparison with other parameters over the full range of observed values.[8]

ROC curves have been used primarily in the evaluation of clinical laboratory tests. A major difficulty of this type of analysis is that patients must be separated into "disease" and "no disease" groups by independent means. For this study we have used 24-hour pH monitoring as our definitive diagnostic test. However, it too will have a certain sensitivity and specificity, both of which we have previously estimated to be greater than 90%.[9,10] Clearly, if the "gold standard"

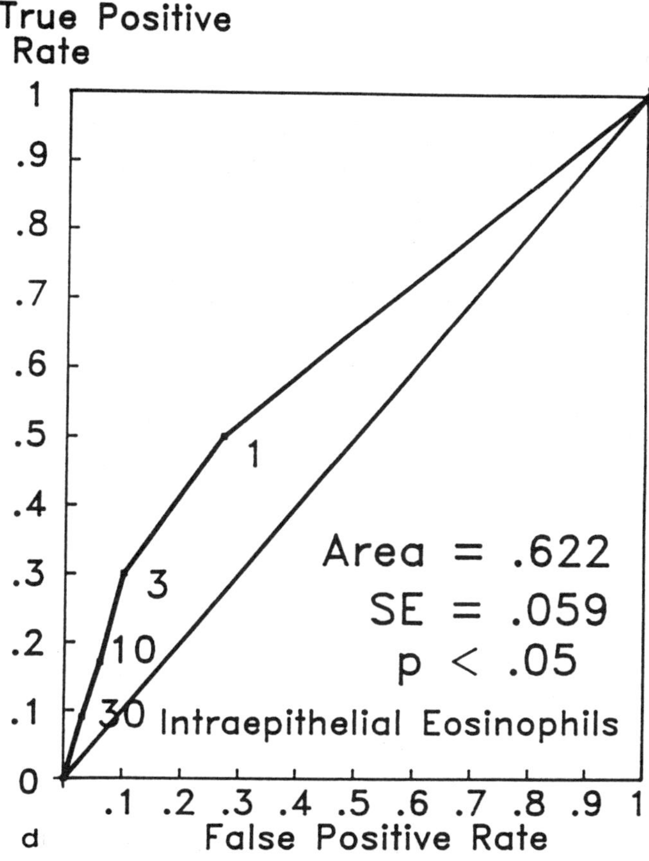

Figure 1D: *Continued*

is not perfect, then the accuracy of any compared test could be under- or overestimated.

The curves for individual histologic parameters show that the best combination of sensitivity and specificity for indicators of squamous epithelial hyperplasia is at the cutoff values of 65% for papillary height and 10% for basal zone thickness, values similar to those suggested by previous authors.[1-3] At these points, the sensitivity of each parameter is approximately 75% and the specificity is 65% to 70%. The results for intraepithelial inflammation also parallel previous experience, with only 50% of acid refluxers having IEP or IEE. Note, however, that for low-grade inflammation, i.e., one inflammatory cell

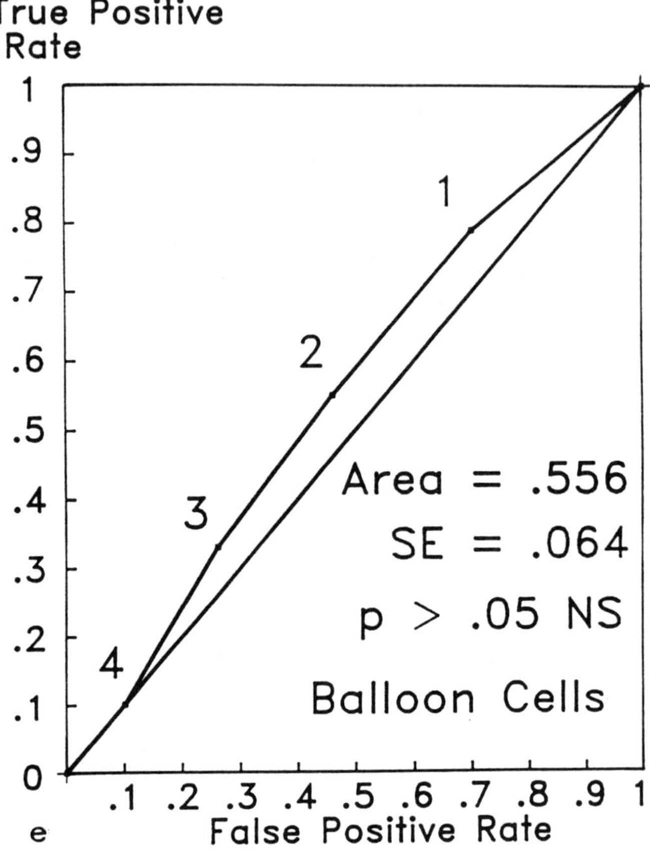

Figure 1E: *Continued*

per tissue section, the specificity of IEP for acid reflux is 82%, while IEE has a specificity of 75%. If the cutoff value is shifted to three or more inflammatory cells per section, the specificity climbs to greater than 90%, but the sensitivity drops to around 30%. Thus, intraepithelial inflammatory cells are useful if present, but the parameters for squamous hyperplasia provide better separation of acid-refluxers from nonreflux populations.

When the histologic parameters are combined, the prediction becomes more accurate. With two or more parameters above their point of maximum likelihood, the accuracy is clinically useful with a sensitivity of 78% and a specificity of 70%.

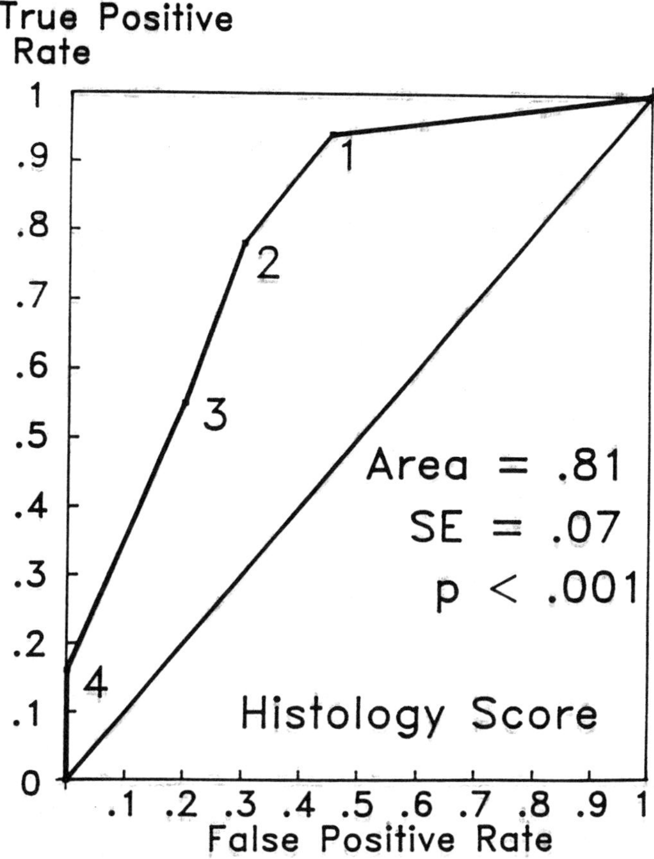

Figure 2: Receiver Operator Characteristic curve for the number of histologic abnormalities that indicate acid gastroesophageal reflux disease, using a score of one unit for each abnormal parameter: papillary height, basal zone hyperplasia, intraepithelial polymorphs, and intraepithelial eosinophils.

Three aspects of this study may limit its accuracy. First, the lack of a diagnostic gold standard for reflux esophagitis. We believe 24-hour pH monitoring is the single best test of excess esophageal acid exposure, but differences in protective factors or differences in the nature of the refluxate may mean that a similar degree of exposure to pH < 4 causes esophagitis in one patient but not in another. Second, our disease-free population is not composed of normal volunteers. They are symptomatic patients with normal levels of esophageal acid exposure. This group could include patients with esophagitis due to pills, infection, or other factors. This highlights the point that histologic abnormalities are markers of tissue injury, but not necessarily markers of the etiology of disease. Balloon cells in particular appear to be a sensitive and early marker of esophageal injury[11] and their detection may be more useful in practice than is shown in this study.

Finally, the specific location of esophageal biopsies is not known in our patients. Most investigators feel that biopsies from the distal 2 cm of the esophagus cannot be used to diagnose reflux esophagitis because of the effects of physiological reflux.

Conclusions

Histologic abnormalities can be useful predictors of acid gastroesophageal reflux disease. While no one parameter is ideal, abnormalities in any combination of two or more parameters are highly specific for gastroesophageal reflux disease and sensitive enough to be of clinical value. A positive histologic result in the presence of a negative 24-hour pH study should prompt a search for an alternative cause of esophagitis.

References

1. Ismael-Beigi F, Horton PF, Pope CE: Histological consequences of gastroesophageal reflux in man. Gastroenterology 58:163, 1970.
2. Ismael-Beigi F, Pope CE: Distribution of the histological changes of gastroesophageal reflux in the distal esophagus of man. Gastroenterology 66:1109, 1974.
3. Behar J, Sheahan DC: Histologic abnormalities in reflux esophagitis. Arch Pathol 99:387, 1975.
4. Heilmann KL, Siewert JR, Ottenjann R, et al: Histomorphology of esophageal reflux disease: Results of biopsy histology in a multicenter trial with cimetidine. In: Diseases of the Esophagus, Siewert JR, Hölscher AH (eds), Springer Verlag, 1987, p 1130.
5. Jessurum J, Yardley JH, Giardiello FM, et al: Intracytoplasmic plasma proteins in distended esophageal squamous cells (balloon cells). Mod Pathol 3:175, 1988.
6. DeMeester TR, Wang C-I, Wernley JA, et al: Technique, indications and clinical use of 24-hour esophageal pH monitoring. J Thorac Cardiovasc Surg 79:656, 1980.
7. Johnson LF, DeMeester TR: Development of the 24-hour intraesophageal

pH monitoring composite scoring system. J Clin Gastroenterol 8(Suppl): 52, 1986.
8. Beck JR, Shultz EK: The use of relative operating characteristic (ROC) curves in test performance evaluation. Arch Pathol Lab Med 110:13, 1986.
9. DeMeester TR: The limitations of 24-hour pH monitoring of the esophagus. In: Esophageal Disorders: Pathophysiology and Therapy, DeMeester TR, Skinner DB (eds), New York, Raven Press, 1985, p 109.
10. Fuchs KH, DeMeester TR, Albertucci M: Specificity and sensitivity of objective diagnosis of gastroesophageal reflux disease. Surgery 102:575, 1987.
11. Smyrk T, Brewer A, Bailey RT, et al: Balloon cells are an early finding in pill-induced esophageal injury. Mod Pathol 2:89a, 1989.

9

Lower Esophageal Sphincter Opening Pressure and Volume Define the Gastric Component of the Reflux Barrier

P. Carvalho, Philip E. Donahue, I. Miidla,
Y.-S. Shen, C. Thomas Bombeck, Lloyd M. Nyhus

Introduction

Gastroesophageal reflux (GER), regurgitation of gastric contents from the stomach into the esophagus, occurs as a result of differences in pressure between these segments of the gastrointestinal tract. Since intraesophageal pressure is negative and intragastric pressure is positive, there is a pressure gradient which, in the absence of a reflux barrier, forces gastric contents into the esophagus. Physiological reflux occurs when the gastroesophageal pressure gradient (GEPG) overcomes the effective pressure of the reflux barrier. The existence of a multifactorial reflux barrier is well recognized. However, since Fyke et al.[1] identified the lower esophageal sphincter (LES), this structure has been considered to be the most important factor in reflux prevention. In the past two decades, the LES component of the esophageal reflux barrier has been the focus of studies of GER.

The gastric components of the reflux barrier (GCRB), such as the gastric cardia muscle, intragastric pressure, and gastric distension,

Little AG, Ferguson MK, Skinner DB: Diseases of the Esophagus, Vol. II: Benign Diseases. Futura Publishing Company, Inc., Mount Kisco, NY, © 1990.

have gained little attention because of the inherent difficulties in their measurement. We aim to examine this portion of the reflux barrier by simultaneously measuring the esophageal component of the reflux barrier (ECRB) and the GCRB, thus elucidating the initiation of reflux episodes and the pathogenesis of gastroesophageal reflux (GER).

Materials and Methods

Ten adult mongrel dogs (US Research Farm, Medina, TN) with a mean weight of 35.4 ± 5.9 kg were studied. Each dog was fitted with a lateral cervical esophagostomy and gastrostomy with a Thomas cannula. Repeated measurements of esophageal function were performed beginning in the fourth postoperative week. The ECRB was evaluated by esophageal manometry, following a 12-hour fast, with dogs restrained in a Pavlov sling. The animals were administered 0.5 mg of intravenous Innovar (Critikon) for sedation. The lower esophageal sphincter pressure (LESp) and lower esophageal sphincter length (LESl) were measured by station pull-back and rapid pull-back methods, using a six-lumen tube, lumen diameter 1.0 mm. The tube had openings at 3.0 cm from the tip, located at 0, 60, 120, 180, 240, and 300 degrees around the circumference. Each lumen of the catheter was connected to a Statham PB22 pressure transducer, with electrical signals relayed to a Sensormedics R-612, eight-channel dynograph, in-line with a Sensormedics computer system (Sensormedics Corp, Anaheim, CA). The catheter was perfused by a pneumohydraulic pump using an Arndorfer capillary perfusion apparatus with a perfusion rate of 0.7 ml/min.

The LES level was determined by introducing the catheter via the esophagostomy into the stomach, and "pulling back" in 1.0-cm increments. Once the sphincter level was known, the catheter was reintroduced below and a rapid pull-back (RPB) at 1.0 cm/sec was done three separate times. To provide a constant speed of 1.0 cm/sec, a custom-made linear pull-back device, powered with a high-torque hysteresis synchronous motor was used. LESp and LESl were calculated for each RPB by averaging three RPB values. LES opening pressure (LESOp) and LES opening volume (LESOv) are defined as the intragastric pressure and intragastric volume which force the LES to open from below allowing GER. Simultaneous measurements of esophageal pH values and intragastric pressure during a rapid infusion of dilute acid solution into the Thomas cannula were performed. GER was defined as a fall of esophageal pH below 4.0. At the time of GER, the LESOp and the LESOv were recorded. A pH electrode was introduced through the cervical esophagostomy, and positioned 5.0 cm above the LES. The reference electrode was attached to a rear leg, with its surface covered; 20% sodium chloride jelly was used to maintain electrical contact. The pH probe output was connected to a portable Synectics pH monitor. The Thomas cannula was opened, washed with water, and a two-channel cap was attached. One channel was used for infusion of 0.1 N HCl solution by a Harvard infusion pump at 100 ml/min. The second channel was used for continuous intragastric pressure recording by means of a Statham pressure transducer connected to a Dynagraph.

The test was repeated following administration of atropine. Atropine was chosen because of its known effect on the gastroesophageal junction. We determined the dose of atropine which would result in a 75% decrease in the LESp, in order to simulate LES failure. The first day, an intravenous infusion of 150 µg/kg of atropine was administered over 20 minutes. Thereafter, the dose was increased by 50 µg/kg until the desired decrease in LESp was manometrically observed.

The timed reflux test was performed on different days than the LESOp test days. Since dogs have very little interdigestive acid secretion, a dilute acid solution (0.1 N HCl) was infused into the stomach through the Thomas cannula at the rate of 2.5 ml/min. The reflux test was performed for 3 hours. The first hour was a control period, while the second and third hours were the timed reflux test following the administration of the atropine. The number of reflux episodes (#RE), the number of reflux episodes longer than 5 min (#RE>5), the longest reflux episode (Long. RE), the number of reflux episodes per hour (Reflux Index), the total time that intraesophageal pH was below 4.0 (TT pH<4), and the percent time that intraesophageal pH was below 4.0 (%TT pH<4) were calculated using a Synectics Esophagogram computer program.

Statistical analysis was performed with each animal serving as its own control. The data were treated by analysis of variance (ANOVA). Subsequently, paired two-tailed Student's *t*-tests were performed. A complementary regression analysis was used to measure the relationship between any two variables. The results were expressed as means and standard error of means (SEM).

Table I
Esophageal and Gastric Components of Reflux Barrier: Results of pH-Metry and Gastric Infusion Studies

	Control (N = 10)	*Atropine (N = 10)*	*p Value*
LESp (mmHg)	24.94 ± 2.76	6.22 ± 1.21	.0002
LESl (cm)	2.33 ± 0.11	1.36 ± 0.07	.0001
LESOp (mmHg)	15.98 ± 2.28	6.13 ± 0.61	.0008
LESOv (ml)	1032.5 ± 179.12	471.5 ± 107.8	.0009
RE	0.2 ± 0.13	6.1 ± 2.20	.02
#RE >5 min	0.0 ± 0.0	1.6 ± 2.20	.00004
LRE (min)	0.1 ± 0.1	22.9 ± 6.13	.004
TT pH <4 (min)	0.1 ± 0.09	34.6 ± 8.02	.001
FT pH <4 (%)	0.21 ± 0.19	28.97 ± 6.70	.001
RI (Reflux/hr)	0.15 ± 0.12	3.98 ± 1.19	.01

Lower Esophageal Sphincter Pressure (LESp); Length (LESl); Opening Pressure (LESOp); Opening volume (LESOv); # of Reflux Episodes (#RE); # of Reflux Episodes Longer than 5 min (# RE >5 min); Longest Reflux Episode (LRE); Total Time pH <4 (TT <4); Fraction Time pH <4 (FT pH <4); and Reflux Index (RI),

Results

ANOVA revealed significant differences between values in control and atropine periods. Atropine (0.381 ± .013 μg/kg) impaired the ECRB and GCRB, allowing gastroesophageal reflux. The ECRB, shown by changes in LESp and LESl, was altered as shown in Table I. The respective decreases in LESp and LESl were 75.06% and 41.6%, and LESOp dropped from 15.98 mmHg to 6.13 mmHg and LESOv from 1032.5 ml to 471.5 ml—decreases of 61% and 55%, respectively. Regression analysis revealed a strong correlation between LESp and LESl (r = .82), and a moderate correlation between LESOp and LESOv (r = .67).

GER was reliably produced by atropine, as shown in Table I. Prior to atropine administration, only one reflux episode was recorded (in a single dog), most probably representing physiological reflux. Following the administration of atropine, all dogs showed abnormal reflux.

Discussion

The ECRB and the GCRB were both affected by atropine infusion, which induced reflux. Thus, our pharmacological model produced

GER without destroying the anatomic integrity of the gastroesophageal junction. The similarity of this model to human GER disease is reflected by both the LES pressure and the percent time of reflux parameters.

The possibility of measuring a GCRB offers a potential explanation for observations in the clinical motility laboratory. For example, esophageal manometry alone does not provide enough discriminating information about patients or the severity of their underlying disease, as the results in nonrefluxing controls have substantial overlap with patients with disease. Similarly, Bancewicz et al.[2] emphasize that there is no correlation between the success of an antireflux procedure and an increase in LES pressure, a finding previously described by Ellis.[3] This suggests that changes in LES pressure and length following floppy Nissen fundoplication do not control reflux. Instead, fundoplication improves the function of a deficient LES.

In addition, we recently reported evidence that the GCRB is indeed a separate component of the reflux mechanism, as endoscopic sclerosis of the gastric cardia in dogs prevented reflux without measurable changes in LES pressure and length.[4] These experiments are the first to show a separation of the ECRB and the GCRB and that strengthening of the GCRB alone is a potential treatment for GER disease.

The regression analysis data reported herein provide further evidence that the ECRB and the GCRB work in concert to prevent reflux. We acknowledge that the major problem in measuring these factors is that there may be overlapping functions, or other variables which confound the data. The mild correlation between LESOp and LESOv reflects this possibility, which we proposed intuitively, knowing the function of gastric reflexes such as receptive accommodation in response to changes in volume. The best conclusion from these is that the LES opening test is an overall or "summary" measurement of all gastric components of the reflux barrier including the balance between gastric wall tension, the gastroesophageal junction, intragastric volume and the receptive relaxation reflex.

While Pettersson et al.'s[5] theory that the immediate cause of GER was related to the effects of gastric distension on the LES set the stage for the current work, the concept of a GCRB is more recent. Pettersson suggested that as gastric wall tension increases, the lowermost portion of the LES is pulled apart, shortening and weakening the squeeze-pressure function of the LES. Next, Samelson et al.[6] demonstrated that a silicone antireflux prosthesis prevents GER by limiting distraction of the lower portion of the LES as does fundoplication; in fact, all antireflux procedures have a similar effect. Interestingly, these current studies are not the first to implicate the proximal gastric wall as a component of the antireflux mechanism; Gahagan suggested that the gastric sling fibers might serve this function over 25 years ago.[7]

Recently a "new" factor, transient relaxation of the LES (TRLES), has been invoked as a mechanism of GER. Dent et al.[8] suggested that gastric distension is the most important stimulus for provoking TRLES, possibly mediated by a neural mechanism. Our group demonstrated that balloon gastric distension increases mean LES pressure, the frequency of LES relaxation, and the gastroesophageal pressure gradient (GEPG). Thus, during LES relaxation an increased GEPG easily overcomes the reflux barrier. This finding explains why the amount of reflux increases postprandially in both physiological and pathological states.

In conclusion, this work provides a model for the evaluation of GER, as well as for investigation of the ECRB and GCRB. The GCRB can be considered an essential component of reflux prevention and should be considered as such in future discussions of the reflux barrier.

References

1. Fyke FE, Code C, Schlegel T: The esophageal sphincter in healthy human beings. Gastroenterologia 86:135–150, 1956.
2. Bancewicz J, Mughal M, Marples M: The lower esophageal sphincter after floppy Nissen fundoplication. Br J Surg 74:162–164, 1987.
3. Ellis F: The effect of fundoplication on the lower esophageal sphincter. Surg Gynecol Obstet 143:1–5, 1976.
4. Donahue PE, Carvalho P, Yoshida J, Miidla I, et al: Endoscopic sclerosis of the cardia affects gastroesophageal reflux. Surg Endosc 3:11–12, 1989.
5. Pettersson G, Bombeck CT, Nyhus LM: The lower esophageal sphincter: Mechanism of opening and closure. Surgery 88:307–319, 1980.
6. Samelson S, Bombeck CT, Siewert R, et al: A new concept in the surgical treatment of gastroesophageal reflux. Ann Surg 197:254–257, 1983.
7. Gahagan TH: The function of the musculature of the esophagus and stomach in the esophagogastric sphincter mechanism. Surg Gynecol Obstet 114:293, 1962.
8. Dent J, Holloway RH, Toouli J, Dodds WJ: Mechanisms of lower esophageal sphincter incompetence in patients with symptomatic gastroesophageal reflux. Gut 29:1020–1028, 1988.

10

Mechanisms of Increased Lower Esophageal Sphincter Pressure Following Intraduodenal Peptone Infusion in Dogs

Anthony D. Sandler, Mardi R. Karin,
Jerry F. Schlegel, James W. Maher,
James E. McGuigan

Introduction

The lower esophageal sphincter (LES) plays an important role in the prevention of gastroesophageal reflux. Previous studies suggest that the postprandial increase in lower esophageal sphincter pressure (LESP) is produced by the synergistic interaction of neural and hormonal components.[1,2] Peptone perfusion of the excluded duodenum produces an increase in LESP,[3] suggesting a possible duodenal phase in the regulation of postprandial LESP. This study was undertaken to investigate the role of cholinergic, adrenergic, and hormonal mediators in the response of the LES to intraduodenal peptone infusion.

Supported by NIH grants DK37256-02 and AM13711-18.
Little AG, Ferguson MK, Skinner DB: Diseases of the Esophagus, Vol. II: Benign Diseases. Futura Publishing Company, Inc., Mount Kisco, NY, © 1990.

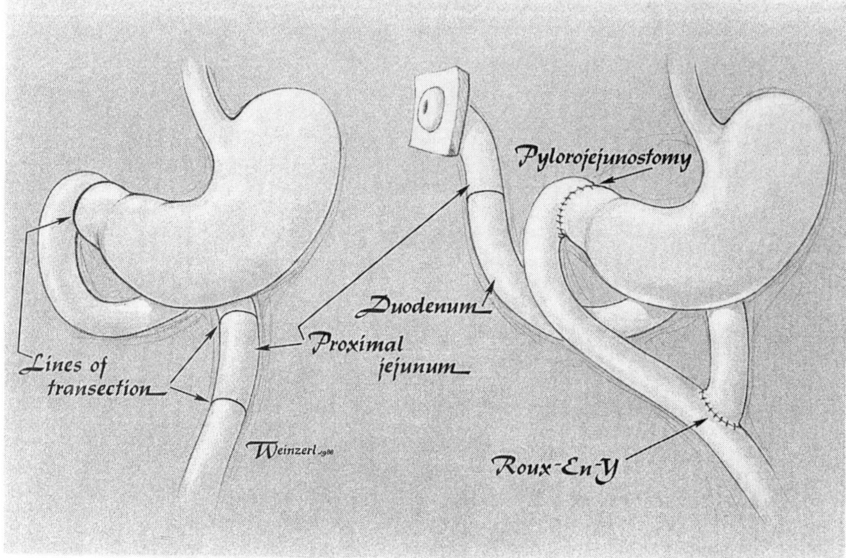

Figure 1: Surgical procedure for duodenal exclusion. Note the end-to-end pylorojejunostomy, Roux-en-Y duodenal diversion and formation of a mucocutaneous fistula with a jejunal segment interposition.

Methods

Experiments were performed on 10 adult mongrel dogs weighing 16–20 kg.

Surgical Procedure

Dogs underwent a cervical loop esophagostomy and duodenal exclusion under general anesthesia. The duodenum was excluded using the method described by Koelz et al.,[3] in which a Roux-en-Y pylorojejunostomy was performed. A mucocutaneous fistula was formed by interposing a 10-cm isoperistaltic jejunal segment between the duodenum and skin. The duodenojejunostomy was performed 36 cm distal to the pylorus (Fig. 1). A 3–4 week postoperative recovery period was allowed before testing began.

Manometric Technique

LESP was measured with a six-lumen esophageal manometry probe passed into the stomach via the cervical loop esophagostomy. LESP determinations were obtained using a slow "pull-back" technique. The LESP was taken as the mean end expiratory pressure at the point of respiratory reversal in all six leads. Pressures were expressed in cm H_2O in relation to end expiratory gastric pressure.

Duodenal Peptone Infusion

A 16-French Foley catheter was inserted through the mucocutaneous fistula for the infusion of peptones. Following insertion, the balloon was inflated prior to measuring the resting lower esophageal sphincter pressure. One hundred milliliters of a 20% peptone solution (1.6 osmoles, pH 5.7, Na+ 203 meq, K 350 meq and Cl^- 135 meq) was instilled into the excluded duodenum over a 10-minute period. The catheter was left in place for the duration of the experiment.

Radioimmunoassay (RIA)

Peripheral venous blood samples were taken concurrently with lower esophageal sphincter pressure determinations before and after peptone infusion at the various time intervals. Measurement of gastrin and pancreatic polypeptide (PP) blood levels were made by radioimmunoassay. Both hormones have been shown to increase LESP.[4-6] The technique for performing these assays has been previously described.[7,8]

Protocols

Control Studies

Following recovery from the surgical procedure, three of the dogs underwent LESP measurements in a fasted unmedicated state before and after infusion of 100 ml saline solution into the excluded duodenum. All 10 dogs then underwent LESP measurements under the same conditions following infusion of 100 ml peptone solution. LESP measurements were made at 15-minute intervals for a 60-minute period after intraduodenal infusion of the peptone solution. Studies were then repeated on a separate day following either truncal vagotomy or pretreatment with a pharmacological antagonist.

Vagotomy Studies

Experiments were repeated in four dogs following bilateral transthoracic truncal vagotomy at the level of T6 with transabdominal pyloroplasty (TVP).

Atropine Studies

To determine the effect of cholinergic muscarinic blockade, 0.5 mg of atropine was administered as a single subcutaneous injection in five dogs prior to testing.

6-Hydroxydopamine (6OHDO) Studies

To obtain pharmacological sympathetic denervation, a single intraperitoneal injection of 6OHDO at a dose of 16.5 mg/kg was administered 24–72 hours prior to testing in three dogs.

Somatostatin (GHRIH) Studies

Six dogs were tested following infusion of synthetic somatostatin intravenously at 4 μg/kg/min for the duration of the experiment. GHRIH was used to suppress enteral hormone secretion in this study, and thus determine the role of humoral mediators.

Statistical Analysis

Measurements of LESP, PP, and gastrin blood levels were made at each time interval in all dogs. The results are expressed as the mean plus or minus the standard error of the mean (SEM). Statistical analysis was made using the Student's *t* test and analysis of variance (ANOVA). Differences were considered to be significant at $p < 0.05$.

Results

Control Studies

LES Pressure

Saline infusion into the excluded duodenum did not produce a change in LESP. Peptone infusion into the excluded duodenum resulted in a significant increase in LESP at all time intervals measured ($p < 0.005$). An increase of 11 ± 3.2 cm H_2O, 21.4 ± 3 cm H_2O, 28.3 ± 4.2 cm H_2O, and 29.9 ± 3 cm H_2O was observed at the 15, 30, 45, and 60 minute periods, respectively ($n = 10$).

PP and Gastrin Levels

Pancreatic polypeptide increased from a fasting blood level of 67 $\pm$ 6.4 pg/ml to 145 ± 21 ($p < 0.05$); 100 ± 10 ($p < 0.05$); 108 ± 20 ($p < 0.05$); and 104 ± 11 ($p > 0.05$) pg/ml at the 15, 30, 45, and 60 minute periods, respectively, following intraduodenal peptone infusion. The mean fasting gastrin level was 36.5 ± 5.4 pg/ml. Levels following peptone infusion at the respective time intervals were 47.3 ± 6; 43.8 ± 5; 44.2 ± 5.3 and 41.5 ± 7.2 pg/ml. These levels were not statistically different from the fasting gastrin level prior to peptone infusion ($p > 0.2$).

Vagotomy Studies

LES Pressure

Transthoracic truncal vagotomy and transabdominal pyloroplasty (TVP) blocked the increases in LESP following intraduodenal peptone infusion. No significant changes in LESP were observed at any of the time intervals ($p > 0.4$).

PP and Gastrin Levels

The basal PP blood level was 107 ± 30.2 pg/ml. This was not statistically different from basal levels prior to vagotomy. The levels increased to 243 ± 32; 161 ± 32; 171 ± 50 and 113 ± 22 following peptone infusion at the 15, 30, 45, and 60 minute periods, respectively. Only the increase at the 15-minute interval was statistically significant ($p < 0.005$). The mean fasting plasma gastrin level was 115 $\pm$ 36.5 pg/ml. Following peptone infusion, the mean plasma gastrin levels increased to 273 $\pm$ 65.3; 196 $\pm$ 66; 138.7 $\pm$ 47.6 and 122 $\pm$ 32.9 pg/ml at the 15, 30, 45, and 60 minute periods, respectively. The 15, 30, and 60 minute plasma levels were significantly increased when compared to the corresponding periods in the control studies prior to vagotomy ($p < 0.05$).

Atropine Studies

LES Pressures

Pretreatment with subcutaneous atropine blocked the LESP response to intraduodenal peptone. There was no significant increase in LESP at any of the time intervals. LESP increased by 3.7 $\pm$ 3.6, 8.5 $\pm$ 6.6, 11.9 $\pm$ 5.8, and 13.9 $\pm$ 7.5 cm H_2O at the 15, 30, 45, and 60 minute periods, respectively ($p > 0.2$).

PP and Gastrin Levels

Following peptone infusion in the atropine-treated animals, there were no changes in either PP blood levels ($p > 0.3$) or in gastrin blood levels ($p < 0.1$).

6-Hydroxydopamine Studies

LES Pressure

In the dogs pretreated with 6-hydroxydopamine, a significant increase in LESP was observed at the 15, 30, 45, and 60 minute periods following peptone perfusion of the excluded duodenum ($p < 0.05$).

PP and Gastrin Levels

PP plasma levels in the fasted dogs pretreated with 6OHDO (119 $\pm$ 13 pg/ml) were significantly greater than the levels assayed in the control period (67 $\pm$ 6 pg/ml) ($p < 0.01$). No differences were noted between the postpeptone infusion levels in this group and the plasma levels at the corresponding control periods (p>0.1). Similarly, gastrin blood levels were not significantly different from levels assayed in the control (p>0.2).

Somatostatin Studies

LES Pressure

Following peptone infusion, a significant increase in LESP was observed at all time intervals. Increases of 12.2 ± 5.3, 22.7 ± 4.8, 31.9 ± 4.7, and 32.7 ± 4.1 cm H_2O was observed at the 15, 30, 45, and 60 minute periods, respectively (p<0.05).

PP and Gastrin Levels

GHRIH suppressed the peptone-induced release of PP that was observed during the control experiments. PP blood levels in response to peptone infusion were not significantly different from the fasting level (p>0.5). The PP levels were significantly less than the levels at all corresponding time intervals in control animals (p<0.05). Following GHRIH, the mean resting gastrin blood level decreased by 13 ± 2.5 pg/ml (p<0.01). No changes in gastrin blood levels were observed in these animals following peptone infusion (p>0.2).

Discussion

This study demonstrates that intraduodenal peptone infusion produces a significant increase in LESP, confirming previous observations by Koelz et al.[3] The duodenum is known to have marked effects on upper gastrointestinal motility and secretions.[9-11] These effects are mediated by both enteral hormone secretion and/or neural pathways.[9-11]

The possibility exists that enteric hormones may modulate changes in LES pressure. Gastrin and pancreatic polypeptide (PP) must be considered as possible candidates for mediating the LES response under examination. Both enteric hormones are released postprandially, and administration of these peptides has been shown to stimulate an increase in LESP.[4-6]

In the present study, the slow but sustained increase in LESP observed after intraduodenal peptone infusion suggests a hormonally mediated effect. However, truncal vagotomy blocked the increase in LESP observed in response to intraduodenal peptone infusion. This observation suggests that either a vagally denervated LES does not respond in a normal fashion to possible hormonal stimuli, or that the effect of intraduodenal peptone on LESP is neurally mediated via the central nervous system.

Atropine pretreatment blocked the increases in LESP seen following intraduodenal peptone infusion. Besides blocking cholinergic neurotransmission at muscarinic receptors on the LES smooth muscle, atropine may also act by blocking both the release and receptor action of enteral hormones. Atropine has been shown to block the increase in PP secretion that occurs following a meal,[12] as well as the stimulation of lower esophageal sphincter pressure by administration of PP.[6] In the present study, atropine blocked the increase in PP blood levels ordinarily seen following peptone infusion. It is also of note that previous studies have shown that both vagotomy and atropine pretreatment block the postprandial increase in LESP.[13]

Pharmacological sympathetic denervation with 6OHDO had no effect on the observed increases in LESP following intraduodenal peptone infusion; thus sympathetic efferent pathways are probably not involved. The increase in LESP is not mediated by intramural neural pathways between the duodenum and esophagus as these are severed by the duodenal exclusion procedure performed in these experiments.

Somatostatin treatment abolished the increase in PP blood levels following peptone infusion, but a significant increase in LESP was still observed under these conditions. This finding conflicts with previous studies from this laboratory, demonstrating elimination of the LES response to both intraduodenal peptone and feeding following treatment with somatostatin.[14] Studies in the baboon have also shown that GHRIH abolished the increase in LESP ordinarily seen in response to both intragastric alkali and glycine by the apparent suppression of a hormonally mediated mechanism.[15] The authors are at a loss to explain this variation in data; however, the current study suggests that the hormones assayed are not essential in producing the LES response to intraduodenal peptones.

In conclusion, the mechanism by which intraduodenal peptone infusion LESP increases in dogs may be centrally mediated and appears to be dependent on vagal innervation and cholinergic neurotransmission. If humoral mediators do play a role, this study suggests that pancreatic polypeptide is of minor importance and that the vagally denervated LES does not react in a normal fashion to the hormonal response. These findings are consistent with the hypothesis that a duodenal phase exists for the regulation of postprandial LESP.

References

1. Olinde AJ, Maher MS, Maher JW, McGuigan JE: The effect of varying levels of vagotomy on postprandial lower esophageal sphincter pressure and pancreatic polypeptide. World J Surg 10:809–813, 1986.
2. Dodds WJ, Hogan WJ, Helm JF, Dent J: Pathogenesis of reflux esophagitis. Gastroenterology 81:376–394, 1981.
3. Koelz HR, Lepsien G, Hollinger AP, Sauberli H, Largiader F, Arnold R, Blum AL, Siewert R: Effect of intraduodenal peptone on the lower esophageal sphincter pressure in the dog. Gastroenterology 75:283–285, 1978.
4. Giles GR, Mason MS, Humphries C, Clark CG: Action of gastrin on the lower esophageal sphincter in man. Gut 10:730–734, 1969.
5. Coltharp W, Maher JW, Maher MS, Schlegel JF, Sandler AD, McGuigan JE : The effect of truncal vagotomy on the response of the canine lower esophageal sphincter to varying doses of pancreatic polypeptide. Surgery 103:620–623, 1988.
6. Rattan S, Goyal RK: Effect of bovine pancreatic polypeptide on the opossum lower esophageal sphincter. Gastroenterology 77:672–676, 1979.
7. Chance RE, Moon NE, Johnson MG: Human pancreatic polypeptide (HPP) and bovine pancreatic polypeptide (BPP). In: Methods of Hormone Radioimmunoassay, 2nd Ed., Jaffe BM, Behlman HR (eds), New York, Academic Press, Inc, 1979, pp 657–672.
8. McGuigan JE, Wolfe MM: Gastrin radioimmunoassay. Clin Chem 28:368, 1982.
9. Cooke AR: Duodenal acidification: Role of the first part of duodenum in gastric emptying and secretion in dogs. Gastroenterology 67:85–92, 1974.
10. Preshaw RM, Cooke, AR, Grossman MI: Quantitative aspects of the responses of the canine pancreas to duodenal acidification. Am J Physiol 210:629–634, 1966.
11. Konturek SJ, Johnson LR: Evidence for an enterogastric reflex for the inhibition of acid secretion. Gastroenterology 61:667–674, 1971.
12. Taylor IL, Impicciatore M, Carter DC, et al: Effect of atropine and vagotomy on pancreatic polypeptide response to a meal in dogs. Am J Physiol 235:443–447, 1982.
13. Maher JW, Crandall V, Woodward ER: Effects of cholinergic blockade on postprandial and acid-stimulated lower esophageal sphincter pressure. Am Surg 44:758–760, 1978.
14. Maher JW, Olinde AJ, Coltharp WC, McGuigan JE: The role of the duodenum in regulation of postprandial lower esophageal sphincter pressure (LESP): Evidence for hormonal control. Gastroenterology 86:1171, 1984.
15. Bybee DE, Brown FC, Georges LP, Castell DO, McGuigan JE: Somatostatin effects on lower esophageal function. Am J Physiol 237(1):E77-E81, 1979.

11

Interaction of Gastroesophageal Reflux and Esophageal Motility in Healthy Men Undergoing Combined 24-Hour Mano/pH-metry

Rudolf Bumm, Hubertus Feussner, Carsten Emde, Arnulf H. Hoelscher, Jörg Ruediger Siewert

Introduction

Some healthy volunteers occasionally exhibit extensive gastroesophageal reflux (GER)[1] and should, therefore, possess mechanisms for clearance of refluxed materials from the distal esophagus. A mechanism for esophageal clearance would be of considerable interest in patients with GER disease, where motility disorders have been postulated.[2] Most previous studies on esophageal acid clearance have been performed using stationary manometry and/or scintigraphic methods in combination with acid/marker instillation. It is only recently that lightweight solid-state recorders[3] enabled long-term recordings of intraesophageal pH and pressure. Moreover, an advanced computer program for data retrieval of long-term combined mano/pH-metry (MP24) has been developed and validated.[4] With this technique, the circadian motility pattern of normal man has been defined.[5]

Little AG, Ferguson MK, Skinner DB: Diseases of the Esophagus, Vol. II: Benign Diseases. Futura Publishing Company, Inc., Mount Kisco, NY, © 1990.

Based on this study, MP24 seemed to be ideally suited to identify the effects of GER on circadian esophageal motility.

The aim of the present study, therefore, was (1) to develop a method for combined analysis of intraesophageal pH and manometry and (2) to study the interaction between GER and esophageal motility in healthy volunteers with considerable GER periods, and in particular to measure esophageal basal motor activity shortly before, during, and shortly after GER during day and night.

Materials and Methods

Study Population

Seven healthy volunteers (four male, three female, median age 28 years) without history of heartburn or esophageal disorder were included in this study. As a prerequisite, all volunteers had shown a total reflux time of more than 2% during a MP24 examination.

MP24 System

The recording system comprised a measuring assembly, a data logger, and a computer program for analysis of pH and manometric data. The measuring assembly consisted of a probe with three intraluminal pressure transducers (16CT/s-3, Gaeltec Ltd., Dunvegan, Scotland) located 0, 5, and 10 cm from the tip and a pH glass electrode (44M4, Ingold, Urdorf, Switzerland). Data sampling rates of 10 Hz (pressure) and 0.2 Hz (pH) were chosen. All data from a 24-hour examination were stored digitally without data reduction in a portable data logger (Autronic GmbH, Karlsruhe, FRG). Data were permanently stored on 3.5" diskettes.

Study Protocol

The measuring assembly was placed 5 cm above the lower esophageal sphincter (LES), which had been determined in a previous manometry, at 3 P.M. on the examination day. Standardized meals, which had to be eaten within 30 minutes, were given at 6 P.M. (day 1) and 12 noon (day 2). Smoking was forbidden throughout the examination, but the subjects were allowed free access to tap water. Drinking of acid juices was not permitted.

Analysis of pH Data

A reflux episode was assumed if intraesophageal pH dropped below 4.0. The end of a reflux episode was assumed if pH rose above 4.0. For each of the individuals, the number of GER episodes, the total GER time (% of examination time), and the daily, postprandial, and nocturnal GER time was evaluated. Times of meal intake were excluded from the present analysis.

Analysis of Manometric Data

In each of the three pressure channels, the number of esophageal contractions, and for each contraction, the peak amplitude (hPa), duration (s), upstroke contractility (hPa/s), and area under the curve (hPa*s) were evaluated. In addition, the program allowed for classification of esophageal contractions into simultaneous, peristaltic, and segmental waves. Program algorithms were identical to those recently published (Emde)[3] and validated (Bumm)[4] including continuous pressure baseline adapation and identification of pressure artifacts.

Combined Analysis of Intraesophageal pH and Pressures

For this purpose, each of the 24-hour examinations was divided into distinct periods (Fig. 1): PRE-period (2 minutes before GER), REFL-period (during GER), POST-period (2 minutes after GER), and NO-period (without any GER). In case of two consecutive reflux episodes with a time interval of less than 2 minutes, this interval was excluded from the present analysis in order to avoid an overlay of PRE- and POST-period. Every registered contraction was assigned to one of the four periods. For each period, individual mean values for amplitude, duration, contractility, and area were calculated. In addition, the overall frequency of contraction (number/minute period duration) and the frequency of simultaneous, peristaltic, and segmental contractions were evaluated. Finally, for each volunteer, an individual

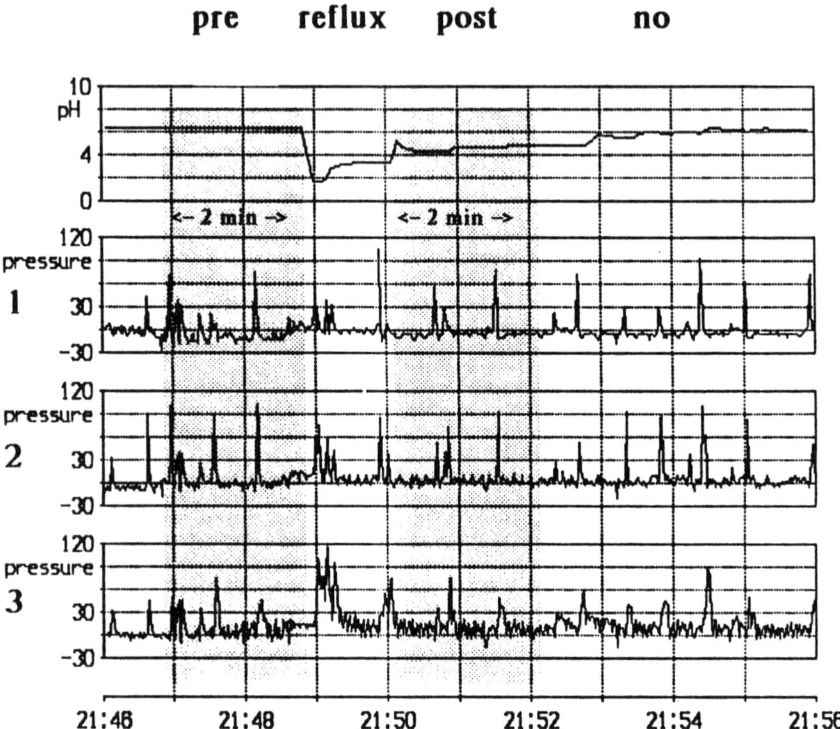

Figure 1: Association of GER periods and esophageal manometry. An original MP24 recording (one pH-channel, three pressure channels) is depicted. Marked is the time period within 2 minutes before reflux (PRE), during GER (REFL), 2 minutes after GER (POST), and without GER (NO).

reflux/motility plot was prepared; frequency of contractions during each GER episode was plotted against duration of the GER episodes.

Statistics

In order to take into consideration circadian changes of esophageal motility, the data were generally calculated for day (7 A.M.–3 P.M., 3 P.M.–10 P.M. excluding meals) and night (10 P.M.–7 A.M.). Data from the individuals were compared using nonparametric test statistics (Sign test, Wilcoxon's test for paired samples, where appropriate). A probability of p≤0.05 was regarded as significant. Frequency of

Table I
Characteristics of GER in Seven Healthy Volunteers

Volunteer	pH <4.0 Total (%)	pH <4.0 Day (%)	pH <4.0 Post-Prandial (%)	pH <4.0 Night (%)
Vol. 1	2.1	0.8	7.3	0.2
Vol. 2	3.0	5.0	3.2	0.2
Vol. 3	16.6	1.3	2.1	44.3
Vol. 4	6.6	0.0	1.9	16.5
Vol. 5	4.9	3.0	11.3	1.3
Vol. 6	2.6	0.8	8.1	1.0
Vol. 7	12.9	10.4	13.9	3.3
median	4.9	1.3	7.3	1.3

GER time (total, day, postprandial, and night) is expressed in % of total examination time.

contractions and duration of GER was correlated by linear regression analysis.

Results

Characteristics of GER

Median GER time in the seven volunteers was 4.9% (Table I). Although two of the examined volunteers displayed extensive nocturnal GER, relative frequency of GER was highest postprandially.

Frequency of Esophageal Contractions

Figure 2 shows the frequency of esophageal contractions registered during daytime in all seven volunteers and expressed per minute of GER-related periods. During the daytime, esophageal motility increased during PRE- and REFL-period and was highest during POST-period ($p < 0.05$) compared to basal motor activity.

At night (Fig. 3), frequency of contractions increased during PRE- and POST-periods ($p < 0.05$ versus NO), whereas REFL-periods were not

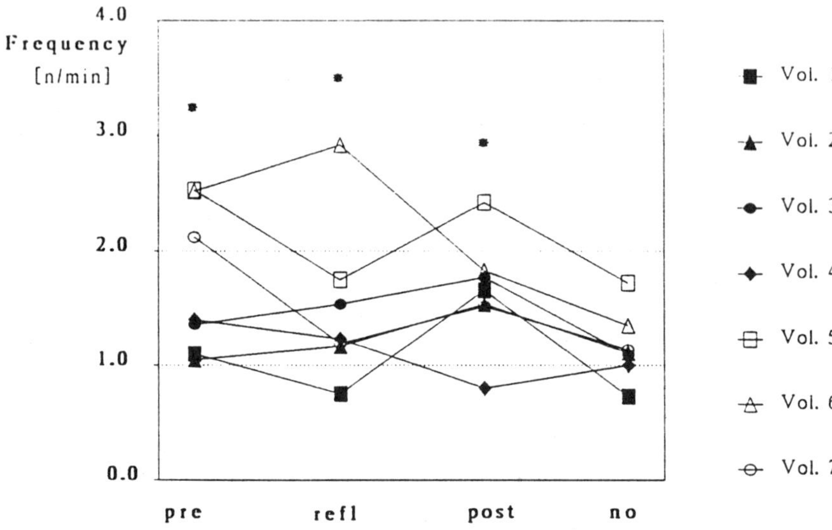

Figure 2: Frequency of esophageal contractions during GER-related periods (day). Given are data for each volunteer, expressed as number of contractions per minute GER period.

different from NO-periods. In fact, esophageal contractions were consistently less frequent during REFL- compared to POST-period ($p < 0.05$).

Type of Contractions

We evaluated the type of esophageal contractions for day- and night time and, in particular, during GER-related periods. During the day (not shown), the type of esophageal contractions did not differ between PRE-, REFL-, POST- and NO-period. Figure 4 shows the percentage of peristaltic contractions registered at night and during each of the GER-related periods. The percentage of peristaltic contractions decreased during PRE-period ($p < 0.05$ versus NO) and increased during POST-period ($p < 0.05$, POST versus NO). The type of esophageal contractions did not differ, however, if REFL-period and NO-period were compared.

Shape of Contractions

The shape of esophageal contractions during day and night is summarized in Table II (proximal pressure channel). No significant

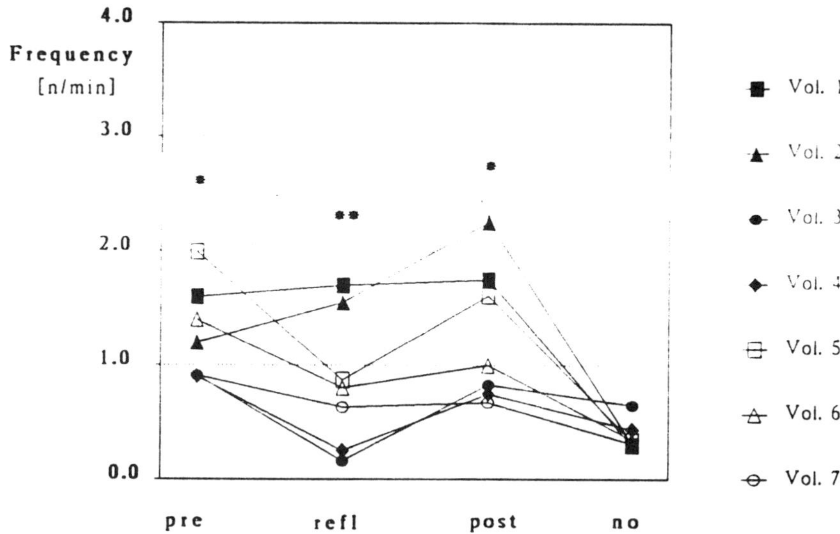

Figure 3: Frequency of esophageal contractions during GER-related periods (night). Given are data for each volunteer, expressed as number of contractions per minute GER period.

differences existed between PRE-, REFL-, POST-, and NO-periods (not shown) for contractions registered on each of the pressure channels.

Duration of GER and Esophageal Motility

Figure 5 shows a summary plot of all GER episodes registered in the seven subjects and the corresponding frequency of esophageal contractions registered during the particular GER episode. Two facts can be read from this graph. First, GER duration and esophageal activity were closely related; long GER episodes had a low esophageal motor activity, whereas short GER periods were accompanied by high motor activity. Second, the data points were concentrated near the y-axis, indicating a predominance of short GER episodes with high motor activity in this volunteer study. Transformation of these data by $y = 1/y$ resulted in a second distribution which, when linear regression analysis was applied, demonstrated a linear dependency (rho = 0.84).

In order to illustrate the individual courses from each volunteer, equivalent graphs were created for each of the seven volunteers (Fig.

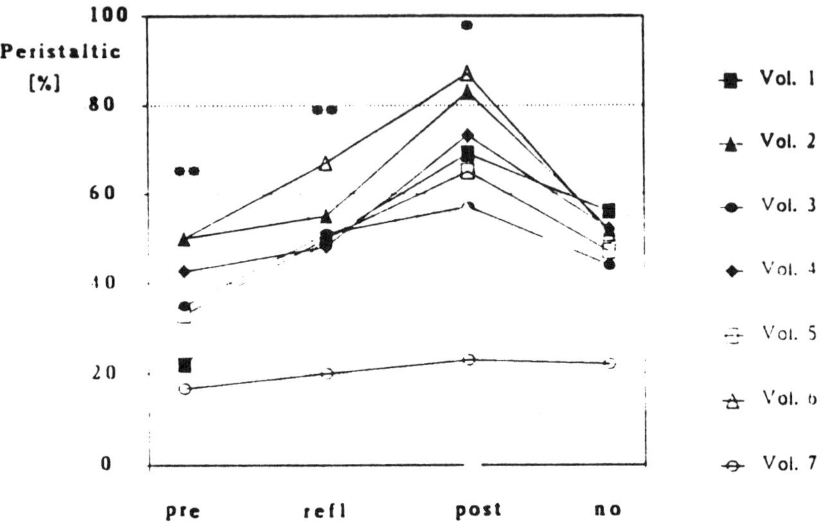

Figure 4: Type of contractions during GER-related periods (night). Given are data for each volunteer expressed as percentage of all of contractions registered during GER periods.

6). In all but one volunteer (vol. 5, rho = 0.19), duration of GER versus 1/frequency was closely correlated (rho 0.77–0.97).

Discussion

The aim of this study was to analyze the interplay between GER and esophageal motor activity in healthy volunteers. We studied a

Table II
Number and Shape of Esophageal Contractions Registered on the Most Proximal Pressure Channel

Period	No. of Contrac- tions	Ampli- tude (hPa)	Dura- tion (s)	Contrac- tility (hPa/s)	Area (hPa*s)
DAY	857	66.3	3.45	39.2	124.2
range	600–1330	42.2–82.1	2.9–4.5	32.1–76.4	74.5–179.3
NIGHT	205	71.7	4.7	40.1	162.9
range	171–240	49.4–99.0	4.1–5.9	26.4–89.4	90.4–199.0

Given are medians and range from seven healthy volunteers for day and night.

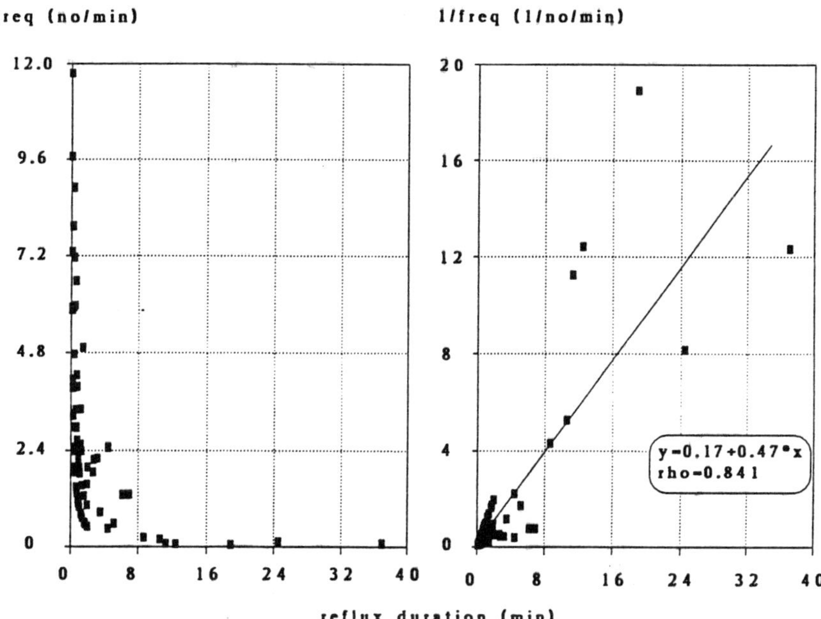

Figure 5: Frequency of clearance motility vs. duration of single reflux episodes derived from seven healthy volunteers. (Left) Each square represents one reflux episode. (Right) Transformation of frequencies (y-axis) into 1/frequency and linear regression of resulting data.

group of volunteers with considerable "physiological" GER, because they (a) demonstrated a sufficient number of GER episodes for further analysis, (b) were not symptomatic and therefore likely to present motility phenomena of the normal human esophagus, and (c) should possess a protective mechanism for clearance of refluxed material from the distal esophagus.

We have used a new ambulatory recording technique which, for the first time, allows circadian studies on esophageal manometry and pH-metry and should, therefore, be ideally suited to define the interplay of GER and esophageal motor function. This was made possible by the use of recently developed, lightweight data loggers and the availability of an advanced computer program for analysis of the large amounts of data generated by such recordings.[3] Furthermore, the ability of the program to detect and classify esophageal contractions had been recently validated in a study involving several working groups in the field of gastrointestinal motility.[4]

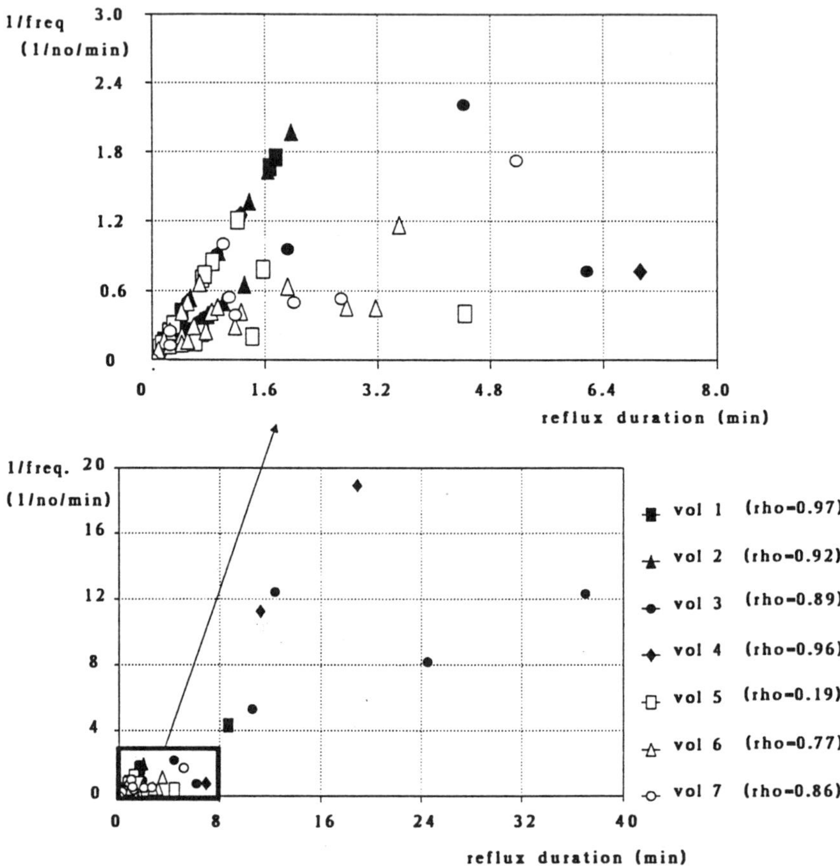

Figure 6: Frequency of clearance motility and duration of gastroesophageal reflux episodes in seven healthy volunteers. Frequency was transformed into 1/frequency (y-axis); rho of linear regression analysis from each individual is given at the right.

Previous work of Dent et al.[6] and a pilot study[7] had given evidence for a contractile response of the human esophagus to GER, but in both series only a few volunteers had developed relevant GER which, therefore, made statistical evaluation difficult. From the present study, however, there is strong evidence for a regulatory interplay of esophageal motor activity and GER in healthy man. Analysis of the results showed that esophageal contractions during the day were more frequent during GER but also in the periods before and after GER, indicating a "clearance motility response." Surprisingly, this response seemed to differ at night when the frequency of contractions was increased shortly after GER, but not during or before GER. This indicates that the clearance mechanism could be influenced by the degree of consciousness in the individuals.

Most interestingly, the duration of GER correlated directly with the esophageal motor activity in the present study. There were no prolonged GER episodes with notable esophageal motor activity (and vice versa). For each of the studied subjects we found a characteristic GER/frequency distribution with a close correlation in all but one subject.

In addition, we noticed a change in type of contraction during the course of GER. Before GER, contractions were less peristaltic, during GER they were indifferent, and after GER they were more peristaltic than during basal esophageal motor activity. It has to be noted, however, that these changes were observed only during the night, not during the day. It may well be that potential changes in the type of contractions were suppressed by basal esophageal activity and therefore were not obvious during the day, but unmasked during the night, when the esophagus was at rest. The low peristaltic activity before GER is consistent with another study[6] in which GER episodes were commonly preceded by incomplete peristaltic sequences in connection with transient LES relaxations.

Unexpectedly, neither amplitude, duration, contractility, nor area of esophageal contractions changed during the course of GER. It has to be noted, however, that comparison of medians between the individuals may not be appropriate and the number of studied subjects may have been too small to identify distinct changes in these parameters. Nevertheless, the clearance/motility response to GER in the normal esophagus seems to be primarily mediated by changes of frequency and type, not by changes in shape of contractions. There is incomplete knowledge on the precise mechanism of how GER effects motility in the normal esophagus. It is well known that instilled fluid bolus may by itself initiate secondary esophageal peristalsis. In addition, lowering of intraesophageal pH decreases the volume of fluid needed for initiation of peristalsis.[8] Instillation of acid into the distal esophagus increases the pulmonary resistance and alters pulmonary function parameters in control subjects,[9] perhaps mediated by a vagal pathway.[9] Data from the present study suggest that the response to GER underlies circadian changes which could be also expressed as changes in consciousness. This study provides the first detailed description of the interplay between GER and circadian esophageal motility in healthy subjects. The data presented suggest a specific motility response to GER, which could be precisely quantified by the methods described. It will be of interest to study the clearance motility response of the esophagus in patients with GER disease in whom motility disorders have been postulated.

References

1. Smout AJ, Breedijk M, Van der Zouw, et al: Physiological gastroesophageal reflux and esophageal motor activity studied with a new system for 24-hour recording and automated analysis. Dig Dis Sci 34(3):372, 1989.
2. Kahrilas PJ, Dodds WJ, Hogan WJ, et al: Esophageal peristaltic dysfunction in peptic esophagitis. Gastroenterology 91:897, 1986.
3. Emde C, Armstrong D, Bumm R, et al: Twenty-four hour continuous ambulatory measurement of esophageal pH and pressure: A digital recording system and computer aided manometry analysis (CAMA). JAMA (in press).
4. Bumm R, Emde C, Armstrong D, et al: Ambulatory esophageal manometry: Comparison of expert analysis and computer aided manometry analysis (CAMA). Gastroenterology (in press).
5. Armstrong D, Emde C, Bumm R, et al. Twenty-four hour pattern of esophageal motility in healthy volunteers. Dig Dis Sci (in press).
6. Dent J, Dodds WJ, Friedman RH, et al: Mechanism of gastroesophageal reflux in recumbent asymptomatic human subjects. J Clin Invest 65:256, 1980.
7. Bumm R, Emde C, Bauerfeind P, et al: Nocturnal gastroesophageal reflux and motility of the tubular esophagus: The question of hen and egg. Gastroenterology 94:A54, 1988.
8. Corazziari E, Prozzessere C, Dani, et al: Intraluminal pH and esophageal motility. Gastroenterology 75:275, 1978.
9. Deschner KW, Benjamin SB: Extraesophageal manifestations of gastrointestinal reflux disease. Am J Gastroenterol 84:1, 1989.

12

Gastroesophageal Reflux and Esophageal Body Function: Correlation with Severity of Mucosal Changes

Steven J. Walker, Alfonso M. Maiorana,
Suriya Chakkaphak, Mark K. Ferguson,
David B. Skinner, Alex G. Little

Introduction

Gastroesophageal reflux is a multifactorial disease.[1] Studies in a large number of patients have shown that overall there is an inverse relationship between lower esophageal sphincter pressure (LESP) and the degree of reflux.[2,3] Whether sphincter hypotension or excessive reflux was the initiating event is in most instances unknown. However, Eastwood et al.[4] have shown that increasing degrees of experimentally induced mucosal damage can result in a progressive reduction in sphincter pressure. An important factor in preventing reflux damage is the ability of the esophagus to clear noxious material that has escaped the primary antireflux mechanisms at the gastroesophageal junction.[5,6] Clearance may be impaired in patients with esophagitis, but whether a similar progressive relationship exists among the severity of mucosal damage, the extent of acid reflux, and the degree of esophageal body motor dysfunction is not known.

Little AG, Ferguson MK, Skinner DB: Diseases of the Esophagus, Vol. II: Benign Diseases. Futura Publishing Company, Inc., Mount Kisco, NY, © 1990.

Table I
Characteristics of the Patients and Controls

	Patients	*Controls*
Number	60	10
Males:females	33:27	5:5
Mean age	52 years (range 20–84)	35 years (range 22–56)

Method

The study population is comprised of 60 consecutive patients with reflux symptoms and abnormal acid reflux on pH monitoring, and 10 asymptomatic controls (Table I). Symptoms of heartburn, regurgitation, and dysphagia were assessed on a scale of 0 (no symptoms) to 3 (frequent severe symptoms).[7] All patients underwent fiberoptic esophagogastroduodenoscopy (endoscopy) under sedation (diazepam) and were divided into three groups on the basis of their endoscopic appearance (Table II).[8] Biopsies were taken in selected patients to exclude malignant disease and confirm the presence of columnar-lined (Barrett's) esophagus.

Standardized manometry was performed in patients and controls using a triple-lumen assembly of 1.1 mm diameter polyvinyl catheters perfused at 0.6 ml/minute by a low compliance pneumohydraulic infusion pump.[9] Radially oriented side ports were spaced 5 cm apart. The individual catheters were attached to Bell and Howell (type 4-327-I) transducers and the changes in pressure were recorded using a four-channel pen recorder running at 2.5 mm/second (Hewlett-Packard). Swallowing was detected by an additional oropharyngeal perfused catheter. Subjects were studied off all relevant medication and after an overnight fast.

The pressure and length of the lower esophageal sphincter (LES) were determined using the "station pull-through" technique.[10] The amplitude of pressure in the sphincter was measured as the difference between the end-expiratory intragastric pressure and the end-expiratory intrasphincteric pressure.

Motility in the esophageal body was studied with the catheter positioned to record pressure at 5, 10, and 15 cm above the LES. The patient performed 10 wet swallows (5 ml water) at 30-second intervals.[11] The wave amplitude was calculated as the difference between

Table II
Study Groups

	N	Mean Age (range)	Characteristics
Controls	10	35 (22–56)	Asymptomatic, normal pH results
Group I	18	48 (30–69)	Grades 1 and 2 endoscopic esophagitis
Group II	22	52 (20–84)	Grade 3 endoscopic esophagitis
Group III	20	54 (34–75)	Barrett's esophagus

mean basal pressure and maximum peak pressure (mmHg). The wave duration was determined by drawing a line through the maximum upstroke and downstroke of each primary contraction and then determining the intersection of these lines with the basal pressure and measuring the interval between these two points (seconds). The velocity between the 15- and 10-cm positions, and 10- and 5-cm positions was calculated from the time interval between the onset of each pair of waves (cm/second).[12]

Recordings were assessed for the frequency and type of abnormal wave forms, including nonpropagated, simultaneous, spontaneous, or repetitive contractions.[12–14] For a wave to be classified according to one of these categories, the abnormality had to be detected by all three recording channels. All manometry tracings were assessed by an independent researcher unaware of the subject's status.

Esophageal acidity was measured during 24 hours of standardized ambulatory pH monitoring (Synectics) using an antimony electrode positioned 5 cm above the manometrically determined LES. Analysis was at pH<4 for total percentage reflux time.[15] Results were compared by unpaired *t*-test and Chi-squared test.[12]

Results

Our results confirm that worsening degrees of esophagitis are associated with increasing patient age, greater levels of acid reflux, and decreasing LES pressure (Tables II, III). In this study, there were no significant differences in LES length among the different groups. Reflux symptoms increased with progressive mucosal injury. Patients

Table III
Mean Total % Reflux Time pH <4 (pH), Lower Esophageal Sphincter Pressure (LESP mmHg), Length (LESL cm), and Symptom Scores (0–3)

	pH (± SD)	LESP (± SD)	LESL (± SD)	HB	REG	DYS
Controls	0.7 (0.5)	15.4 (5.3)	3.3 (0.7)	—	—	—
Group I	14.8 (11.3)*	12.3 (6.2)	3.1 (1.4)	2.1	1.5	0.7
Group II	18.8 (9.4)*	8.9 (3.0)*@	3.9 (1.6)	2.4	2.1	1.2
Group III	27.7 (23.7)*@	7.5 (6.8)*@	3.5 (1.8)	1.9@+	1.3	1.3

* = p < 0.05 vs. Controls; @ = p < 0.05 vs. Group I; + = p < 0.05 vs. Group II.
All patients had more frequent reflux symptoms than controls (p < 0.05).
Chi-squared test for symptoms using individual scores.
HB = heartburn; REG = regurgitation; DYS = dysphagia.

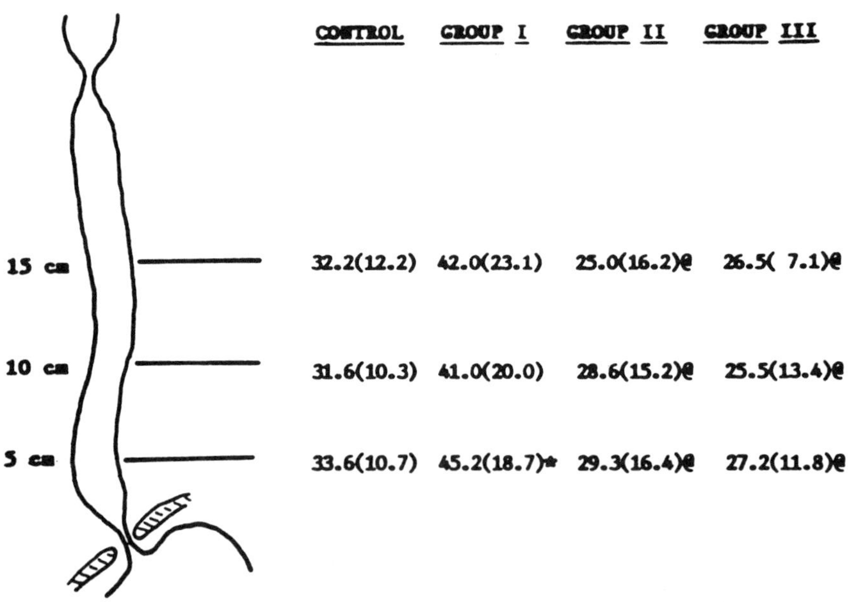

Figure 1: Mean amplitude (± standard deviation) of primary peristaltic waves recorded at the three esophageal levels in patients and controls (mmHg).

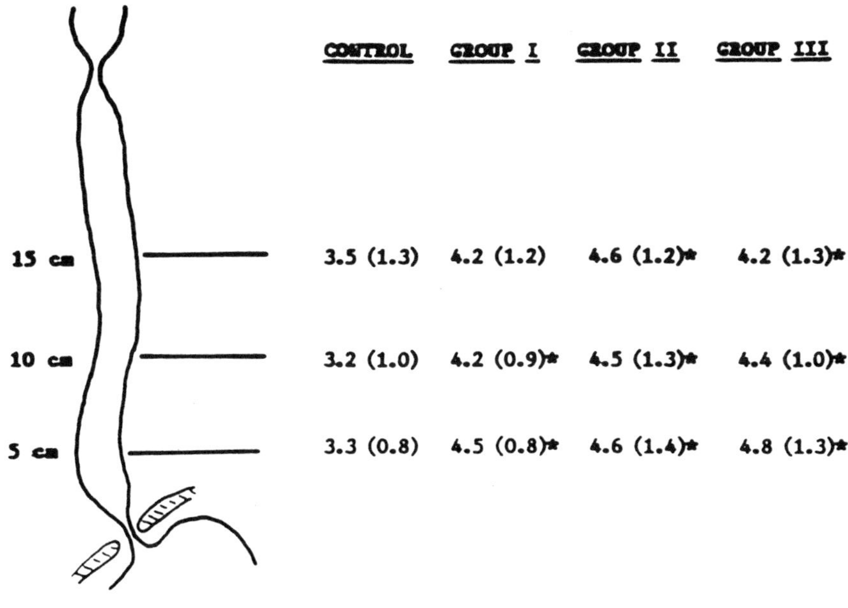

Figure 2: Mean duration (± standard deviation) of primary peristaltic waves recorded at the three esophageal levels in patients and controls (seconds).

with Barrett's esophagus, however, had lower scores for heartburn and regurgitation but more severe dysphagia. The mean values of wave amplitude, duration, and velocity are compared in Figures 1, 2, and 3. They show that the contraction amplitude is decreased in groups II and III patients compared to both controls and group I patients at the three levels examined in this study. Contraction duration is increased and velocity is diminished, however, in all three patient groups compared to controls.

No abnormal motility patterns were observed in the esophageal body in the control subjects. It will be seen from Table IV that patients with severe mucosal damage (group II) or Barrett's esophagus (group III) had a higher frequency of repetitive, nontransmitted, and simultaneous contractions than patients in group I. The number of spontaneous contractions was greater in the latter group. In addition, the number of nonclassifiable contractile abnormalities generally increased with the degree of esophagitis.

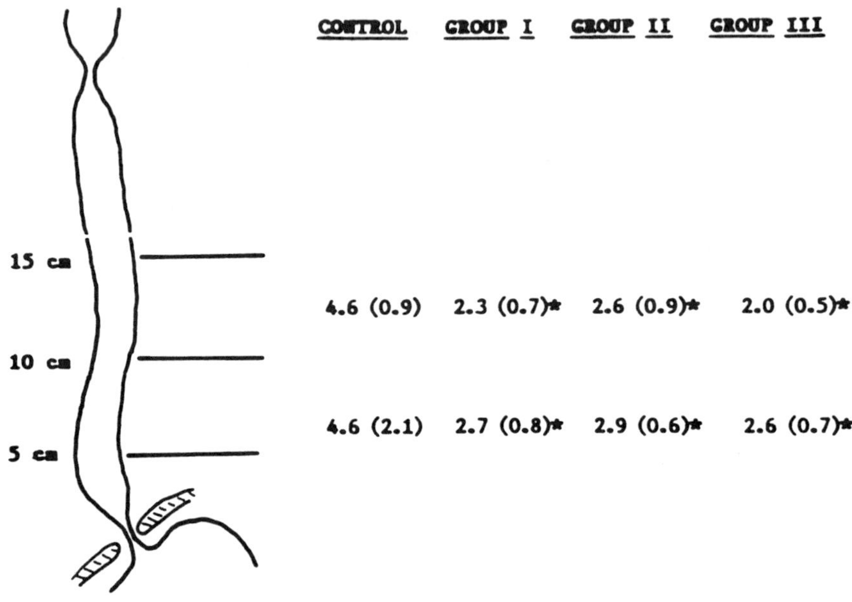

Figure 3: Mean velocity ($\pm$ standard deviation) of primary peristaltic waves recorded at the three esophageal levels in patients and controls (cm/second).

Table IV
Contractile Abnormalities According to Degree of Esophagitis

	Repetitive	Nontransmitted	Spontaneous	Simultaneous
Control	—	—	—	—
Group I	0	1	6	6
Group II	1	7	2	22*@
Group III	3	10*@	3	15*@ +

$*$ = $p < 0.05$ vs. Controls; @ = $p < 0.05$ vs. Group I; + = $p < 0.05$ vs. Group II.

Discussion

This study has shown that worsening esophagitis is associated with increased acid reflux and abnormal motility. In mild esophagitis, the initial abnormalities are an increase in wave duration and a reduction in velocity of travel with preservation of the "squeeze." With worsening degrees of mucosal damage, the strength of the esophageal squeeze diminishes and contraction pressure wanes. Those subjects with severe esophagitis appear to have similar abnormalities to patients with a Barrett's esophagus. However, in going from control subjects to these latter two groups, there appears to be a stepwise progression both in the abnormal wave parameters and in the number of abnormal contractions. These manometric features are nonspecific and it is therefore not possible from the results of this study to precisely correlate motility patterns with mucosal damage. At present, it would seem unlikely that these features would be of diagnostic value.

We speculate that the increase in amplitude of primary contractions seen in group I patients represents an attempt by the still relatively healthy esophagus to clear itself of noxious material. This may be lost with further mucosal damage. Similarly, the higher number of spontaneous contractions might suggest an increased sensitivity to acid exposure.

When more damage occurs, as seen in groups II and III patients, motor activity is disrupted as manifested by the appearance of repetitive, simultaneous, and nontransmitted contraction waves. It is interesting that esophageal body motility is similar in patients with advanced esophagitis and those with a Barrett's epithelium as the latter typically have no inflammation in the columnar-lined segment.[16] Again, the relationship between reflux and Barrett's epithelium remains enigmatic.

These progressive alterations in the motility pattern of the esophageal body, though presumably caused by acid reflux, potentiate mucosal injury by impairing esophageal clearance of refluxed material. It is not at present known whether these changes can be reversed, but our results support therapeutic, pharmacological attempts at improving motility in medically treated patients with esophagitis.

References

1. Dodds WJ, Hogan WJ, Helm JF, et al: Pathogenesis of reflux esophagitis. Gastroenterology 81:376, 1981.

2. Fisher RS, Malmud LS, Roberts GS, et al: The lower esophageal sphincter as a barrier to gastroesophageal reflux. Gastroenterology 72:19, 1977.

3. O'Sullivan GC, DeMeester TR, Joelsson BE, et al: Interaction of lower esophageal sphincter in the abdomen as determinants of gastroesophageal competence. Am J Surg 143:40, 1982.

4. Eastwood GL, Castell DO, Higgs RH: Experimental esophagitis in cats impairs lower esophageal sphincter pressure. Gastroenterology 69:146, 1975.

5. Skinner DB, Booth DJ: Assessment of distal esophageal function in patients with hiatal hernia and/or gastroesophageal reflux. Ann Surg 172:627, 1970.

6. Little AG, DeMeester TR, Kirchner PT, et al: Pathogenesis of esophagitis in patients with gastroesophageal reflux. Surgery 88:101, 1980.

7. DeMeester TR, Johnson LF, Joseph GJ, et al: Patterns of gastroesophageal reflux in health and disease. Ann Surg 184:459, 1976.

8. Savary M, Miller G: The Esophagus: Handbook and Atlas of Endoscopy, Verlag Gassman AG, Solothurn, Switzerland, 1978, p 119.

9. Arndorfer RC, Stef JJ, Dodds WJ, et al: Improved infusion system for intraluminal esophageal manometry. Gastroenterology 73:23, 1977.

10. Winnans CS, Harris LD: Quantitation of lower esophageal sphincter competence. Gastroenterology 52:773, 1967.

11. Vanek AW, Diamant NE: Response of the human esophagus to paired swallows. Gastroenterology 92:643, 1987.

12. Kahrilas PJ, Dodds WJ, Hogan WJ, et al: Esophageal peristaltic dysfunction in peptic esophagitis. Gastroenterology 91:897, 1986.

13. Weihrauch TR: Esophageal Manometry. Methods and Clinical Practice, Baltimore-Munich, Urban & Schwarzenberg Inc., 1981, p 80.

14. Clouse RE, Staino A: Contractile abnormalities of the esophageal body in patients referred for manometry: A new approach to manometric classification. Dig Dis Sci 28:784, 1983.

15. Johnson LF, DeMeester TR: Twenty-four-hour monitoring of the distal esophagus. Am J Gastroenterol 62:325, 1974.

16. Paull A, Trier JS, Dalton MD, et al: The histologic spectrum of Barrett's esophagus. N Engl J Med 295:276, 1976.

13

Which Region of the Stomach is Responsible for Delay in Gastric Emptying of Solids in Patients with Gastroesophageal Reflux Disease?

Glyn G. Jamieson, J.C. Myers, P.J. Collins,
Thomas C.B. Dehn, G.J. Maddern, M. Horowitz

Introduction

It is now established that some patients with gastroesophageal reflux disease (GERD) have delayed gastric emptying of liquids and/or solids. However, the relative proportions of patients with delayed emptying and the significance of any delay remain controversial issues.[1] Gastric emptying is a complex process and many factors influence it. Therefore, some of the differences that have been recorded are probably related to the different techniques being used to assess gastric emptying.

The aim of this study was to examine the gastric emptying of a group of patients with proven GERD. In those patients in whom emptying was delayed, we sought to determine if the delay was in

Little AG, Ferguson MK, Skinner DB: Diseases of the Esophagus, Vol. II: Benign Diseases. Futura Publishing Company, Inc., Mount Kisco, NY, © 1990.

the proximal stomach, in the transfer of food from proximal to distal stomach, or delay in the distal stomach; or indeed, was the delayed emptying a combination of all three possibilities? At the present time there is relatively little known about gastric redistribution and emptying of simultaneously ingested solid and liquid meal components.[2,3]

Methods

We used a recently developed technique to assess the emptying from the proximal stomach and from the distal stomach.[3] The basic technique in these patients has been described previously in detail.[4] In short, it consists of the ingestion of 100 ml of 10% dextrose containing 0.5 mCi (20 MBq) of ^{113m}In-DTPA and 100 g of chicken liver/ beef hamburger, containing 1.5 mCi (60 MBq) of ^{99m}Tc. The patient sits in front of a gamma camera and the radioactive counts are fed into a computer. Several parameters of solid emptying from the whole stomach are measured: (a) the period of time before any food leaves the stomach—the lag period (LP), (b) the percentage of food which is retained in the stomach at 100 minutes, after ingestion of the meal, (c) the rate at which food empties from the stomach.

The new technique allows us to divide the stomach into a proximal and distal region of interest on the basis of the site where food first enters the stomach. It is likely that the proximal area corresponds with the fundus and body of the stomach and the distal area corresponds with the antrum of the stomach.[3] The use of this technique allows us to measure several further parameters of gastric emptying: (a) for the proximal stomach, the percentage of retention of food at 55 minutes, (b) for the distal stomach, the time taken for 90% of the maximum content of the meal to reach the distal stomach (DT 90), and a parameter which gives an indication of food retention in the distal stomach. This latter figure is derived by subtracting the DT 90 from the LP.

Thirty-six consecutive patients with stage 2 or greater reflux disease had emptying assessed by the above technique.

Results

On the basis of previously established normal ranges,[4] the patients were divided into those with normal solid food retention at 100

Table I
Gastric Emptying Results

	"Normal" *Emptiers* *n = 16*	*"Delayed"* *Emptiers* *n = 20*	*p* *value*
Total Stomach			
Lag period (mins)	32 (25–42)	63 (49–72)	0.0001
% retention at 100 mins	37 (33–50)	69 (64–88)	0.0001
Rate of emptying (% min)	0.92 (0.74–1.0)	0.69 (0.41–0.88)	0.0136
Proximal Stomach			
% retention at 55 mins	43 (26–50)	55 (42–66)	0.0075
Distal Stomach			
Time taken to reach maximal content (mins)	32 (18–39)	54 (44–69)	0.0002
Retention time (mins)	0.50 ({−10}+16)	5.50 ({−3}+14)	0.4354

minutes (16 patients—"normal" emptiers), and those with increased retention at 100 minutes (20 patients—"delayed" emptiers).

The gastric emptying results are shown in Table I. The statistic used to assess the p-value was the Mann-Whitney U test.

Discussion

It seems that all investigators find some reflux patients who have delayed emptying of solids. However, some groups have found no overall significant delay in emptying compared with controls,[6–8] and some have found significant delay in patients compared to controls.[4,9–14] Two groups have found that patients with delayed emptying are more likely to have endoscopic esophagitis, suggesting that the emptying problem may play a pathogenetic role in the development of GERD.[4,14] This study appears to show that the delay in emptying in patients with GERD is from the proximal stomach and emptying from the distal stomach is normal. However, the technique used does not allow the measurement of any retropulsion from the antrum and it is possible that antral or pyloric dysfunction may lead to a greater degree of retropulsion in patients with delayed emptying, and this might also explain our results. Abnormalities have been described in both antrum and body of the stomach in patients with GERD.[15–17] Autonomic dysfunction with associated vagal neuropathy in GERD patients has also been described.[18,19]

Whether the dysfunction is occurring in the proximal stomach, the distal stomach, or in both regions, the net result is that food is retained longer in the proximal stomach and this introduces the potential for a greater number of transient lower esophageal sphincter relaxations to occur.[20]

Conclusion

In patients with gastroesophageal reflux disease and delayed emptying from the stomach, the delay in emptying appears to arise from the proximal stomach where the food remains longer and is slower to move into the distal stomach. Once it arrives in the distal stomach, emptying occurs normally. These findings support the concept that delayed gastric emptying of solids may be of pathogenetic significance in gastroesophageal reflux disease.

References

1. Dubois A: Clinical relevance of gastro-duodenal dysfunction in reflux esophagitis. J Clin Gastroenterol 8:17, 1986.
2. Moore JG, Christian BS, Coleman RE: Gastric emptying of varying meal weight and composition in man: Evaluation by dual liquid and solid phase isotopic method. Dig Dis Sci 26:16, 1981.
3. Collins PJ, Horowitz M, Chatterton BE: Proximal, distal and total stomach emptying of a digestible solid meal in normal subjects. Br J Radiol 61:12, 1988.
4. Maddern GJ, Chatterton BE, Collins PJ, Horowitz M, Shearman DJC, Jamieson GG: Solid and liquid gastric emptying in patients with gastro-oesophageal reflux. Br J Surg 72:344, 1985.
5. Jamieson GG, Duranceau AC: Staging of severity of gastro-esophageal reflux. In: Gastro-Esophageal Reflux, Jamieson GG, Duranceau A (eds), Philadelphia, WB Saunders, 1988, pp 105–111.
6. Bost R, Hostein G, Gignoux C, Busquet G, Lachet B, Fournet J: Vidange gastrique d'un repas solide-liquide au cours du reflux gastro-oesophagien chez l'adulte. Gastroenterol Clin Biol 10:322, 1986.
7. Johnson DA, Winters C, Drane WE, Cawtau EL, Karvelis KC, Silverman ED, Spurling TJ, Chobanian SJ, Dubois A: Solid phase gastric emptying in patients with Barrett's esophagus. Dig Dis Sci 6:31–37, 1980.
8. Shay SS, Eggli D, McDonald C, Johnson LF: Gastric emptying of solid

food in patients with gastroesophageal reflux. Gastroenterology 92:459, 1987.

9. McCallum RW, Mensh R, Laing ER: Definition of the gastric emptying abnormality present in gastroesophageal reflux patients. In: Motility of the Digestive Tract, Weinbeck M (ed), New York, Raven Press, 1982 pp 362–365.

10. Collins PJ, McFarland RJ, O'Hare MMT, Shore C, Buchanan KD, Love AHG: Gastric emptying of a solid liquid meal and gastrointestinal hormone responses in patients with erosive esophagitis. Digestion 33:61, 1986.

11. Donovan IA, Harding LK, Keighley MR, Griffin DW, Collis JL: Abnormalities of gastric emptying and pyloric function in uncomplicated hiatus hernia. Br J Surg 64:847, 1977.

12. Valenzuela JE, Dooley C, Ansar IA, Miranda M. Samloff MI: Abnormal esophageal and gastric functions in patients with reflux esophagitis. Gastroenterology 82:1201, 1982.

13. Velasco N, Hill LD, Gannan RM, Pope CE: Gastric emptying and gastroesophageal reflux: Affects of surgery and correlation with esophageal motor function. Med J Surg 144:58, 1982.

14. Little AG, DeMeester TR, Kirschner PT, O'Sullivan GC, Skinner DB: Pathogenesis of esophagitis in patients with gastro-esophageal reflux. Surgery 88:101, 1980.

15. Behar J, Ramsby YG: Gastric emptying and antral motility in reflux esophagitis: Effect of oral metoclopramide. Gastroenterology 74:253, 1978.

14

Respiratory Complications of Gastroesophageal Reflux in Children:
Asthma versus Recurrent Infections

Anne Malfroot, Margherita Giocoli, Isi Dab

Introduction

At present, several investigators agree that gastroesophageal reflux (GER), not to be mistaken for harmless regurgitations, can be responsible for, or aggravate, chronic respiratory disease (RD), both in adults and in children.[1-3] In 1985 we started to study GER in children with chronic RD of unknown origin. A first group of 38 children, showed GER in 63% of the cases and this was considered to be responsible for their respiratory complaints. Indeed, RD was cured in 82% of them after correct treatment of the reflux[4]; however, some problems remain unsolved.

Originally, abnormal GER was defined by gastroenterologists, since they needed criteria to predict the hazard of peptic ulcerations of the esophagus. Gastroenterologists are therefore more concerned by acid refluxes. We wonder whether the same criteria are valid in RD, that is, whether only those refluxes which might induce esophageal ulcerations are dangerous for the respiratory tract, or whether

Little AG, Ferguson MK, Skinner DB: Diseases of the Esophagus, Vol. II: Benign Diseases. Futura Publishing Company, Inc., Mount Kisco, NY, © 1990.

refluxes which are not likely to produce esophageal injury could nevertheless be harmful for the respiratory system. If this is true, we must also define new criteria for GER which would be valid for pulmonology, especially in pediatrics.

Until now, most authors do not differentiate patients with asthma from patients with recurrent infections, and often these respiratory symptoms are not described with precision. After our first series, we had the impression that reflux often causes asthma, but that a smaller number of patients suffered from recurrent infection.

To answer these questions, we completed our first study on a larger number of children and we discovered some differences in the characteristics of refluxes between asthma and recurrent or chronic infections.

Patient Description

The presence of GER was looked for in chronic respiratory patients who fulfilled one or both of the following criteria:

1. All classic complementary examinations yield negative results on sweat tests, tuberculin tests, skin tests for different allergens, specific IgE (RAST). Patients with cystic fibrosis, an immunodeficiency disease, or a bronchopulmonary malformation were excluded, as well as children with a neurological disease.

2. Previous specific treatments such as antibiotics, cromolyn inhalations, and bronchodilators have failed.

On this basis, 269 children have been selected over a period of 4 years. Their ages ranged from 3 months to 16 years. All were referred to our Pediatric Pulmonology and CF Clinic for persistent major respiratory symptoms, mostly starting at birth or lasting at least for more than 6 months. Gastrointestinal disorders such as vomiting, or heartburn in older patients were present in only 10% of the patients and were never a major complaint. According to their main respiratory symptoms, they were separated into two groups: a first group of 151 patients mainly with signs of wheezing and bronchial hyperreactivity, i.e., asthma, and a second group of 118 patients mainly with recurrent pulmonary infections, i.e., chronic or recurrent consolidation on chest X-ray, mostly in the right middle lobe, and/or positive bacterial culture of the bronchial aspiration.

Diagnosis of GER in RD

In RD, the detection of GER requires methods enabling the study of esophageal function over an adequate period of time. Barium swallow is less sensitive as it shows esophageal function only briefly. Esophagoscopy is useful only for the detection of esophageal injury or malformation.

Since there is no absolute standard method that can confirm GER, most authors use more than one technique in combination to enhance the accuracy of the diagnosis of GER. We used esophageal pH monitoring and reflux scintiscanning in combination. Both examinations were performed simultaneously and all medications were interrupted at least 24 hours before investigation (especially theophylline, which could influence the results of the GER investigations).

Prolonged esophageal pH monitoring is probably the best method available at the present time. In our patients, esophageal pH recordings were performed continuously for approximately 20 hours, starting in the afternoon and lasting throughout the night and a part of the next day. All of the episodes with a pH<4 were measured by the method described by Vandenplas et al.[5] A pH tracing (Fig. 1) was considered abnormal if the value of any one of the parameters exceeded the mean + 2 SD of age-matched asymptomatic infants according to the normal values given by Vandenplas et al.[6]

The advantages of the pH monitoring are: (1) the prolonged observation period and (2) the avoidance of postural restrictions (the normal behavior of the children was not disturbed and they played, slept, and were fed as usual).

Gastroesophageal scintiscanning (Fig. 2) is a simple method especially suited for children, not requiring the introduction of an esophageal catheter, which can interfere with normal peristalsis. All esophageal radioactivity peaks can be quantified, and their sum can be expressed as a percent of the total gastric activity, i.e., the isotopic reflux index, a method described by Fisher et al. and Piepsz et al.[7,8]

An advantage of this method is the fact that it allows clear visualization of the reflux episode, whatever the pH level in the postprandial period. This can be important in children in whom acid secretion in the stomach is disturbed or in very young milk-fed infants. It is known that milk slows gastric emptying and that gastric juice can be buffered as long as milk remains in the stomach, sometimes for many hours.[9] However, refluxes with a pH above 4 are not detected by pH measurements. The question is whether these refluxes,

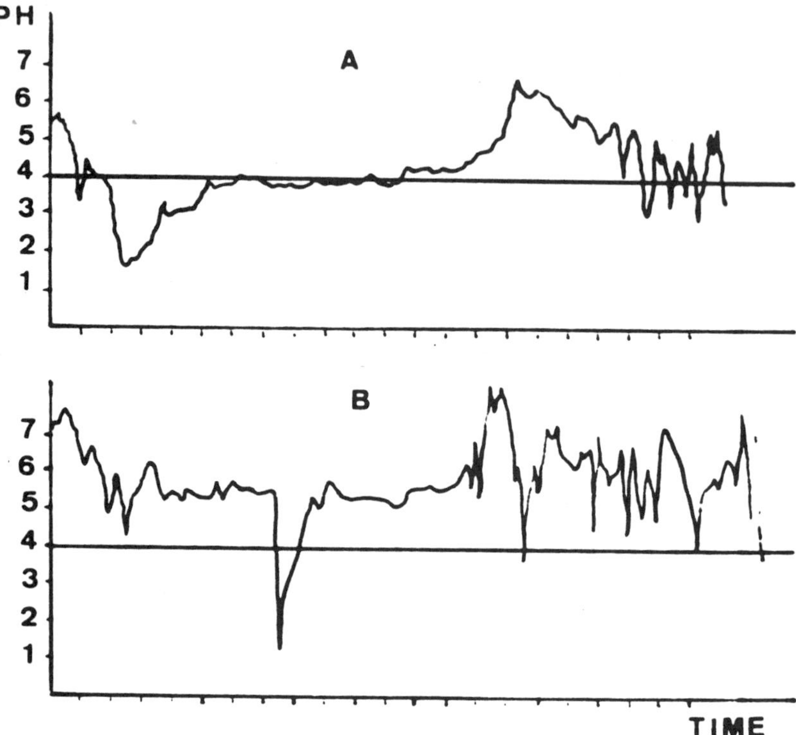

Figure 1: (A) Severely disturbed pH monitoring in a 22-month-old girl with chronic cough and wheezing. Reflux index (the sum of all periods of pH<4 over the whole duration of the investigation time expressed in %) = 49%, the duration of the longest reflux episode = 156 min, the number of refluxes = 51, and the number of refluxes >5 min = 15. (B) During medical antireflux treatment, reflux index decreases to 5%, the longest reflux episode falls to 41 min, the number of reflux episodes becomes 28, and the number of refluxes >5 min is only 1.

which are not meaningful for gastrointestinal disorders because they will not cause esophagitis, could have respiratory consequences.

Another advantage of reflux scintiscanning is the possibility to demonstrate pulmonary aspiration by scanning the chest 4 hours after the test to detect any radioactivity in the lungs. However, in our experience, sensitivity of the scintiscanning method to confirm aspiration is rather low.[4]

A disadvantage of the scintigraphy is the rather short observation time. The esophagus can be observed only during approximately 1

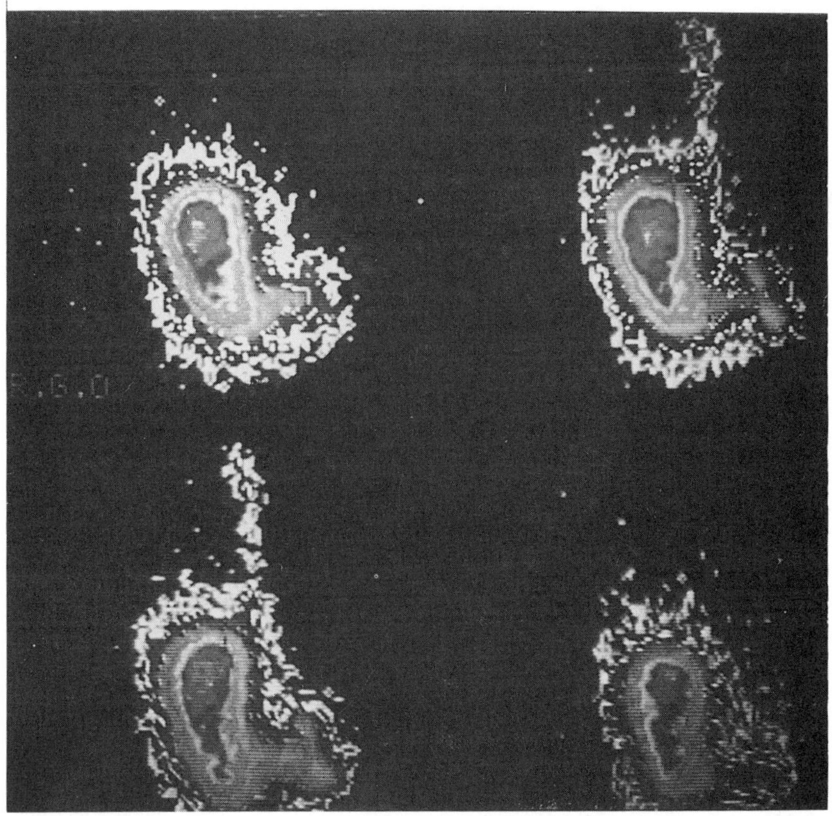

Figure 2: Picture of a gastroesophageal reflux scintigraphy. After the administration of the tracer (^{99m}Tc-sulfur colloid, 0.74 MBq/kg body weight, mixed with milk or pudding) the patient takes the remainder of the meal to clear the esophagus of any residual radioactivity, then he is placed in supine position above a large-field scintillation camera, and 20-sec frames are collected during a period of 1 hour over both the esophagus and the stomach. This figure shows clearly a reflux episode on two of the images.

hour, as the radiotracer progressively leaves the stomach through the physiological gastric emptying. This is insufficient for the diagnosis of refluxes between meals and during the night.

Results

Using pH monitoring and scintiscanning simultaneously in 269 respiratory infants and children, GER was diagnosed in 143 patients

Table I
Respiratory Symptoms and GER Characteristics in 143 Patients

	GER/Total Number of Patients	Acid Refluxes	Nonacid Refluxes	Pulmonary Aspiration
Asthma	96/151 (64%)	86	10	0
Infections	47/118 (39%)	23	24	4
Total	143/269 (53%)	109	34	

(53%). GER was demonstrated by both investigations in 51 cases; it was detected only by pH monitoring in 58 cases, and only by scintiscanning in 34 cases. We concluded that 109 patients had acid refluxes (i.e., 51 plus 58) and that the remaining 34 had nonacid refluxes (Table I). During analysis of respiratory symptoms in the 143 patients in whom GER was detected, we noticed that GER was diagnosed more frequently, with a highly significant difference ($p<0.001$) in the group with asthma (64%) and less frequently in the group with mainly infections (39%). Moreover, we observed that asthma occurred almost exclusively in patients with acid refluxes, and that recurrent infection occurred preferentially in patients with nonacid refluxes, the difference being also highly significant ($p<0.001$) (Table I). Pulmonary aspiration, as proven by late scintigraphic images, could be demonstrated in only four patients, all of whom suffered from recurrent infections with normal lung function testing. Figure 3 illustrates the characteristics of the pH monitoring of the patients with nonacid refluxes.

All 143 patients underwent medical antireflux therapy. Only five of them eventually underwent a Nissen fundoplication because of failure of medical treatment. Remission of the RD was observed in 80% of the children in whom GER disappeared by either medical or surgical treatment.

Finally, the esophageal pH tracings of 50 patients in whom pH monitoring and reflux scintigraphy together were considered as normal were reanalyzed more thoroughly. Sixteen patients showed particular tracings: the pH clearly dropped during the night, but just above the level of 4 (Fig. 4). Such tracings have never been observed in asymptomatic children who served to establish the normal values, or in children with only gastrointestinal symptoms. We wondered whether such a tracing could be responsible for RD. Therefore, med-

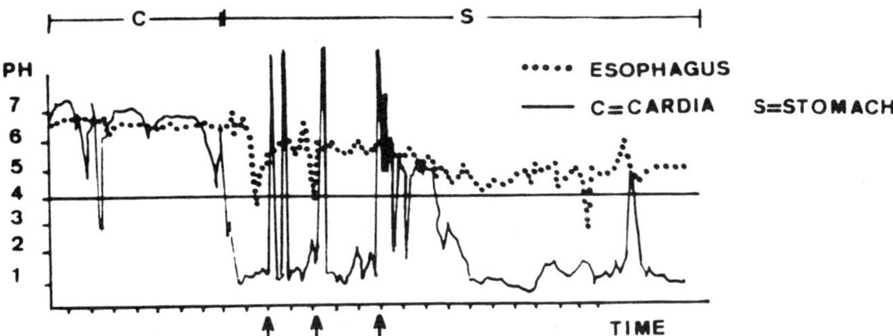

Figure 3: Double pH monitoring tracings performed simultaneously with one electrode in the esophagus and one at the level of the cardia (checked by fluoroscopy) in a 3½-year-old boy suffering from chronic bronchitis with permanent *Hemophilus influnzae* on sputum cultures since the age of 1 year. Esophageal pH tracing is within the age-related normal range. Scintiscanning shows a reflux of 70% of the gastric activity, i.e., nonacid refluxes. The second electrode at the cardia (C) shows a high pH at this level with some short acid reflux peaks. After 8 hours, this electrode is pushed into the stomach (S) and demonstrates a normal gastric acidity, however buffered over short periods by the meals (↑). Buffering of the gastric content during the meals could be an explanation for nonacid postprandial refluxes that were missed by pH monitoring.

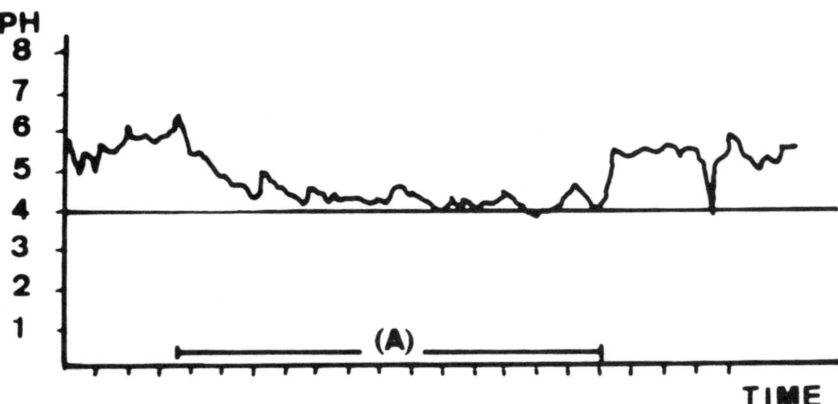

Figure 4: Illustration of a pH tracing considered as normal since pH>4 at any time. All parameters are within normal ranges based on present criteria. However, during the night (A) pH approaches the level of 4.

ical antireflux therapy has been recently started in 3 of these 16 patients and respiratory complaints disappeared. In one of them antireflux therapy was discontinued and RD relapsed immediately.

Discussion

We purposely selected for this study only respiratory patients without any other underlying disorder, such as cystic fibrosis or neurological disease, as it would complicate the interpretation of the results. Indeed, we know by personal observations in a series of babies with cysitc fibrosis[10] that reflux is very frequent in young cystic fibrosis patients. Antireflux therapy can improve the pulmonary and nutritional conditions in these patients but cannot fundamentally cure the disease, and infectious exacerbations will inevitably interfere. This applies also to other disorders, such as children with either severe neurological disease or tracheoesophageal fistula repair or premature babies in whom GER is a very frequent finding. Patients with GER and RD but without any other underlying disorder are more suitable for a correct analysis of the possible relation between these two troubles.

In our group of 269 selected children with chronic RD, a large percentage of GER was observed (53%), despite the fact that gastrointestinal symptoms were mainly absent or only of minor importance. Other studies have reported comparable numbers,[1,2] but these authors looked for GER in selected patients with gastrointestinal complaints and used only pH monitoring with the classic criteria as established by gastroenterologists for the diagnosis of GER. Our observations prove that chronic RD of unknown origin, or not responding to classic therapy, can be due to GER even if gastrointestinal complaints are lacking. We are now convinced that criteria for pathological reflux in RD differ from those in gastrointestinal disorders:

1. Prolonged pH monitoring seems to be the best technique, because it allows observation over a long period of time, but only refluxes with a pH<4 are recognized if criteria are used as established by gastroenterologists. For RD, these criteria probably need to be adjusted. It is possible that a clear decrease of the pH during the night, even if not below 4, should be considered as pathological, as has been demonstrated in 16 of our patients with otherwise normal pH tracings (Fig. 4). Further investigations are in progress to confirm these preliminary findings.

2. The results observed by using the scintigraphic method for GER investigation stress that specific criteria are needed for pediatric pulmonology. In this series of 143 patients, the diagnosis of GER has been confirmed in 34 (31%) by the scintigraphic method only. About 80% of them were cured of their RD after correct antireflux therapy, which represents the same proportion as for the whole group of acid and nonacid refluxes together and provides evidence that also non-acid refluxes can be responsible for respiratory symptoms. The scintigraphic method is not very useful for digestive symptoms since post-prandial nonacid refluxes generally do not result in esophagitis. On the contrary, for RD, the use of the reflux scintiscans will enhance the accuracy of the diagnosis of GER, especially for refluxes not detected by the pH monitoring (Fig. 3).

This series illustrates the variety of the respiratory symptoms caused by GER. It also illustrates that there must be a relationship between the kind of symptoms and the characteristics of GER. Bronchial hyperreactivity and asthma were almost exclusively associated with acid refluxes. We don't know whether this bronchial hyper-reactivity was a primary defect in these patients, or whether it was a consequence of the acid refluxes. Increased bronchial responsiveness to metacholine has been observed in adults after esophageal acid instillation by some authors,[11] while others could not demonstrate a direct correlation between episodes of acid refluxes and deterioration of lung function.[12] On the other hand, chronic or recurrent infections were more frequently, though not exclusively, associated with non-acid refluxes.

Different theories have been suggested to explain the mechanisms by which GER can cause RD. An attractive hypothesis is pulmonary aspiration or microaspiration of the gastric content into the lungs.[13] The frequency of delayed radioactivity detection in the lungs is controversial. Some investigators have reported frequent evidence of aspiration[14] while others have found a low sensitivity of the test as in our series.[15] One can imagine that the amount of radioactivity that enters the lungs is frequently too small to be detected by the camera. Furthermore, pulmonary aspiration doesn't have to occur continuously, but only occasionally. Moreover, continuous pulmonary aspiration is probably incompatible with life. Therefore, pulmonary aspiration must be considered, even if it is not easy to demonstrate with the presently available methods. This applies especially for the nonacid refluxes. In our series of nonacid GER, lung aspiration could be demonstrated in four children, all of whom had recurrent infections.

We conclude that nonacid refluxes can be responsible for RD, probably by lung aspiration, and that this mechanism might explain infectious phenomena. Another possible mechanism by which GER can play a role in RD includes a reflex, mediated by the vagus nerve, triggered by the presence of an acid solution in the lower esophagus and resulting in bronchospasm.[16] This theory is confirmed by our series: in 92% of all patients with asthma and GER, we found acid refluxes, while in only 8% of them, nonacid refluxes were observed. We conclude that asthma is mostly caused by acid refluxes by means of a reflex mechanism. The opposite is less true: acid refluxes do not need to cause only asthma. They can be also responsible for repeated infections (Table I).

In most of patients, respiratory symptoms disappear under correct antireflux treatment. Usually medical treatment is sufficient and should always be tried before resorting to surgery.

ACKNOWLEDGMENTS: The authors are indebted to Yvan Vandenplas who developed pH monitoring in the department, to Amnon Piepsz for providing the scintiscanning images, and to Marie Paule Derde for helping with the statistical evaluation.

References

1. Euler AR, Byrne WJ, Ament ME, et al: Recurrent pulmonary disease in children: A complication of gastroesophageal reflux. Pediatrics 63:47, 1979.
2. Houyoux Ch, Forget P, Lambrechts L, et al: Chronic bronchopulmonary disease and gastroesophageal reflux in children. Pediatr Pulmonol 1:149, 1985.
3. Berquist WE, Rachelewsky GS, Kadden M, et al: Gastroesophageal reflux associated recurrent pneumonia and chronic asthma in children. Pediatrics 68:29, 1981.
4. Malfroot A, Vandenplas Y, Verlinden M, et al: Gastroesophageal reflux and unexplained chronic respiratory disease in infants and children. Pediatric Pulmonol 3:208, 1987.
5. Vandenplas Y, Sacre-Smits L: Seventeen-hour continuous esophageal pH monitoring in the newborn: Evaluation of the influence of position in asymptomatic and symptomatic babies. J Pediatr Gastroenterol Nutr 5:356, 1985.
6. Vandenplas Y, Sacre-Smits L: Continuous 24-hour esophageal pH monitoring in 283 asymptomatic infants (0 to 15 months old). J Pediatr Gastroenterol Nutr 6:220, 1987.

7. Fisher RS, Malmud LS, Roberts GS, et al: Gastroesophageal scintiscanning to detect and quantitate reflux. Gastroenterology 70:301, 1976.
8. Piepsz A, Georges B, Perlmutter N, et al: Gastroesophageal scintiscanning in children. Pediatr Radiol 11:71, 1981.
9. Sonheimer JM, Clarke DA, Gervaise EP: Continuous gastric pH measurement in young and older healthy preterm infants receiving formula and clear liquid feedings. J Pediatr Gastroenterol Nutr 4:352, 1985.
10. Dab I, Malfroot A: Gastroesophageal reflux: A primary defect in cystic fibrosis? Scand J Gastroenterol 23(suppl 143):125, 1988.
11. Herve P, Denjean A, Jian R, et al: Intraesophageal perfusion of acid increases the bronchomotor response to metacholine and to isocapnic hyperventilation in asthmatic subjects. Am Rev Respir Dis 143:986, 1986.
12. Ekström T, Tibbling L: Gastroesophageal reflux and triggering of bronchial asthma: A negative report. Eur J Respir Dis 71:177, 1987.
13. Mendelson CL: The aspiration of stomach contents into the lungs during obstetric anesthesia. Am J Obstet Gynecol 52:191, 1946.
14. Boonyaprapa S, Alderson PO, Garbinkel DJ, et al: Detection of pulmonary aspiration in infants and children with RD: Concise communication. J Nucl Med 21:314, 1980.
15. Heymans S, Kirkpatrick JA, Winter HS, et al: An unproved radionuclide method for the diagnosis of gastroesophageal reflux and aspiration in children. Radiology 131:479, 1979.
16. Mansfield LE, Stein MR: Gastroesophageal reflux and asthma: Demonstration of a possible reflex mechanism. Am Rev Respir Dis 117:72, 1978.

15

Omeprazole or High-Dose Ranitidine in the Treatment of Patients with Reflux Esophagitis not Responding to Standard Doses of H$_2$-Receptor Antagonists

Lars Lundell, I. H. Westin, L. Backman,
L.-C. Enander, O. Fausa, T. Lind, H. Lönroth,
S. Sandmark, B. Sandzén, P. Unge

Introduction

Standard doses of H$_2$-receptor antagonists have repeatedly been shown to leave a considerable number of patients with reflux esophagitis unhealed and with incomplete symptom relief.[1,2] In addition, it has to be established whether an increased dose of an H$_2$-receptor antagonist will be followed by a further improvement in the clinical results. Omeprazole, an inhibitor of H$^+$K$^+$-ATPase in the parietal cell,[3] has been shown to be very effective in promoting healing of esophagitis as well as in relieving symptoms.[4-8] In a prospective, randomized clinical study, we have compared the efficacy of omeprazole (40 mg once daily) with that of a high dose of ranitidine (300

Little AG, Ferguson MK, Skinner DB: Diseases of the Esophagus, Vol. II: Benign Diseases. Futura Publishing Company, Inc., Mount Kisco, NY, © 1990.

mg b.i.d.) given for 4 to 12 weeks in patients still suffering from esophagitis in spite of at least 3 months of full-dose H_2-blocker therapy.

Patients and Methods

Study Design and Patient Selection

The study was performed as a randomized, double-blind, multicenter trial with two parallel groups using a double dummy technique. Only patients with esophagitis of at least grade 2, verified by endoscopy within a week prior to the start of treatment, were eligible to enter the study.[7] Each patient had to be unhealed after at least 3 months' treatment with therapeutic doses of cimetidine (minimum dose = 200 mg daily) or ranitidine (minimum dose = 300 mg daily). The presence of Barrett's esophagus and/or an esophageal stricture was recorded. The definition of healing was a complete epithelialization of all esophageal erosions and/or ulcerations in the squamous epithelium.

Patients were randomly allocated to treatment with 40 mg omeprazole once daily or 300 mg ranitidine twice daily and were initially treated for 4 weeks and then for another two 4-week periods if the esophagitis was unhealed at the respective endoscopic examination. No other medication recommended in the treatment of esophagitis was allowed after commencement of trial medication.

Assessments

A general medical history was obtained before entry. Details on alcohol and tobacco consumption were also recorded. Esophagus, stomach, and duodenum were examined endoscopically in each patient within one week before treatment started. Endoscopy was performed by the same investigator on all occasions whenever possible. Before entry and at the scheduled visits, all patients were questioned concerning the presence and severity of heartburn, regurgitation, dysphagia, and odynophagia. The severity of reflux symptoms was scored from 0 to 3 (0 = no symptoms, 3 = severe symptoms). Other symptoms were recorded only as present or absent. Before inclusion and at 4-week intervals during the study, blood and urine samples were taken for hematological and biochemical analyses. Esophageal biopsy specimens were taken only to exclude malignancy and to verify the presence of columnar lined esophagus. Barrett's esophagus was defined as suggested by Skinner et al.[9]

Statistics and Ethics

We analyzed the healing data according to "intention to treat," which includes all patients entering the study except those withdrawn because of malignant diseases or abnormal findings in the pre-entry laboratory screen or other major violation of the protocol. In the intention to treat analyses, patients in whom an endoscopy was not repeated were considered nonhealed. All decisions to exclude patients from the statistical analyses were taken before breaking the treatment code. The Mantel-Haenszel test was used for analyzing the endoscopic healing data. Reflux symptoms were analyzed with a Wilcoxon rank test with stratification according to pre-entry severity grade of heartburn. The study protocol was approved by the local ethical committees and informed consent was obtained from each patient before entering the study.

Results

Patients

Ninety-eight patients were included in the study and 51 of these were allocated to omeprazole treatment. As seen in Table I, the pre-entry characteristics of the two study groups were very similar.

Healing of Esophagitis

The endoscopic healing rates in patients receiving omeprazole were markedly superior to those given ranitidine (Fig. 1). This difference was statistically highly significant at all time periods studied. After 12 weeks of treatment, 90% of those allocated to omeprazole were healed as compared to only 47% among those given ranitidine ($p<0.0001$). On analyzing the endoscopic healing of esophagitis as related to pre-entry endoscopic grading, 29 of 30 patients with grade 2 esophagitis randomized to omeprazole were healed as compared

Table I
Pre-Entry Characteristics of Patients in Study Groups

Characteristics	Omeprazole n = 51	Ranitidine n = 47
Male/Female	36/15	36/11
Age (mean ± SE) years	58.1 ± 16.2	59.8 ± 16.0
Smokers	11	9
Alcohol consumers	31	24
Duration of esophagitis		
<1.0 year	3	2
1.0–5.0 years	25	15
>5.0 years	23	30
Esophagitis grade		
Grade 2	30	27
Grade 3	17	17
Grade 4	4	3
Barrett's esophagus	8	6
Stricture	3	1

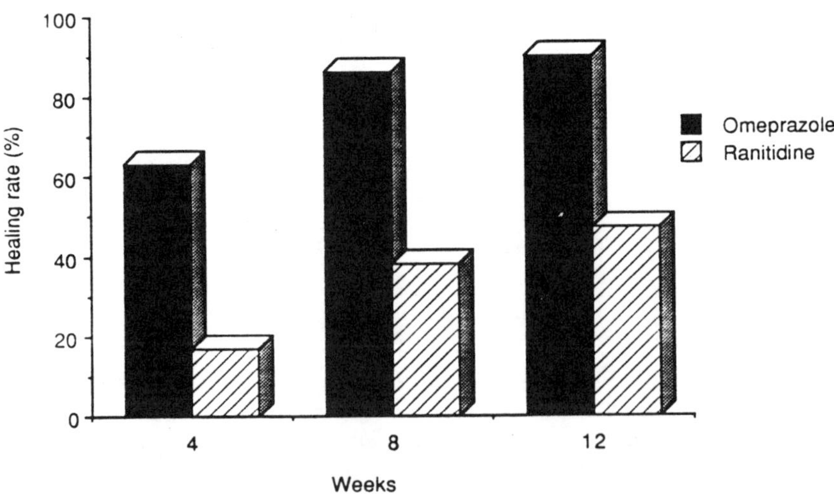

Figure 1: Endoscopic healing of esophagitis. Intention to treat analysis.

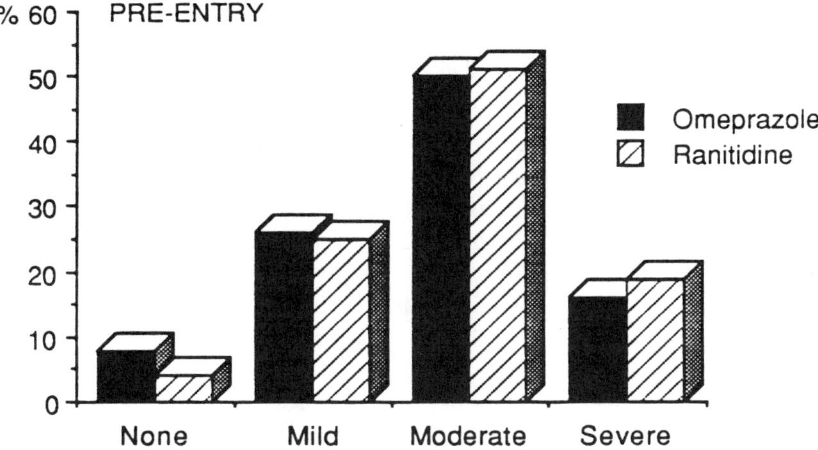

Figure 2: The frequency of heartburn at the pre-entry evaluation and during the study period.

to only 16 of 27 given ranitidine. The corresponding healing figures for 34 patients with pre-entry grade 3 was 14 of 17 of those given omeprazole and 5 of 17 of those randomized to ranitidine.

Reflux Symptoms

Patients allocated to treatment with omeprazole experienced more rapid and profound symptom relief (Fig. 2). After 4 weeks of treatment with omeprazole, 86% were completely free from heartburn compared to only 32% among those given ranitidine (p<0.0001). This large difference in symptom relief remained through the study period.

Safety Assessment

Minor adverse events were recorded in similar frequency in the two groups as well as minor deviations from the reference values in the laboratory screening. There were no clinically and/or statistically significant changes either within each treatment group or between the two groups.

Discussion

Although insufficient for some patients with erosive and/or ulcerative esophagitis, pharmacological acid inhibition induced by histamine H_2-receptor antagonists has been the cornerstone in the medical treatment of this disease.[1] One reasonable explanation for the low endoscopic healing rates may be the predominant influence of 24-hour intragastric acidity in the pathogenesis of reflux disease. Ranitidine (300 mg/day) and cimetidine (1 g/day) increase the median pH of gastric juice from 1.4 to 1.7 and 2.4, respectively.[10] Omeprazole, on the other hand, is known to cause a more sustained and prolonged acid inhibition, although not complete.[11] Twenty-four-hour pH monitoring in the distal esophagus of patients before and during treatment with H_2-receptor antagonists has shown a marginal and/or at best a significant effect on the acid exposure of the esophageal mucosa.[12,13] Corresponding observations during omeprazole treatment have revealed a more profound reduction in the acid reflux to the esophagus.[14]

The optimal dose of an H_2-blocker in patients with reflux esophagitis has to be determined. Increasing the ranitidine dose to 300 mg b.i.d. does not seem to improve the efficacy in the average patient.[13,15] Our results, on the other hand, would suggest that clinical benefit can be achieved by increasing the dose of ranitidine as well as by prolonging the duration of treatment. Still a profound difference in clinical effect was observed among patients allocated to omeprazole treatment and those given 600 mg of ranitidine per day. In conclusion, in patients with reflux esophagitis resistant to medical treatment with standard doses of H_2-receptor antagonist, 40 mg of omeprazole daily is highly effective, obtaining an endoscopic healing rate of 90% with a corresponding effect on symptom relief and being far more effective than a high dose of ranitidine. This goal was achieved without any adverse events or abnormal findings in the laboratory screen.

Repeated observations have indicated a high recurrence rate following cessation of medical treatment of reflux esophagitis either with H_2-blockers or with omeprazole.[7,8,15] These observations highlight the importance of evaluating the effectiveness of any medical regimen as maintenance therapy for patients with reflux esophagitis, particularly in those not suitable for surgical treatment. The design and safety of such a long-term therapy with omeprazole is currently being evaluated.

References

1. Koelz HR: Treatment of reflux esophagitis with H_2-blockers, antacids and prokinetic drugs: An analysis of randomized clinical trials. Scand J Gastroenterol 24(suppl)156:25–36, 1989.
2. Tytgat GNJ, Nio CU: The medical therapy of reflux esophagitis. Clin Gastroenterol 1:791–807, 1987.
3. Wallmark B, Lorentzon B, Larsson H: The mechanism of action of omeprazole: A survey of its inhibitor action in vitro. Scand J Gastroenterol (suppl)108:37–51, 1985.
4. Klinkenberg-Knol EC, Jansen JMBJ, Festen HBM, Meuwissen SGM, Lamers CBHW: Double-blind multicentre comparison of omeprazole and ranitidine in the treatment of reflux esophagitis. Lancet I:349–351, 1987.
5. Havelund T, Laursen LS, Skoupo-Kristensen E, Andersen BN, Pedersen SA, Jensen KB, Fenger C, Hamberg-Sörensen F, Lauritsen K: Omeprazole and ranitidine in the treatment of reflux esophagitis: Double-blind comparative trial. Br Med J 296:89–92, 1988.
6. Vantrappen G, Rutgeerts L, Schurmans B, Coengrachts JL: Omeprazole (40 mg) is superior to ranitidine in short-term treatment of ulcerative reflux esophagitis. Dig Dis Sci 33:523–529, 1988.
7. Sandmark S, Carlsson R, Fausa O, Lundell L: Omeprazole or ranitidine in the treatment of reflux esophagitis: Results of a double-blind, randomized, Scandinavian multicentre study. Scand J Gastroenterol 23:625–632, 1988.
8. Hetzel EJ, Dent J, Reed WD, Narieldala FM, MacKinnon M, McCarthy JH, Michell B, Beveridge BR, Laurence BH, Gibson GG, Grant AK, Schearman DJC, Whitehead R, Buckel BJ: Healing and relapse of severe peptic esophagitis after treatment with omeprazole. Gastroenterology 95:903–912, 1988.
9. Skinner DB, Walther BC, Ridell RH, Schmidt H, Iascone C, DeMeester TR: Barrett's esophagus: Comparison of benign and malignant cases. Ann Surg 198:554–566, 1983.
10. Walt RB, Gomes MFA, Wood C, Logan LH, Pounder RE: Effect of daily oral omeprazole on 24-hour intragastric acidity. Br Med J 287:12–14, 1983.
11. Lind T, Cederberg C, Ekenved G, Haglund U, Olbe L: Effect of omeprazole: A gastric proton pump inhibitor on pentagastrin-stimulated acid secretion in man. Gut 24:270–276, 1983.
12. Johansson KE, Tibbling L: Maintenance treatment with ranitidine compared with fundoplication in gastroesophageal reflux disease. Scand J Gastroenterol 21:779–788, 1986.
13. Schaub N, Meyrick TJ, Misiewicz J, Lovell D, Troutman IF: Investigation of ranitidine 150 mg b.i.d. or 300 mg b.i.d. in the treatment of reflux disease. Hepatogastroenterology 33:206–213, 1986.
14. Ruth M, Ehnbom H, Lundell L, Lönroth H, Sandberg N, Sandmark S: The effect of omeprazole or ranitidine treatment on 24-hour esophageal acidity in patients with reflux esophagitis. Scand J Gastroenterol 23:1141–1146, 1988.

15. Koelz HR, Birchler R, Bretholz A, Brun B, Capitaine J, Gonvers JJ, Halter F, Hammer B, Kauasseh L, Kobler E, Miller G, Münst G, Belloni S, Reallini S, Schmid B, Voirol M, Blum AL: Heaing and relapse of reflux esophagitis during treatment with ranitidine. Gastroenterology 91:1198–1205, 1986.

16

A Double-Blind Comparative Study of Omeprazole Versus Cimetidine in Erosive Reflux Esophagitis

Thomas C. B. Dehn, H. A. Shepherd,
D. Colin-Jones, M. G. W. Kettlewell,
N. J. H. Carroll

Introduction

The treatment of reflux esophagitis by histamine H_2-receptor antagonists is unsatisfactory since many patients remain symptomatic and unhealed endoscopically despite 6–8 weeks of treatment.[1-3] Omeprazole has been shown to be more effective than ranitidine[4-6] and placebo[7] both in the short-term treatment of reflux esophagitis and in treatment of esophagitis resistant to long-term high-dose cimetidine therapy.[8] No study has compared the efficacy and rates of healing of esophagitis in patients receiving omeprazole and the recommended dose of cimetidine.

Patients and Methods

Out-patients, aged between 18 and 80 years, with symptomatic, gastroesophageal reflux, confirmed both endoscopically and histo-

Little AG, Ferguson MK, Skinner DB: Diseases of the Esophagus, Vol. II: Benign Diseases. Futura Publishing Company, Inc., Mount Kisco, NY, © 1990.

logically, were randomized to receive 8 weeks of continuous treatment with omeprazole 40 mg once daily or cimetidine 400 mg four times daily using a double-blind, double-dummy technique.

Study Protocol

Esophagitis was graded endoscopically as grade I (erythema), grade II (isolated round and linear erosions incompletely involving the lower 2 cm of esophagus), grade III (erosions above 2 cm or involving the entire circumference), grade IV (benign ulcer), and grade V (stricture). Esophageal biopsies were also graded: grade I (basal cell hyperplasia without inflammatory infiltration), grade II (I plus extension of papillae and mild inflammatory infiltration), grade III (massive polymorphonuclear infiltration), and grade IV (III plus ulceration). Patients were included in the study when both endoscopic esophagitis was grade I or worse and pre-entry esophageal biopsies were histologically grade I or worse, and when none of the exclusion criteria were met. Patients were seen pre-entry and at 2-week intervals thereafter and symptoms of heartburn, regurgitation, and dysphagia were graded. Diary cards (to record reflux symptoms and daily antacid consumption) and the trial medication remaining were collected. New cards and drugs were then issued. Endoscopy was undertaken before entry, after 4 weeks of treatment and was repeated at 8 weeks if healing (defined as complete re-epithelialization) was incomplete or histologic grades ≥ 2 were reported. Quadrantal biopsies were obtained from inflamed epithelium and a reference biopsy taken 5 cm proximal to the upper margin of the inflamed epithelium.

Outpatient 24-hour esophageal pH metry was undertaken before entry and during the fifth week of treatment (Oxford Medilog 1000) recorder and radiotelemetry capsule (RTC) (Remote Control Systems, London). Ethical approval was obtained from the participating hospitals and verbal informed consent from each patient.

The statistical analyses were performed on a per protocol basis, and parametric (Student's t-test) and nonparametric (Mantel Haensel, Chi-square, Mann Whitney U-test, Wilcoxon test) methods used as appropriate.

Results

Between November 1985 and September 1987, 67 patients were studied. Table I illustrates the pre-entry characteristics of these pa-

Table I
Patient Demographics

	Omeprazole (n = 31)	Cimetidine (n = 36)
Sex M:F	21:10	23:8
Age, years: mean (range)	54 (21–74)	39.6 (24–78)
Duration of reflux symptoms (months)	24 (2–600)	36 (1–600)
Smokers	29	36
Alcohol drinkers	31	34
Previous gastrointestinal hemorrhage/ esophageal stricture	3	6
Previous antireflux/antacid therapy	13	23
Pre-entry endoscopy		
Grade 1 esophagitis	2	5
2 esophagitis	10	8
3 esophagitis	16	21
4 esophagitis	3	2
Pre-entry symptoms		
Heartburn	89%	97%
Regurgitation	75%	74%
Dysphagia	46%	35%

tients. Two patients (1 omeprazole, 1 cimetidine) were withdrawn for protocol violations, one patient (cimetidine) for lack of compliance, and three patients (1 omeprazole, 2 cimetidine) for adverse events. Thus the per protocol analysis at 4 weeks included 28 patients on omeprazole and 31 patients on cimetidine.

Table II illustrates the severity score for heartburn. After 2 weeks' treatment, heartburn was absent in 21/28 (75%) omeprazole compared to 13/31 (42%) cimetidine patients (p = 0.0064). After 4 weeks, heartburn was absent in 26/28 (93%) and 17/31 (55%; p = 0.0011) of patients, respectively, and remained substantially unchanged at the 8-week assessment. There was no significant difference between treatments in the relief of symptoms of either regurgitation or dysphagia. Table II also illustrates the pre-entry occurrence of symptomatic regurgitation and dysphagia. At 4 weeks regurgitation was present in 3/28 (11%) omeprazole and 9/31 (29%) cimetidine patients (p = 0.09); dysphagia was present in 4/28 (14%) and 6/31 (19%; p = 0.6).

Between days 0–15, the median number ($\pm \frac{1}{2}$ interquartile range) of diary card reports of daytime reflux symptoms were 0.21 ± 0.14 (omeprazole) and 0.38 ± 0.37 (cimetidine; p = NS). After 4 weeks there

Table II
Effect of Omeprazole and Cimetidine Treatment on Symptoms of Heartburn, Regurgitation, and Dysphagia

	Number of Patients (%)					
	Heartburn		*Regurgitation*		*Dysphagia*	
	Om	*Cim*	*Om*	*Cim*	*Om*	*Cim*
Entry						
None	3 (11%)	1 (3%)	7 (25%)	8 (26%)	15 (54%)	20 (65%)
Mild	7	13	11	14	4	7
Moderate	9	9	9	7	4	2
Severe	9	8	1	2	6	2
	NS		NS		NS	
Week 2						
None	21 (75%)	13 (42%)	24 (86%)	21 (68%)	24 (86%)	29 (94%)
Mild	7	14	4	7	0	0
Moderate	0	4	0	3	0	0
Severe	0	0	0	0	0	0
	$p = 0.0064$		NS		NS	
Week 4						
None	26 (93%)	17 (55%)	25 (89%)	22 (71%)	24 (86%)	25 (81%)
Mild	2	11	3	8	4	5
Moderate	0	3	0	1	0	1
Severe	0	0	0	0	0	0
	$p = 0.011$		NS		NS	
Week 6						
None	24 (96%)	19 (63%)	22 (88%)	21 (70%)	24 (96%)	28 (93%)
Mild	0	8	3	8	1	2
Moderate	1	3	0	1	0	0
Severe	0	0	0	0	0	0
	$p = 0.0054$		NS		NS	
Week 8						
None	23 (92%)	17 (59%)	23 (92%)	27 (93%)	24 (96%)	27 (93%)
Mild	2	11	2	1	1	2
Moderate	0	1	0	1	0	0
Severe	0	0	0	0	0	0
	$p = 0.0056$		NS		NS	

Om = Omeprazole; Cim = Cimetidine.

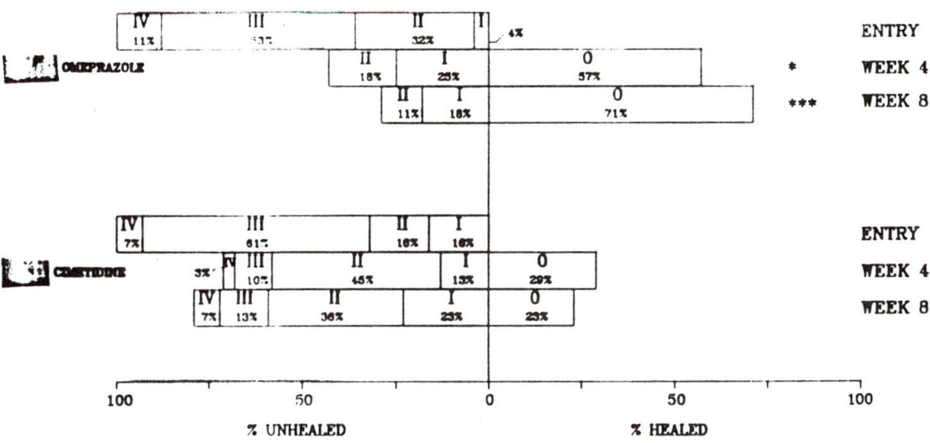

Figure 1: Cumulative endoscopic grading scores at entry and after 4 and 8 weeks' treatment with omeprazole or cimetidine. The percentage of patients for each grade (Roman numerals) is shown. Significance between treatments at 4 and 8 weeks is indicated; *p=0.029, ***p<0.001. (Reproduced by permission of the Editor of *Gut*.)

was a significant reduction between treatment groups in the record of daytime reflux symptoms to 0.0 ± 0.12 (omeprazole) and 0.32 ± 0.27 (cimetidine) (p=0.004). Nocturnal symptoms were also significantly reduced in omeprazole patients but not in the cimetidine group. These differences were mirrored in the reduction of daily antacid tablet consumption.

Figure 1 illustrates the endoscopic grading of esophagitis. After 4 weeks, healing had occurred in 16/28 (57%) omeprazole and 9/31 (29%) cimetidine patients (p=0.029). After 8 weeks, cumulative healing rates were 20/28 (71%) and 7/31 (23%; p=0.0001). Over the 8-week treatment period, endoscopic appearances remained unchanged in two patients on omeprazole and in five on cimetidine. The endoscopic grade worsened during treatment in five patients receiving cimetidine.

Before treatment, there was no difference in the results of the median (range) worst histologic scores taken from esophageal biopsies; 4 (1–4) in both treatment groups (p=NS). At 4 weeks the median worst scores were 1 (0–4) omeprazole vs. 3 (0–4) cimetidine (p=0.0028). At the final endoscopy, the median worst scores were 1 (0–4) omeprazole vs. 2 (0–4) cimetidine (p=NS).

Eighteen patients (9 omeprazole, 9 cimetidine) completed 24-

Table III
Effect of Omeprazole and Cimetidine Treatment on Percentage Esophageal Acid Exposure to pH<4

Total Acid Exposure %—All Patients

| | *Daytime* | | *Night-time* | | *Overall* | | |
	Day 0	*Day 29*	*Day 0*	*Day 29*	*Day 0*	*Day 29*	*N*
Cimetidine							
Mean	10.48	10.50	7.66	11.56	9.51	10.78	9
Range	(3.25–21.98)	(2.97–34.00)	(0–30.94)	(0–40.23)	(1.91–21.19)	(2.38–36.42)	
Omeprazole							
Mean	11.25	0.74**	11.31	7.50	11.43	3.37**	9
Range	(2.07–36.10)	(0–5.89)	(0–40.56)	(0–55.07)	(1.83–37.86)	(0–23.10)	

Total Acid Exposure %—Healed Patients

| | *Daytime* | | *Night-time* | | *Overall* | | |
	Day 0	*Day 29*	*Day 0*	*Day 29*	*Day 0*	*Day 29*	*N*
Cimetidine							
Mean	8.74	5.28	7.00	7.44	8.11	5.95	5
Range	(3.25–12.52)	(2.97–7.29)	(0–30.94)	(0–32.00)	(1.91–19.94)	(2.38–16.37)	
Omeprazole							
Mean	6.53	0.08*	7.25	0.00	6.99	0.05*	6
Range	(2.07–11.23)	(0–0.25)	(0–16.08)	(0–0.02)	(1.83–11.23)	(0–0.14)	

Total Acid Exposure %—Unhealed Patients

| | *Daytime* | | *Night-time* | | *Overall* | | |
	Day 0	*Day 29*	*Day 0*	*Day 29*	*Day 0*	*Day 29*	*N*
Cimetidine							
Mean	12.66	17.02	8.48	16.70	11.27	16.81	4
Range	(4.35–21.98)	(8.26–34.00)	(2.29–19.93)	(1.64–40.23)	(3.98–21.19)	(7.82–36.42)	
Omeprazole							
Mean	20.70	2.07	19.42	21.28	20.30	10.01	3
Range	(5.85–36.10)	(0.04–5.89)	(5.15–40.56)	(2.95–55.07)	(8.35–37.86)	(1.07–23.10)	

Values are mean and range * p < 0.05, ** p < 0.001.

hour pH metry both pre-entry and after 4 weeks' treatment. There were no significant differences in the recorded pH parameters at the pre-entry tests. Daytime esophageal acid exposure was significantly less at 4 weeks in the omeprazole-treated patients (Table III, Fig. 2).

Both day and night-time esophageal acid exposure was abolished in the six patients on omeprazole in whom endoscopic esophagitis

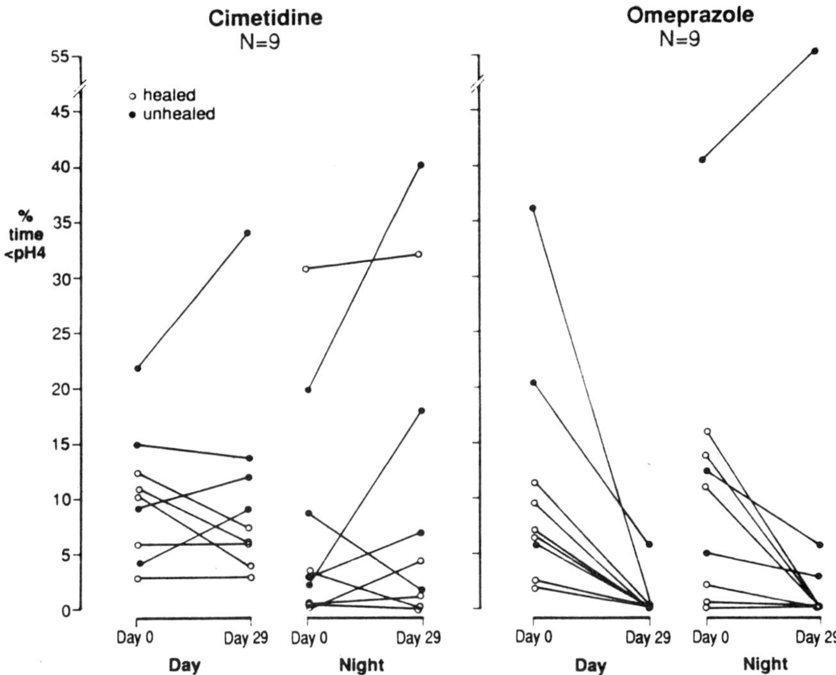

Figure 2: Results of 24-hour pH metry before and after 4 weeks' treatment with cimetidine (N = 9) or omeprazole (N = 9). Patients with endoscopic healing at 4 weeks are represented by open circles and those with persistent endoscopic esophagitis are represented by filled circles. Percentage time below pH4, vertical axis. Night time = time between retiring to bed and arising in the morning. (Reproduced by permission of the Editor of *Gut*.)

had healed. In those five patients with endoscopic healing after 4 weeks' cimetidine treatment, a daytime acid (pH<4) exposure in excess of 5% was recorded in three and night-time exposure in excess of 2% persisted in two patients.

In the three endoscopically unhealed patients receiving omeprazole, mean daytime esophageal acid exposure fell from 20.7 to 2.1%, but remained >5% in only one patient. Mean night-time acid exposure did not change (19.4% vs. 21.3%), remaining above 2% in all three patients and being reduced in only one patient. In the four endoscopically unhealed patients receiving cimetidine, daytime esophageal acid exposure increased in three patients and night-time exposure increased in three of the four patients.

Discussion

Patients were well matched in all aspects of their esophageal reflux disease. Only 7/67 (10%) patients had endoscopic grade I esophagitis; the remaining 90% had erosive or ulcerative esophagitis.

Our results, in agreement with others,[2-6] demonstrate that heartburn is relieved more rapidly and more effectively with omeprazole than with H_2-blocker therapy. Moreover, in our study 41% of cimetidine patients had no relief of this symptom throughout the study period.

Endoscopic healing rates of esophagitis in patients treated with omeprazole for 4 weeks have been reported to vary between 76% and 85%,[4-6] although two reports[4,6] included the presence of endoscopic erythema as evidence of healing, and Van Trappen[6] defined healing as the disappearance of esophageal ulceration. The latter definitions and the higher dose of omeprazole (60 mg) used by Klinkenberg-Knol[3] would explain the reported differences in endoscopic healing rates. Further advantages of omeprazole therapy are that, during the study, no patient receiving omeprazole had worsening endoscopic grading of esophagitis and, moreover, the endoscopic grading remained unchanged in only two patients. Of the 31 patients receiving cimetidine, endoscopic grading worsened in five and remained unchanged in five.

Histologic grading of esophagitis is improved to a greater extent with omeprazole therapy by comparison to ranitidine.[5,9] Our study has also demonstrated that after 8 weeks of therapy, histologic gradings are similar in the two groups. This implies that both drugs produce histologic healing of esophagitis, but omeprazole, at 40 mg daily, achieves healing more rapidly.

A major factor in the cause of reflux esophagitis is inappropriate exposure of the distal esophagus to gastric acid.[10] Esophageal pH metry provides a useful indicator of the degree and pattern,[11] although caution must be used in interpreting the results because of variation within individuals.[12] Our results demonstrate that omeprazole is far more effective in increasing the pH of gastroesophageal refluxate by comparison to cimetidine. Moreover, omeprazole treatment completely abolished acid reflux in six of the nine patients receiving that drug who underwent pH recordings.

In those patients in whom endoscopic healing was recorded, omeprazole reduced esophageal acid exposure to a much greater degree than cimetidine (Table III, Fig. 2). Nocturnal acid reflux, because of its prolonged contact with and poor clearance[13] from the distal esophagus, is believed to be extremely injurious to the esophageal epithelium.[8,14] This view is supported by the fact that in three of the four patients receiving cimetidine, and without endoscopic healing, nocturnal acid exposure increased substantially. In only one of three patients receiving omeprazole, and in whom endoscopic healing had not occurred, did nocturnal esophageal acid exposure fall. Thus, omeprazole does not entirely abolish nocturnal esophageal acid exposure in all patients, even when a higher dose (60 mg) is administered.[4]

This study has demonstrated the superiority of omeprazole 40 mg once daily over cimetidine, 400 mg four times a day, in the treatment of erosive reflux esophagitis. In those few patients who prove refractory to healing, use of esophageal pH profiles may indicate a requirement for the short-term administration of a higher dosage of omeprazole[4] for more prolonged therapy at a lower dose[15] or for antireflux surgery.

ACKNOWLEDGMENTS: We are most grateful to the following for their help in this project: Dr. C. Mason (Oxford), Dr. A. Vincenti (Winchester), and Dr. J. Burston (Portsmouth) for undertaking the historic studies; Dr. Veronica Sprott and Dr. J. Snook (Portsmouth) for help with the clinical studies and Mrs. Julie Marks (Oxford) for assistance with pH monitoring and endoscopy. We acknowledge the Editor of Gut *for allowing us to reproduce material published in that journal, and the Oxford District Health Authority for financial support.*

References

1. Wesdorp E, Bartlesman J, Pape K, Dekker W, Tytgat GN: Oral cimetidine in reflux oesophagitis: A double-blind controlled trial. Gastroenterology 74:821, 1978.
2. Wesdorp ICE, Dekker W, Klinkenberg-Knol EC: Treatment of reflux esophagitis with ranitidine. Gut 24:921, 1983.
3. Klinkenberg-Knol EC, Jansen JMBJ, Festen HPM, et al: Double-blind multicentre comparison of omeprazole and ranitidine in the treatment of reflux oesphagitis. Lancet 1:349, 1987.
4. Keolz HR, Birchler R, Bretholz, et al: Healing and relapse of reflux esophagitis during treatment with ranitidine. Gastroenterology 91:1198, 1986.
5. Havelund T, Laursen LS, Skoubo-Kristensen E, et al: Omeprazole and ranitidine in the treatment of reflux oesophagitis: Double-blind comparative trial. Br Med J 296:89, 1988.
6. Van Trappen G, Rutgeerts L, Schurmans P, et al: Omeprazole (40 mg) is superior to ranitidine in short-term treatment of ulcerative reflux esophagitis. Dig Dis Sci 33:523, 1988.
7. Dent J, Hetzel DJ, Reed W, Narielvala FM, Mitchell BL, McCarthy JH:

Healing of peptic esophagitis with omeprazole. Gastroenterology 1392:90, 1986.

8. Bardhan KD, Morris P, Thompson M, et al: Omeprazole in the treatment of erosive esophagitis refractory to high-dose cimetidine. Gastroenterology 92:1306, 1987.

9. Whitehead R, Hetzel DJ, Dent J, Reed W, Narielvala FM, Mackinnon M: Histological healing of peptic esophagitis with omeprazole. Gastroenterology 92:1693, 1987.

10. Richter JE, Castell DO: Gastroesophageal reflux: Pathogenesis, diagnosis and therapy. Ann Intern Med 97:93, 1982.

11. Demeester TR, Johnson LF, Joseph C-J, Toscano MS, Hall AW, Skinner DB: Patterns of gastroesophageal reflux in health and disease. Ann Surg 4:459, 1976.

12. Walker SJ, Holt S, Hartley MN, Sanderson CJ, Stoddard C: The reproducibility of ambulatory pH monitoring. Br J Surg 75:1240, 1988.

13. Orr WC, Johnson LF, Robinson MG: Effect of sleep on swallowing, esophageal peristalsis and acid clearance. Gastroenterology 86:814, 1984.

14. Johnson LF, Demeester TR, Haggitt RC: Esophageal epithelial response to gastroesophageal reflux: A quantitative study. Dig Dis Sci 23:498, 1978.

15. Klinkenberg-Knol EC, Festen HPM, Meuwissen SGM: Omeprazole compared to ranitidine in effect on 24-hour pH in the distal esophagus of patients with reflux esophagitis: A double-blind trial. Gastroenterology 92:1471, 1987.

16. Dent J, Klinkenberg-Knol E, Elm G, Eriksson K, Rikner L, Solvell L: Omeprazole in the long-term management of patients with reflux esophagitis refractory to histamine H_2-receptor antagonists. Gastroenterology 1(Suppl 1):A847, 1988.

17

Treatment of Gastroesophageal Reflux Disease:
An Effective Twice-Daily Cimetidine Regimen for Heartburn Relief

William O. Frank, Jeffery D. Wetherington,
Robert H. Palmer, Michael D. Young

Introduction

Gastroesophageal reflux disease (GERD) is an ill-defined disorder associated with the reflux of gastric contents into the esophagus. It may be manifested by symptoms, typically heartburn and/or esophagitis. This multicenter, randomized, double-blind, placebo-controlled trial was conducted to evaluate the efficacy of cimetidine 800 mg b.i.d. in relieving symptoms associated with GERD.

Methods

Study Design

Each investigator obtained Institutional Review Board approval prior to initiating the study, and informed consent was signed by

Little AG, Ferguson MK, Skinner DB: Diseases of the Esophagus, Vol. II: Benign Diseases. Futura Publishing Company, Inc., Mount Kisco, NY, © 1990.

each patient prior to enrollment. Subjects were adults, 18 years of age or older, who had a history of heartburn, defined as a burning, retrosternal pain made worse by position or eating. Patients were excluded for a history of gastric or esophageal surgery other than oversewing of a gastric ulcer, significant underlying disease, or therapy which would interfere with evaluation of treatment, hypersensitivity or adverse reaction to cimetidine or ranitidine, a history of substance abuse, investigational drug use within 1 month prior to entry, or pregnancy or lactation.

The study began with a 1-week screening phase during which they recorded the frequency and severity of daytime and nighttime heartburn in order to establish a minimum baseline of symptoms. Antacid use was prohibited during the screening phase. Patients who recorded at least eight heartburn episodes during the screening phase and had heartburn on the day before the clinic visit or who had continuous heartburn for 24 hours underwent esophageal pH monitoring[1] to verify acid reflux.

Patients who had postprandial gastroesophageal acid reflux (esophageal pH<4 lasting ≥10 seconds) for 5% or more of the 3-hour monitoring period then had an endoscopy. Both of these evaluations were performed within a 3-day period. After endoscopy, patients with nonerosive GERD (normal endoscopic appearance of the esophagus or only friability or erythema) were randomized to 6 weeks of treatment with coded medication. Patients with erosive GERD (ulcers and/or erosions) were eligible to participate in a second similar study of more prolonged treatment (12 weeks). Patients were excluded from both studies if endoscopy revealed concurrent gastric or duodenal ulcers, overt gastrointestinal bleeding, scleroderma, or overlying candidiasis and/or herpetiform lesions.

Patients were randomized to receive cimetidine 800 mg b.i.d. (n = 140) or placebo (n = 145) for a 6-week treatment period. Antacid consumption was monitored and restricted to eight tablets of Maalox #2 per day. Patients recorded assessments of daytime and nighttime heartburn severity on diary cards twice daily during treatment. Endoscopy was repeated at week 6 or whenever the patient was discontinued from the study.

Efficacy Assessments

Efficacy analyses were performed using an intent-to-treat approach. Patients without on-therapy data for a specific analysis were excluded from that analysis. Patients without daytime or nighttime heartburn on entry into the trial (i.e., on the last observation during the screening phase) were excluded from an evaluation of the effectiveness of the coded medication in the relief of such symptoms.

The first 24 hours with complete freedom from heartburn was defined as consecutive daytime and nighttime heartburn assessments of "none" on the patient diary card. Life-table methods based on the product limit estimator and the log rank test were used to compare median values of the time to the first 24 hours completely free of heartburn for each treatment group.

Relief was defined as a decrease in heartburn severity of at least one grade. Patients with diary card assessments for each of the first 7 days of treatment were used to determine the proportion of patients with relief or complete freedom from heartburn for each of the first 7 days of treatment, and these proportions were then averaged over the first 7 days. Separate analyses were completed for daytime and for nighttime heartburn. The differences between groups were evaluated using a weighted least-squares approach to the analysis of categorical data.[2,3]

The proportions of patients in each group with relief or complete freedom from heartburn at the end of treatment were compared using two-way contingency tables and chi-square statistics.

The proportion of study days with complete freedom from heartburn was calculated for each patient as the ratio of the number of study days with complete freedom from heartburn over the number of study days with assessments.

Results

Most of the 285 randomized patients were white and ranged in age from 18 to 89 years. Randomization of patients resulted in treatment groups which were comparable at baseline for demographic characteristics and disease severity. Seventeen placebo and 18 cimetidine patients withdrew prior to completing the study.

Cimetidine was statistically superior to placebo in alleviating daytime heartburn as measured by each of the parameters shown in Table I. This response was not affected by gender, smoking status, baseline heartburn severity, age, or prior use of antacids.

Fewer patients in both groups reported nighttime heartburn, and differences between the groups were not significant. The average

Table I
Symptomatic Response in Nonerosive GERD

Parameter	Placebo	Cimetidine 800 mg b.i.d.
Median time to achieve 24 hours with complete freedom from heartburn (days)	15	6**
During days 1–7, mean proportion of patients (%) with:		
• Relief of heartburn	44	54*
• Complete freedom from heartburn	16	26**
At week 6 or end-point, proportion of patients (%) with:		
• Relief of heartburn	61	72*
• Complete freedom from heartburn	33	47**
Mean proportion of days with complete freedom from heartburn for days 1–42 (%)	26	36**

* $p < 0.05$; ** $p \leq 0.01$.

number of antacid tablets consumed each week was small in both groups and was significantly smaller in the cimetidine group (1.9 ± 1.9; mean ±SD) than in the placebo group (3.0 ± 5.2) during week 1 ($p<0.02$).

The proportion of patients developing erosions or ulcers during treatment was twice as great in the placebo group (13/128, 10%) as in the cimetidine group (6/121, 5%). While the number of patients was too small for the difference to be statistically significant, the data suggest that cimetidine may be effective in preventing the development of lesions in patients with symptomatic GERD.

Three placebo and two cimetidine patients were discontinued for possible adverse drug experiences. *Placebo:* petechia and rash; impotence; and palpitation. *Cimetidine 800 mg b.i.d.:* diarrhea, nausea and vomiting, fever, nausea, and urinary tract infection. The overall type and incidence of adverse experiences were similar among groups and are consistent with the known safety profile of cimetidine.

Discussion

In this study, cimetidine 800 mg b.i.d. was shown to be effective in relieving heartburn associated with GERD. All patients had clinically important heartburn documented during the screening phase, and all had reflux demonstrated by esophageal pH monitoring. The cimetidine group used significantly fewer antacid tablets, in keeping with the demonstrated efficacy.

Cimetidine was superior to placebo in all of the efficacy parameters measured. The time to the first 24 hours without heartburn and the average proportion of days during the first week with either relief or complete absence of heartburn are early measures of efficacy, while the proportion of patients with relief at end-point and the overall proportion of days during the study with relief are measures of prolonged efficacy. With cimetidine, 50% of patients had achieved 24 hours of complete relief by 6 days, and by 6 weeks, 72% had relief of heartburn; this was complete in approximately two-thirds of those patients.

The patients in this study had reflux characterized by heartburn without lesions in the esophagus. However, symptoms do not reliably distinguish patients with lesions from those without lesions, and it would be desirable to be able to treat patients with heartburn without requiring esophagoscopy to ascertain the status of the esophageal mucosa. Therefore, it is important to know whether patients with esophageal ulcers or erosions have a similar symptomatic response. In a companion study, patients with symptoms who had esophageal

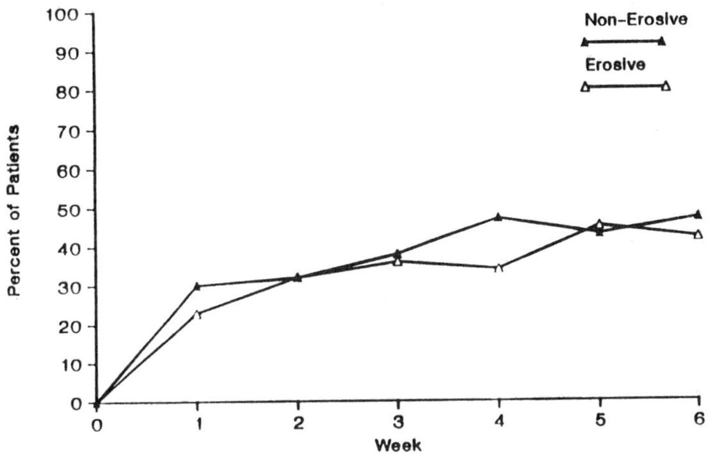

Figure 1: See text, page 162, for description.

ulcers and/or erosions were treated with a similar protocol, and the symptomatic response was almost identical. Figure 1 shows the proportion of patients treated with cimetidine 1600 mg/day who were completely without daytime pain each week for 6 weeks and compares the response of patients without lesions (from the present study, solid triangles) with that of patients with ulcers and/or erosions (from the companion study, open triangles). It is clear that the symptomatic response is similar in the two groups.

Conclusion

This study has demonstrated that cimetidine 800 mg b.i.d. provides rapid and sustained symptomatic relief in patients with heartburn secondary to GERD. Relief is comparable regardless of baseline demographic characteristics, including the presence or absence of erosive esophagitis.

References

1. Fink SM, McCallum RW: The role of prolonged esophageal pH monitoring in the diagnosis of gastroesophageal reflux. JAMA 252:1160, 1984.
2. Koch GG, Landis JR, Freeman JL, et al: A general methodology for the analysis of experiments with repeated measurement of categorical data. Biometrics 33:133, 1977.
3. Grizzle JE, Starmer CF, Koch GG: Analysis of categorical data by linear models. Biometrics 25:489, 1969.

18

Can Failure of Medical Treatment Be Predicted in Gastroesophageal Reflux Disease?

Antony P. Barlow, Lloyd R. Jenkinson, Christopher S. Ball, Tracey L. Norris, Anthony Watson

Gastroesophageal reflux is now the most frequently diagnosed upper gastrointestinal disorder. Its importance is reflected by a recent study which reported a 6-month prevalence of dyspepsia within the community of 38%, with over two-thirds of these patients complaining of heartburn.[1] Improved diagnosis of reflux esophagitis has been accompanied by advances in medical treatment, particularly since the introduction of H_2-receptor antagonists in the 1970s. Most clinical trials have demonstrated significant symptomatic benefit from the short-term use of either cimetidine or ranitidine, but unfortunately their success in healing erosive esophagitis has been less favorable. After 6–12 weeks of treatment with an H_2-receptor antagonist, healing of esophagitis can be expected in 33%–57% of patients,[2-7] although approximately 50% of studies report no significant benefit over placebo.[8,9] Furthermore, relapse after cessation of medical therapy is common and does not seem to be prevented by the use of long-term maintenance therapy.[6]

Little AG, Ferguson MK, Skinner DB: Diseases of the Esophagus, Vol. II: Benign Diseases. Futura Publishing Company, Inc., Mount Kisco, NY, © 1990.

Table I
Patient Characteristics in Phase I and Phase II

	Phase I (R 150 mg b.i.d.)		Phase II (R 300 mg b.i.d.)	
Male:Female	13:19		11:7	
Age (years)	60	(35–74)	67	(37–77)
Smokers	7	(22%)	2	(11%)
Esophagitis:				
Grade I	18		7	
Grade II	9		6	
Grade III	5		5	
Acid Exposure:				
% Total Time pH<4	10.5	(5–51)	9.1	(5–39)
LES Competence:				
Pressure (mmHg)	7.5	(2–13)	6.0	(2–14)
Abdominal length (cm)	1.0	(0–2)	1.5	(0–3)
Overall length (cm)	3.3	(2–5)	4.0	(2–6)
Amplitude Esophageal Body:				
7 cm above LES (mmHg)	38	(20–100)	38	(20–83)
2 cm above LES (mmHg)	53	(16–100)	44	(12–80)

Values expressed as medians with 10th and 90th percentiles. R = ranitidine; LES = lower esophageal sphincter.

Despite these observations, many patients are treated for prolonged periods with H_2 blockers and somewhat arbitrary criteria are used in considering referral for antireflux surgery. As there may be merit in identifying at an early stage those patients who are likely to fail on medical therapy, this study was designed to identify those physiological parameters that might predict likely failure of medical therapy and to evaluate the success of surgery in those who ultimately require an antireflux repair.

Patients and Methods

Fifty patients with symptomatic gastroesophageal reflux of at least 3 months' duration and with endoscopic evidence of esophagitis (grades I–III) entered the study. Those with stricture or Barrett's esophagus were excluded. None had had previous upper gastrointestinal surgery or had taken antisecretory medication within 2 weeks of entering the study.

The study was conducted in two parts. During phase I, 32 patients were treated with ranitidine 150 mg b.i.d., and in phase II, 18 patients received ranitidine 300 mg b.i.d. Each patient cohort had similar reflux parameters (Table I). All patients underwent endoscopy, 24-hour ambulatory esophageal pH monitoring, and esophageal manometry before commencing therapy and at eight weekly intervals while on treatment. Therapy was deemed successful when there was satisfactory control of symptoms with healing of endoscopic esophagitis. The duration of treatment was dependent upon its success, but was for a minimum of 2 months and a maximum of 6 months.

After completion of the medical therapy trial, patients were followed for a mean period of 21 months and maintenance therapy (ranitidine 150 mg or 300 mg daily) was prescribed according to the recurrence of symptoms. Antireflux surgery, using a previously described technique,[10] was offered to those who had failed to respond adequately to the trial of medical therapy and to those who had symptomatic relapse while on maintenance therapy, providing there were no contraindications to surgery. Three months after surgery, patients were restudied as detailed above.

Results

The trial of medical therapy produced satisfactory control of symptoms and healing of esophagitis in 16 patients (32%). However, 34 patients (68%) had persistent esophagitis at the end of the treatment period and a further two patients, in whom treatment had initially been successful, had further troublesome symptoms with recurrent esophagitis despite maintenance therapy. These patients were deemed to have failed on medical therapy. Maintenance therapy was, however, successful at relieving symptoms in 12 of 16 patients who either refused surgery or were considered unsuitable for it (Table II).

Those patients who failed on medical treatment were characterized by greater esophageal acid exposure, which was significant for the total period and the upright period, and by an increased prevalence of severe esophagitis (grade II or III) at the beginning of the study (Table III).

Esophageal function studies showed that these patients had a significantly lower LES (lower esophageal sphincter) pressure, with a shorter abdominal and overall length of sphincter although this failed to reach significance. In addition, these patients had a greater

Table II
The Outcome of Medical Therapy for Gastroesophageal Reflux

	Phase I *(R 150 mg bid)*	*Phase II* *(R 300 mg bid)*
Successful Therapy	12 (38%)	4 (22%)
no maintenance	4	3
satisfactory maintenance	6	1
unsatisfactory maintenance	2	0
Failed Therapy	20 (62%)	14 (78%)
surgery before trial ends	2	3
surgery after trial ends	8	5
satisfactory maintenance	7	5
unsatisfactory maintenance	3	1

R = ranitidine.

Table III
Physiological Reflux Characteristics of Those Who Succeeded
or Failed Medical Therapy

	Successful *Therapy*	*Failed* *Therapy*	*p*
Esophagitis:			
Grade I	10	15	
Grade II	3	12	<0.05
Grade III	1	9	
Acid Exposure:			
% Total time pH <4	8.2	10.8	<0.05
% Upright time pH <4	8.9	14.1	<0.05
% Supine time pH <4	2.8	8.1	NS
LES Competence:			
Pressure (mmHg)	10.0	5.5	<0.01
Abdominal length (cm)	1.8	1.2	NS
Overall length (cm)	4.0	3.0	NS
Amplitude Esophageal Body:			
7 cm above LES (mmHg)	38.0	34.0	NS
2 cm above LES (mmHg)	57.0	30.0	<0.05

LES = lower esophageal sphincter; NS = not significant.

incidence of low amplitude contractions in the distal esophagus. Consequently, of those who failed on medical therapy, 72% had a defective lower esophageal sphincter and 50% ineffective distal esophageal clearance, compared with 29% and 14%, respectively, of those with a successful response (Table III).

Twenty patients (56%) who failed on medical therapy underwent an antireflux repair. There was one death from a myocardial infarction 23 days after surgery and one patient was lost to follow-up. Antireflux surgery resulted in a significant reduction in esophageal acid exposure (% total time pH<4: 11.9 vs. 1.0, p<0.001). In 13 of 16 patients, (81%) esophageal acid exposure was reduced to less than 5% of the total time. This control of acid reflux was reflected by the successful control of reflux symptoms in 17 of 18 patients (94%) and healing of esophagitis in 16 of 18 patients (89%).

Discussion

Successful antireflux therapy should control reflux symptoms, heal esophagitis, and prevent development of the complications of stricture and Barrett's esophagus. This study supports others which show that treatment with an H_2-receptor antagonist is unsatisfactory for many patients with reflux esophagitis who have not responded to standard recommendations relating to diet, posture, smoking, and administration of antacids.

Robertson[11] showed that patients who fail to respond to medical therapy continue to have pathological esophageal acid exposure while on treatment. This study suggests that the inability to prevent acid reflux in many patients is a reflection of the importance of the lower esophageal sphincter and the pump function of the esophageal body in the etiology of the condition. Those patients who are most likely to fare poorly with therapy aimed only at reduction of gastric acid secretion are those with a defective LES and ineffective esophageal clearance. The presence of these factors accounts for the greater esophageal acid exposure and the more severe esophagitis of those who failed medical therapy. This is supported by Lieberman,[12] who found a correlation between recurrence of esophagitis and LES pressure. In contrast, Barlow[13] has shown that 48% of those who reflux through a normal sphincter have gastric hypersecretion and can be predicted to do well with antisecretory therapy.

In patients with abnormal LES and esophageal body function,

healing of esophagitis is only likely to occur if the gastric pH is consistently raised to pH 5 or above, a level at which pepsin no longer produces mucosal damage. Such reduction of gastric acidity is possible with omeprazole, thus explaining its therapeutic benefit over conventional H_2-receptor antagonist therapy.[14,15] Nevertheless, manometric recordings during omeprazole therapy show that reflux continues,[16] which may account for the reported recurrence rate of 82% on cessation of treatment.[17]

Antireflux surgery, which aimed to augment sphincter pressure and increase its intra-abdominal length, successfully prevented reflux, controlled symptoms, and healed esophagitis in more than 80% of a resistant group of refluxers who had failed medical therapy. Therefore, patients who can be predicted to fare poorly with medical therapy because of a defective LES and ineffective esophageal pump function should be identified at an early stage and encouraged to have antireflux surgery.

References

1. Jones R, Lydeard S: Prevalence of symptoms of dyspepsia in the community. Br Med J 298:30, 1989.
2. Wesdorp ICE, Dekker W, Klinkenberg-Knol EC: Treatment of reflux esophagitis with ranitidine. Gut 24:921, 1983.
3. Goy JA, Maynard JH, McNaughton WM, et al: Ranitidine and placebo in the treatment of reflux oesophagitis. Med J Aust 2:558, 1983.
4. Hine KR, Holmes GKT, Melikian V, et al: Rantidine in reflux esophagitis. Digestion 29:119, 1984.
5. McCallum RW, Eshelman F, Nardi R: A double-blind multicenter trial to compare the efficacy of ranitidine and placebo in the short-term treatment of gastroesophageal reflux disease. Gastroenterology 86:1179, 1984.
6. Koelz HR, Birchler R, Bretholz A, et al: Healing and relapse of reflux esophagitis during treatment with ranitidine. Gastroenterology 91:1198, 1986.
7. Pace F, Bianchi Porro G, Sangaletti O: Ranitidine therapy in peptic esophagitis: Doubling the dose or duration of treatment? Gut 29:A1446, 1988.
8. Behar J, Brand DL, Brown FC, et al: Cimetidine in the treatment of symptomatic gastroesophageal reflux. Gastroenterology 74:441, 1978.
9. Richter JE: A critical review of current medical therapy for gastroesophageal reflux disease. J Clin Gastroenterol 8(Suppl 1):72, 1986.
10. Watson A, Jenkinson LR, Norris TL: Lower esophageal sphincter characteristics after a simplified anti-reflux procedure. In: Diseases of the Esophagus, Siewert JR, Holscher AH (eds), Berlin, Springer-Verlag, 1987, p 1178.
11. Robertson DAF, Aldersley MA, Shepherd H, et al: H_2-antagonists in the

treatment of reflux esophagitis: Can physiological studies predict the response? Gut 28:946, 1987.

12. Lieberman DA: Medical therapy for chronic reflux esophagitis. Arch Intern Med 147:1717, 1987.

13. Barlow AP, DeMeester TR, Ball CS, et al: The significance of the gastric secretory state in gastroesophageal reflux disease. Arch Surg 124:937–940, 1989.

14. Klinkenberg-Knol EC, Jansen JMBJ, Festen HPM, et al: Double-blind multicentre comparison of omeprazole and ranitidine in the treatment of reflux oesophagitis. Lancet i:349, 1987.

15. Havelund T, Laursen LS, Skoubo-Kristensen E, et al: Omeprazole and ranitidine in treatment of reflux oesophagitis: Double-blind comparative trial. Br Med J 296:89, 1988.

16. Downton J, Dent J, Heddle R, et al: Elevation of gastric pH heals peptic esophagitis: A role for omeprazole. J Hepatol Gastroenterol 2:317, 1987.

17. Hetzel DJ, Dent J, Reed WD, et al: Healing and relapse of severe peptic esophagitis after treatment with omeprazole. Gastroenterology 95:903, 1988.

19

Factors Affecting Long-Term Results of Medical Therapy of Gastroesophageal Reflux

Clemente Iascone, P. Ginevri, M. Caporossi,
P. Addario Chieco, R. Arca, M. Picchio, C. Maffi,
Aldo Moraldi, Sergio Stipa

Introduction

Gastroesophageal reflux disease (GERD) is frequently observed in the general population, since up to 7% of adults experience heartburn and regurgitation at least once a day.[1] In some patients, symptoms may progress to chronic GERD which requires medical treatment. In our institution in the last decade, indications for antireflux surgery have been progressively decreasing and conversely a greater number of patients have been medically treated. In this study, a series of 120 consecutive patients with documented GERD were reviewed with the following purposes: (1) to assess the need for surgical correction of reflux disease in an unselected patient population; (2) to determine the effectiveness of long-term medical and surgical therapy of GERD; and (3) to detect those factors, if any, affecting the clinical outcome of these patients.

Little AG, Ferguson MK, Skinner DB: Diseases of the Esophagus, Vol. II: Benign Diseases. Futura Publishing Company, Inc., Mount Kisco, NY, © 1990.

Patients and Methods

From 1981 to 1988, abnormal reflux was documented by endoscopy and/or pH test in 221 out of 674 patients referred for evaluation of symptoms of gastroesophageal reflux. One hundred and twenty patients, personally followed by the authors, were reviewed retrospectively. There were 47 males and 33 females with a mean age of 47 ± 13 years. The frequency and severity of esophageal (heartburn, regurgitation, and dysphagia) and gastric symptoms (nausea, vomiting, postprandial fullness, and early satiety) were assessed before treatment and during the follow-up in all patients on the basis of a detailed questionnaire.

Barium swallow, endoscopy, and esophageal manometry[2] were performed in all patients. Twenty-four-hour esophageal pH recordings[3] and esophageal scintigraphy[4] were performed in 57 and 56 patients, respectively.

In all patients, medical management was based on postural and dietary manipulation and pharmacological support which consisted of a combination of antacid/alginic acid and H_2-blockers (ranitidine: 300–450 mg/daily for the first 8–12 weeks and 150 mg/daily at bed time before being discontinued, when possible). Promotility agents were added to the basic regimen if gastric emptying symptoms were prominent or if delayed gastric emptying was objectively documented. During the follow-up period, symptom scores were derived from detailed patient interviews; clinic visits or telephone contact were utilized according to the patient's clinical situation. Endoscopic examinations were not performed routinely; indications for endoscopy were severe relapse of symptoms and surveillance of complex reflux problems (peptic stenoses, Barrett's epithelium).

Seventeen patients have been lost to follow-up (14%) and 23 patients underwent surgical treatment; in the remaining 80 patients on medical therapy, a 6 to 12 months follow-up was achieved in 31% of subjects, a 2 to 3 year follow-up and a 4 to 7 year follow-up was obtained in 41.5% and 27.5% of patients, respectively. For the purpose of analysis, results of therapy were scored as follows: (1) *Excellent:* absent esophageal symptoms ± one occasional gastric symptom; (2) *Very good:* one occasional esophageal symptom ± occasional gastric symptoms; (3) *Good:* one moderate esophageal symptom or several occasional esophageal symptoms; (4) *Fair:* one moderate esophageal symptom + several occasional symptoms; (5) *Failure:* unchanged or worsened symptoms.

Table I
GER Surgical Therapy (1981–1988):
Long-Term Results (23 Belsey Mark IV)

		Patient Opinion		
		Cured	*Improved*	*Unchanged*
Excellent + Very Good	17 (74%)	10	7	—
Fair	1 (4%)	—	1	—
Failure	5 (22%)	—	—	5

Results

Patient Outcome

Twenty-three patients out of 103 eligible for the study (22%) were submitted to antireflux surgery with a standard Belsey repair shortly after being evaluated and were not included in the medical therapy group. There were six patients with peptic stenosis, four with previous failed antireflux surgery, and 13 subjects submitted to a primary repair following failed medical treatment lasting 3 to 10 years. Seventy-four percent of patients had very good or excellent results (Table I).

Very good to excellent results were achieved in 39 out of 80 patients (49%) on medical treatment. In 27% of the 39 patients, therapy was discontinued, in 38% and 35%, respectively, regular consumption of antacids or H_2-blockers was required for symptom-free daily life. By self-assessment, 82% of these patients considered themselves improved and 18% to be cured. Good results were obtained in 22 patients (27%). None discontinued therapy; H_2-blockers or antacids were required in 64% and 36% of patients, respectively. Ninety-one percent of these patients thought they were improved and 9% believed they were unchanged.

Unsatisfactory results (fair results + failures) were observed in 19 patients (23%), in spite of a full dosage of H_2-blockers in 72% of them and antacid treatment in 22%. However, 39% of subjects declared themselves to be improved and 61% complained of unchanged symptoms.

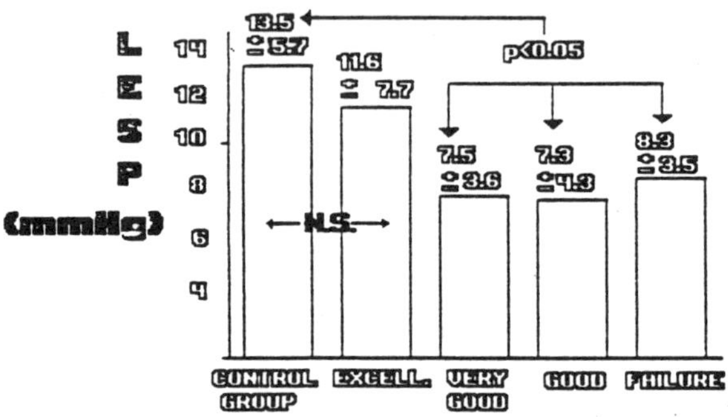

Figure 1: The figure shows the pressure of LES in subjects with proven reflux on medical therapy compared to that of a control group. Patients with less satisfactory results of medical therapy showed a pretreatment LES pressure significantly lower than that of normals.

Factors Affecting the Patient Outcome

On manometry, the overall length of LES, the length of the sphincter exposed to positive abdominal pressure and LES pressure (LESP) did not significantly differ between all groups of patients. However, in subjects with failures, good or very good results, LESP was significantly more hypotensive than that of normal controls (p<0.05). Only patients with an excellent outcome showed a LES pressure comparable to that of normals (Fig. 1).

Nonspecific motility abnormalities of the body of the esophagus were detected in 31% of patients with very good or excellent results, in 41% of subjects with good results, and in 61% of patients with unsatisfactory results (p<0.05).

Similarly, on scintiscan, an abnormal retention of radioisotope in the esophagus was found in 29% of patients with very good or excellent results, and in 63% and 60%, respectively, of patients with good or unsatisfactory results (p<0.03 and p<0.05, respectively).

Comment

In our institution, the frequency of surgery for chronic GERD (ratio of patients operated to patients with proven reflux per year) has been progressively decreasing from a 50% rate in 1981–1983 to 0% in 1987–1988. The availability of several effective drugs may explain this finding and suggests that antireflux surgery may be unnecessary in many patients. In our series, antireflux surgery was performed in 22% of patients enrolled in the study with a 74% very good to excellent late outcome. None required any drugs to maintain a satisfactory clinical situation. It must be stressed that the presence of complex reflux problems greatly affected the incidence of unsatisfactory results, since surgical failures were observed in three sclerodermic patients, in one patient with peptic stenosis, and in two patients with uncomplicated reflux.

In the medically treated group, 49% of subjects obtained a very good to excellent outcome and only 27% of them were able to discontinue the pharmacological support on long-term follow-up. Few reports in the literature[5,6] have evaluated patients with chronic reflux for extended periods, treated medically; in a small and strictly controlled series, Liebermann[5] reports that 75% of patients were taking daily doses of an H_2-blocker at least once daily on long-term follow-up. In our study, follow-up controls and drug therapy were managed in a manner similar to common clinical practice. In spite of this, only 52% of patients required H_2-blockers and 34% had symptoms controlled with antacids alone; furthermore, symptomatic results were comparable to those reported in smaller and controlled series.[7–10]

Satisfactory control of reflux symptoms seems to be related to the mechanical characteristics of the esophagus at the time of the first observation: only in patients who have excellent results with medical treatment is LESP similar to that of normal subjects. In addition, the presence of nonspecific motility disorders of the body of the esophagus on manometry and clearing defects detected with esophageal scintigraphy may affect long-term results of medical treatment.

In a recent report,[5] low LESP was associated with an early relapse of symptomatic reflux in patients on medical therapy. In our series, in 14 patients, LESP, length of abdominal sphincter, and esophageal body motility were within normal limits; 80% had very good to excellent results with medical treatment. On the other hand, in 10 subjects, a hypotensive LES was associated with a short abdominal sphincter and motility disorders of the body of the esophagus; 80% had unsatisfactory symptomatic results from medical therapy. This suggests that patients with combined mechanical defects of the esophagus do not improve significantly in spite of intensive and long-term medical therapy and probably should be candidates for surgical correction of reflux.

Conclusion

Our study showed that in an unselected population of patients with proven GERD, antireflux surgery was performed in 22% of subjects. Results of medical therapy are gratifying in about 50% of patients, but they are not comparable with long-term results of antireflux surgery yet, since the great majority of medically treated patients require chronic drug usage. The late outcome of medically treated patients seems to be related to the presence or absence of motility abnormalities and clearance problems of the esophagus.

References

1. Nebel OT, Forbes MF, Castell DO: Symptomatic gastroesophageal reflux: Incidence and precipitating factors. Am J Dig Dis 21:953, 1976.
2. Winans CS, Harris LD: Quantitation of lower esophageal sphincter competence. Gastroenterology 52:773, 1967.
3. Johnson LF, DeMeester TR: 24-hour pH-monitoring of the distal esophagus: Quantitative measure of gastroesophageal reflux. Am J Gastroenterol 62:325, 1974.
4. Moraldi A, Iascone C, Zerilli M, et al: Patterns of radioisotopic esophageal transit in patients with symptoms of gastroesophageal reflux. In: Diseases of the Esophagus: Pathophysiology, Diagnosis, Conservative and Surgical Treatment, Siewert JR, Hoelsher AH (eds), Monaco, Springer-Verlag, 1988, p 827.
5. Liebermann DA: Medical therapy for chronic reflux esophagitis: Long-term follow-up. Arch Intern Med 147:1717, 1987.
6. Behar J, Brand DL, Brown FC, et al: Cimetidine in the treatment of symptomatic gastroesophageal reflux: A double-blind controlled trial. Gastroenterology 74:441, 1978.
7. Bovero E, Cheli R, Barbara L, et al: Short-term treatment of reflux oesophagitis with ranitidine 300 mg nocte: Italian multicentre study. Hepato-Gastroenterol 34:155, 1987.
8. Sontag S, Robinson M, McCallum RW, et al: Ranitidine therapy for gastroesophageal reflux disease: Results of a large double-blind trial. Arch Intern Med 147:1485, 1987.
9. Simon B, Mueller P: Comparison of the effect of sucralfate and ranitidine in reflux esophagitis. Am J Med 83(suppl 3B):43, 1987.
10. Tytgat GNJ: Clinical efficacy of sucralfate in reflux esophagitis: Comparison with cimetidine. Am J Med 83(suppl 3B):38, 1987.

20

A Comparison of Surgically Treated Reflux Patients in Two Surgical Centers

John Bancewicz, Hugoe R. Matthews,
Tim O'Hanrahan, Ian Adams

Introduction

The indications for antireflux surgery and the optimum operation are still matters for debate. Part of the difficulty is that some patients with gastroesophageal reflux are more complicated to operate on than others. Surgery may be entirely straightforward if the cardia is anatomically normal and there is only mild esophagitis. However, a difficult dissection is often required in cases with panmural esophagitis and esophageal shortening. That severe esophagitis might affect the outcome of antireflux surgery was recognized by Skinner and Belsey in 1967.[1] Apart from this report, there is remarkably little methodical documentation of the relationship between the manifestations of reflux and the outcome of surgery.

We have developed a simple classification that can be used to assess the outcome of antireflux surgery in different types of patients. The early application of this classification in two busy surgical units has shown major differences in the patient populations that may have important implications for future studies of reflux surgery.

Little AG, Ferguson MK, Skinner DB: Diseases of the Esophagus, Vol. II: Benign Diseases. Futura Publishing Company, Inc., Mount Kisco, NY, © 1990.

Methods

Information was available from two separate groups of patients in each center:

1. *Previous operations for gastroesophageal reflux.* A total of 321 patients were studied, 100 from Birmingham and 221 from Manchester. All were first operations for reflux. The Birmingham cases included five resections and 95 Belsey Mark IV procedures. The Manchester cases comprised 212 Nissen fundoplications and nine Collis-Nissen procedures.
2. *Esophageal lab patients.* In order to try to assess the referral practice of the two units, 50 consecutive patients attending each esophageal laboratory were studied.

AFP Classification of Gastroesophageal Reflux

The following descriptive classification of gastroesophageal reflux was applied. It includes anatomical, functional, and pathological features as a means of grading severity. Each of the three elements was given four grades as shown below:

A = Anatomy

    0 No hiatal hernia on routine radiology (no provocative maneuvers) or endoscopy.

    1 Sliding hiatal hernia which reduced on screening or spot film radiology.

    2 Sliding hiatal hernia which was not seen to reduce on screening or spot films.

    3 Mixed sliding and paraesophageal hernia or pure paraesophageal hernia.

F = Function (pH Assessment)

    0 No pathological reflux on 24-hour pH testing.

    1 Reflux related to meals.

    2 Upright reflux not related to meals.

    3 Supine reflux with or without upright reflux. The letters L

(low), N (normal), or H (high) can be added to the code in this section to denote diminished, normal, or increased pressures in the body of the esophagus on manometry, e.g., F3 L.

P = Pathology

0 No macroscopic mucosal abnormality.

1 Macroscopic esophagitis consisting of at least linear streaks in the distal esophagus.

2 Concentric fibrosis (= stricture).

3 Longitudinal fibrosis (= short esophagus) or penetrating ulcer.

The letters CLO can be added to the code in this section to indicate the presence of a columnar-lined esophagus. PS may denote previous surgery. Thus, full coding might read as follows: A2, F3, N, P1, CLO, P. X is used to indicate missing data elements.

Results

Operations

There were several major differences between the two centers. Of the Manchester cases, 57.9% had no hiatal hernia in contrast to only 11% of the Birmingham cases. Likewise, 57.4% of the Manchester cases did not have macroscopic esophagitis as compared to 26.8% in Birmingham. The incidence of esophageal shortening was 4% in Manchester and 17% in Birmingham.

Only 47% of the Birmingham cases had a 24-hour pH study but 78.7% had grade 3 reflux compared with 45% in Manchester. Thus, overall, the Manchester cases had much earlier disease than the Birmingham cases.

Lab Patients

Analysis of the patients referred for laboratory investigation suggested that the differences were due to different referral patterns and perhaps also to different perceptions of the value of esophageal investigation. The Manchester series had a predominance of patients with severe functional disturbance but less in the way of anatomical or pathological change. It would appear, therefore that the two surgeons were choosing their operative candidates from two quite different populations.

Discussion

We feel that the differences we have documented between our two centers may be relevant to the difficulty of interpretation of published surgical data. They also emphasize the need for more standardized methods of assessment before and after operation.

We do not have at present a full explanation for the differences that we have found. There may be rather different indications for operation in the two centers, but we do not think that this is likely to produce such a large discrepancy. A more likely explanation may be that there are different referral patterns. This is supported by the differences in the patients investigated in our esophageal laboratories. It is interesting to speculate how these different referral patterns may have developed. We suspect that they may have as much to do with the attitudes and expectations of our colleagues in other specialties as with our own diagnostic and therapeutic expectations.

We strongly recommend that some form of descriptive classification should be used to describe the patient population in future studies of gastroesophageal reflux. The AFP classification that we have used here takes into account the major components of reflux and is easy to apply. It may also be suitable for studies of the pathophysiology of reflux disease.

References

1. Skinner DB, Belsey RH: Surgical management of esophageal reflux and hiatus hernia: Long-term results with 1030 patients. J Thorac Cardiovasc Surg 53:33, 1967.

21

The Belsey Mark IV Antireflux Procedure:
Indications and Long-Term Results

Toni Lerut, W. Coosemans, R. Christiaens,
Jacques Aime Gruwez

Introduction

For about three decades, surgical techniques to treat gastroesophageal reflux (GER) whether or not associated with hiatal hernia (HH) have been routinely used. Mainly three techniques have emerged: the Nissen fundoplication,[1] the Belsey Mark IV,[2] and the Hill[3] procedure. Although many variations have been described, they remain the classic techniques today.

In contrast with early experiences, indications for surgery are narrowing. This has to be explained by better diagnostic possibilities (e.g., the use of 24-hour pH monitoring) and the use of more potent drugs (e.g., H_2 blockers and more recently omeprazole) increasing the possibilities of conservative treatment.

A direct consequence of this evolution is a more critical judgment of antireflux surgery in terms of reflux control and undesired side effects and, on the other hand, an increasing number of more complex, drug-resistant, or complicated cases for which surgery remains the last chance. In other words, while the overall number of operations decreases, the degree of difficulty of this surgery is increasing.

Little AG, Ferguson MK, Skinner DB: Diseases of the Esophagus, Vol. II: Benign Diseases. Futura Publishing Company, Inc., Mount Kisco, NY, © 1990.

Table I
Belsey Mark IV Procedure Additional
Pathology: Complications in 73 Patients

	No. of Patients
Esophagitis grade III	22
Esophagitis grade IV	6
Barrett's esophagus	26
Reintervention	10
Duodenal Ulcer (HSV)	10
Bleeding	13
Small Benign Tumors	2

In view of this, we have analyzed our experience with the Belsey Mark IV procedure.

Patient Material and Method

From 1977 until December 1987, the Belsey Mark IV procedure was performed on 117 patients, 72 males and 45 females with a mean age of 48.6 years (12–72 years). Symptoms were present in 90% of patients for at least 1 year, and in 41 patients (35%) for at least 5 years. In all but four patients with a complicated paraesophageal hernia, decision for surgery was based on a conservative therapy-resistant reflux. The decision is based on clinical history, X-ray examination, endoscopy, to a certain extent on manometry (70 patients), and the Bernstein test (19 patients). Since 24-hour pH monitoring was introduced, this examination has become more and more the most decisive technical examination (68 patients).

However, in 73 patients (62%) there was additional pathology and/or some complication of GER (Table I): esophagitis grade III, 22 patients; grade IV, 5 patients; Barrett, 26 patients; reintervention for failed antireflux surgery, 10 patients; synchronous duodenal ulcer or hypersecretion necessitating high selective vagotomy (HSV), 10 patients; bleeding, 13 patients (seven with mixed type hiatal hernia, two with a paraesophageal hernia, two with concomitant bleeding duodenal ulcer); concomitant esophageal leiomyoma, two patients.

Table II
Belsey Mark IV Procedure Follow-up
Mean Duration: 4.5 Years all ≥1 year

	Objective Findings		
	No. of Patients		*No. of Patients*
Endoscopy	82	Pathologic	16 (20%)
		8 <Preoperative	
		5 Esophagitis grade I	
X-ray	89	Pathologic	16 (18%)
24 hr pH	62	Pathologic	13 (20%)
Manometry	44	↓ LES	8 (18%)

Objective recurrence (≥2 Pathological criteria): 2 ⎱ 11 (9.5%)
Subjective recurrence: 9 (Objective in 8) ⎰

Results

There was one early mortality due to bleeding and fistula. This is the only patient in which a symptomatic fistula was seen although a second patient showed on X-ray a subclinical small extravasation for which no further treatment was required. Five patients developed a wound infection. Pulmonary complications were seen in 11 patients: pneumonia in three, pleural effusion in two, dyspnea in four, pulmonary embolism in one. In one patient, an obstructing piece of meat had to be evacuated endoscopically and one patient developed esophageal moniliasis. A total of 20 patients developed some postoperative complication.

There was one late mortality 8 months postoperatively in a patient who developed necrosis of the fundus requiring resection, esophagostomy, and gastrostomy; this patient died from a cardiac infarction before continuity could be restored.

All surviving patients have been followed at least for 1 year and the mean follow-up is 4.5 years. After 1 year, a re-evaluation was proposed consisting of an X-ray, endoscopy, manometry, and 24-hour pH study (Table II).

X-ray was accepted by 89 patients and in 16 (18%) reflux or hiatal hernia was suggested. In 82 patients, endoscopy was performed which was pathological in 16 (20%) although in eight patients esophagitis was markedly decreased compared to the preoperative ex-

Table III
Belsey Mark IV Procedure Follow-up:
Undesirable Side Effects

	No. of Patients
Gastrointestinal 9 patients (8%)	
Dysphagia	2
Gas bloat	5
Delayed gastric emptying	1
Biliary vomiting (B II)	1
Other 11 patients (9.5%)	
Post-thoracotomy pain	8
Dyspnea	3

amination; esophagitis grade I was present in five of the eight patients.

Twenty-four-hour pH monitoring was done in 62 patients and showed pathological reflux in 13 (20%). Manometry was accepted by 44 patients and showed a low LES in eight patients (18%). As a whole, 13 patients appeared to have one pathological test, all 13 having the full range of examinations. Two patients had respectively two and three pathological tests and were considered to have recurrent disease although clinically asymptomatic (Table II).

From a clinical point of view, nine patients had symptoms suggesting recurrent reflux disease (8%) being objectively proven in eight. Adding the two above-mentioned asymptomatic recurrences brings the total of objective and subjective recurrences to 11 (9.5%). Undesired gastroesophageal side effects were noticed in nine patients (8%), dysphagia in two, gas bloat in five, delayed gastric emptying in one, biliary vomiting (after B II gastrectomy) in one. Post-thoracotomy pain requiring treatment was seen in eight (7%) patients, and three patients complained of dyspnea with effort (Table III).

The final score (Table IV) combining the patient's (subjective) and the doctor's (objective) opinion showed 70 patients (61%) who were completely asymptomatic without any side effects. Nineteen (16.5%) patients had very good results having one pathological (objective or subjective) finding but clinically asymptomatic for reflux. Thirteen patients (11.3%) had good results with either two pathological non-disturbing findings (of which one was an objective finding) or one

Table IV
Belsey Mark IV Procedure: Final Score

Results	No. of Patients
Excellent	70 (61%)
Very good	19 (16.5%)
Good	13 (11%)
Bad	13 (11%)

disturbing side effect. Finally, there were 13 patients (11%) in whom the results were judged unsatisfactory because of recurrent disease (subjective or objective) in 11 patients or because of a disabling undesired side effect in two (dysphagia and delayed gastric emptying).

Discussion

Provided there are appropriate indications, it is clear that today in about 90% of cases, good control of reflux can be obtained using one of the classic techniques.[4] This is also our experience with a 92.5% clinical and 90.5% clinical and objective control. Our results with Belsey Mark IV are comparable to those in the literature using the same or other techniques. Siewert obtained good results in 89%[5] and DeMeester in 91%,[6] both using Nissen fundoplication. Hill obtained 89%[7] good results with his technique and Maher had 82%[8] with the same technique.

There are few publications mentioning results after a very long follow-up. Orringer[9] analyzed Belsey's material of 892 patients with a 3–15 year follow-up and found 84% good reflux control.

Ackermann[10] has published a follow-up study on 268 patients (probably Nissen's patients) and mentions 78.5% good results 10–20 years after a Nissen fundoplication. Negré[11] has 81% good results with the same technique in a similar study. Those results mainly use a clinical assessment. DeMeester[12] analyzed clinical (subjective) and technical (objective) data by using a scoring system to evaluate the results after randomizing the three classic techniques. In this study, Nissen's fundoplication obtains the highest score, but one can question whether all three different techniques were equally mastered as only 15 patients were operated with each of the different techniques.

Since the results of reflux control are about equal to those of different techniques, it becomes clear that undesired side effects are playing a more and more important role in choosing a certain technique.

As shown in the literature undesired side effects are indeed frequent. Especially Nissen's fundoplication seems to be compromised by these complications. Siewert[13] found an incidence of 24% swallowing problems, gas bloat, or postprandial epigastric fullness in 38%, inability to vomit in 12.6%; and only 41% of the patients were completely asymptomatic after a Nissen operation.

Negré[11] reports meteorism in 35% and inability to vomit in 30%, and Ackermann[10] noticed gas bloat in 18.7%, dysphagia in 30.5%, epigastric pain in 27.3%, diarrhea in 7%, dumping in 7% 10–20 years postoperatively. Although the floppy Nissen modification seems to reduce to some extent the side effects,[6] they remain a drawback of this operation.

As to the Hill procedure, there are no clear data dealing with undesirable side effects. Hill[7] reports 89% good results. Maher[8] had 82% good results, and Skinner[14] had 82% good to excellent results. Most of the side effects seen after a Nissen operation are almost nonexistent with the Belsey Mark IV as shown in our series where 77% of the patients were symptom-free with good reflux control and no disturbing side effects. The most important criticism for the Belsey Mark IV is post thoracotomy pain, which has been seen in 7% of our patients and which can be avoided only by reducing traction on the ribs during the operation. In regard to this sort of complication, it must be mentioned, however, that postlaparotomy pain and incisional hernias occur in 5–10% of laparotomies but no study dealing with reflux addresses this complication. The strengths of the Belsey Mark IV procedure are good reflux control and a minimum of undesirable side effects.

Today, with any good antireflux technique, at least 90% good reflux control will be obtained, and thus we believe that there is a need to increase surgical indications especially regarding age limit. Indeed, often the limit for antireflux surgery is set at the age of 65–70 years even if symptoms persist despite drug therapy. Since esophageal resection, a much more extensive operation for esophageal carcinoma, can be performed routinely on patients aged 70 years or even much older with low mortality rates,[15] there seems to be no reason to deprive those patients from a 90% chance for cure in case of drug therapy resistance.

The most important condition for successful treatment remains a rigorous policy of surgical indications. Certainly more and more patients enjoy the results of the still increasing healing capacities of new drugs, reducing the number of patients who will eventually become candidates for surgery. On the other hand, because of this the number of complicated cases in the surgical population is increasing steadily as again clearly shown in our experience where this was the case in two-thirds of the patients. As a direct consequence, refinement of surgical indications and technical skills are required, and this is for a constantly diminishing number of patients. As Rosetti[16] states: A major current problem is the training of the new generation of surgeons because the indication has become less frequent in reflux surgery. Therefore, perhaps patients undergoing antireflux surgery should be centralized so that evaluation of surgical indications, surgical techniques, and results can be analyzed critically on the basis of comparable data which eventually will lead to the further required refinement of technique and consequent optimization of results.

Conclusion

From our experience, it can be concluded that candidates for surgical treatment of GER often present with a wide variety of reflux-related complications or additional pathology. The long-term follow-up shows excellent to good results in 88.5% of patients, the recurrence rate being 9.5%. Standardization of the criteria for indications, grouping of pathology, and evaluation of objective and subjective results including undesirable side effects which can be used universally are required.

References

1. Nissen R: Gastropexy and fundoplication in surgical treatment of hiatus hernia. Am J Dig Dis 6:954, 1961.
2. Skinner DB, Belsey RHR: Surgical management of esophageal reflux with hiatus hernia: Long-term results with 1030 cases. J Thorac Cardiovasc Surg 53:33, 1967.
3. Hill LD: An effective operation of hiatal hernia: An eight-year appraisal. Ann Surg 166:681, 1967.
4. DeMeester TR, Fuchs KH: Comparison of operations for uncomplicated reflux disease. In: Surgery of the Oesophagus, Jamieson GG (ed), London, Churchill Livingstone, Longman Group UK Ltd, 1988, p 299.

5. Siewert R: Operative Behandlung der Refluxkrankheit. Chirurg 49:137, 1978.

6. DeMeester TR, Bonvina L, Albertucci M: Nissen fundoplication for gastroesophageal reflux disease: Evaluation of primary repair in 100 consecutive patients. Ann Surg 204:9, 1986.

7. Hill LD, Vellasco N: The Hill repair. In: Gibson's Surgery of the Chest, Sabiston DC, Spencer FC (eds), Philadelphia, WB Saunders Co, 1983, p 797.

8. Maher JW, Hollenbeck JI, Woodward ER: An analysis of recurrent esophagitis following posterior gastropexy. Ann Surg 187:227, 1978.

9. Orringer MB, Skinner DB, Belsey RHR: Long-term results of the Mark IV operation for hiatal hernia and analysis of recurrences and their treatment. J Thorac Cardiovasc Surg 63:25, 1972.

10. Ackermann CH, Margreth L, Muller C, Harder F: Symptoms 10–20 years after fundoplication. In: Diseases of the Esophagus, Siewert JR, Hölscher AH (eds), Berlin, Springer-Verlag, 1988, p 1198.

11. Negré JB, Markkula HT, Keyrilainen O, Matikainen M: Nissen fundoplication: Result at 10-year follow-up. Am J Surg 146:635, 1983.

12. DeMeester TR, Johnson LF, Kent AH: Evaluation of current operations for the prevention of gastroesophageal reflux. Ann Surg 180:511, 1974.

13. Siewert JR, Lepsien G: Fundoplication (inclusive operation–Belsey, Hill, and Collis). In: Reflux Therapy, Blum AL, Siewert JR (eds), Berlin, Springer-Verlag, 1981, p 283.

14. Skinner DB, Belsey RHR: Long-term results of antireflux surgery. In: Management of Esophageal Diseases, Skinner DB, Belsey RHR (eds), Philadelphia, WB Saunders Co, 1988, p 600.

15. Perrachia A, Bardini R, Ruola, et al: Carcinoma of the esophagus in the elderly (70 years of age or older): Indications and results of surgery. Dis Esoph 1:147, 1988.

16. Rosetti ME: Thirty years of Nissen fundoplication: Development of fundoplication. In: Diseases of the Esophagus, Siewert JR, Hölscher AH (eds), Berlin, Springer-Verlag, 1988, p 1258.

22

Surgical Treatment for Gastroesophageal Reflux: Which Procedure is the Best?

Jean Marie Hay, Guy Zeitoun, Philippe Segol, Didier Pottier

Introduction

Many studies have been published about gastroesophageal reflux (GER). However, the only prospective randomized study performed was by DeMeester,[1] who evaluated the effectiveness of three commonly used antireflux procedures (Hill, Nissen, and Belsey). Evaluation of the surgical results at a mean of 4 months postoperatively concluded that the Nissen repair best controls reflux, but at the expense of temporary postoperative dysphagia and a 50% chance of being unable to vomit after repair. However, no long-term evaluation was done. Our prospective randomized multicenter study was designed to compare the three most frequent antireflux procedures performed in France, namely the Nissen,[2] Toupet,[3] and Lortat-Jacob[4] repairs and to evaluate their results after a 2-year follow-up.

* From a prospective randomized multicenter trial by the French University for Surgical Research. Surgeons and physicians who participated in this trial are: G. Cargill, P. L. Fagniez, Y. Flamant, J. M. Hay, H. Join, D. Keller, J. P. Lenroit, J. N. Maillard, C. Meyer, J. L. Pailler, D. Pottier, P. Segol, and G. Zeitoun.

Little AG, Ferguson MK, Skinner DB: Diseases of the Esophagus, Vol. II: Benign Diseases. Futura Publishing Company, Inc., Mount Kisco, NY, © 1990.

Patients and Methods

From September 1982 to May 1985, 52 patients (34 males, 18 females) with a mean age of 53 and a range of 15 to 70 years were included. Complete evaluation was performed on each patient: (1) preoperatively, to confirm the diagnosis of GER, to determine its cause, to eliminate other possible pathology to account for the patient's symptoms, and to exclude patients who did not meet the criteria for inclusion; and (2) postoperatively, at 2 years follow-up, to evaluate and compare the results of the surgical repairs.

Methods of Evaluation

pH-Metric Test

pH-metric testing was done to link the clinical findings to GER. A standard acid reflux test was performed. If a spontaneous reflux (pH<4) was present, the esophagus was flushed with water, the pH electrode was withdrawn slowly and repositioned 10, 15, 20, and 25 cm above the top of the high pressure zone (HPZ) to determine the height of spontaneous reflux. Where the pH was greater than 4, provocative maneuvers were performed. Results were expressed by a score (Minaire's score)[5] from 1 to 9 based on the frequency, severity, and duration of reflux episodes and then classified as follows: 0–1, none; 2–3, mild; 4–6, moderate; 7–9, severe. Only patients with moderate to severe reflux were included in this trial.

Contrast Radiology

Contrast radiology was done to classify gastroesophageal malpositions and hiatal hernias.

Endoscopy

Endoscopy was done to detect and classify esophagitis.

Esophageal Manometry

Esophageal manometry was done to exclude motility disorders and to assess lower esophageal sphincter (LES) tonicity and the antireflux components of each type of repair (LES length, total esophageal length (TEL), length between the LES and the pressure inversion point (PIP) [LES-PIP]), that is, the decrease of the thoracic segment of the LES after surgical repair.

Criteria of Inclusion and Exclusion

Included in this study were patients with symptomatic reflux and a moderate or severe Minaire's score. Patients who were excluded met one of the following criteria: (1) previous psychiatric history; (2) scleroderma; (3) gastric or duodenal ulcer; (4) previous antireflux surgery or any surgery on esophagus, stomach, or duodenum (including vagotomy); (5) acquired shortened esophagus; (6) other esophageal diseases (i.e., diverticulum, motility disorders); (7) patients who could not undergo a 2-year follow-up examination (e.g., foreigners, cancer patients). Cholelithiasis was not a contraindication for inclusion.

Surgical Procedures

All procedures were performed by an abdominal approach. **Nissen**[2]: Total fundoplication was performed over a #50F bougie to avoid obstruction and postoperative dysphagia. To avoid the so-called "slipped Nissen," the left and right lateral wall of the mobilized abdominal esophagus was sutured to the adjacent gastric fundus wrap. **Toupet**[3]: 180° posterior fundoplication and gastrophrenopexy to the right phrenic crus was performed. **Lortat-Jacob**[4]: Accentuation of the angle of His by placing sutures between the left border of the mobilized esophagus and the right border of the adjacent fundus was performed as well as esophagogastrophrenopexy to the left phrenic crus. *In all procedures:* the esophageal hiatus was narrowed to prevent the fundoplication from slipping into the thorax.

Statistical Methods: Judgment Criteria

Recommendations for prospective multicenter clinical trials were followed. After preoperative medical evaluation, patients were divided into two strata according to reflux severity (moderate, severe). At operation, the surgeon initially evaluated the abdomen with respect to inclusion criteria and operative feasibility for each procedure. If acceptable, the patient was then randomized to a particular procedure using a balanced center-specific randomization procedure. Postoperative endoscopy, pH-metry, and manometry evaluation were blind procedures with respect to the physicians performing these studies. For statistical analysis, Chi-square tests were used for qualitative data comparisons, and Student's *t*-test for quantitative data. For pre- and postoperative data comparisons, each patient was his own control. The number of patients to be included for statistical evidence was calculated from DeMeester's study[1]: 15 patients in each of the three surgical repair groups, 45 patients total.

Results

Fifty-two patients were included as follows: 20 Nissen, 18 Toupet, and 14 Lortat-Jacob repairs. Although consents were obtained from all patients before inclusion, four postoperative asymptomatic patients refused further postoperative evaluation. A fifth patient was lost to follow-up. Of these five patients, two had a Nissen, two had a Toupet, and one had a Lortat-Jacob repair. Thus, this analysis was performed on 47 patients (90%). Each group was comparable with respect to age, sex ratio, clinical symptoms, radiology, endoscopy, manometry, and pH-metry evaluations (Tables I and II). Intra- and postoperative complications did not significantly differ in the three groups. However, three splenic tears occurred during Nissen procedures, leading in one case to a splenectomy. Eleven cholecystectomies were performed but this did not change the morbidity. There were no intra- or postoperative deaths.

Clinical Results

Clinically, the number of symptom-free patients did not differ significantly in the three groups. However, several recurrences of symptoms occurred: one recurrence after Nissen (normal pH-metry), one recurrence after Toupet, and three recurrences after Lortat-Jacob repair. In these four last patients (1 Toupet, 3 Lortat-Jacob), postoperative pH-metry was abnormal and two had esophagitis at en-

Table I
Preoperative Comparability

	Nissen	Toupet	Lortat-Jacob	Total
Patients	18	16	13	47
Age (years)*	49.3 ± 14	53.6 ± 12	57.6 ± 11	53.3 ± 12
Age Range	28–73	31–73	42–74	28–74
Sex Ratio (M/F)	14/4	15/5	7/6	32/15
Radiology				
hiatal hernia	11	12	8	31
malposition	7	4	5	16
Endoscopy				
esophagitis	9	8	7	24
Manometry*				
LES tonicity (cm H_2O)	9.3 ± 11.41	12.7 ± 11.1	10.2 ± 6.8	10.7 ± 9.7
Esoph. length (cm)	39.0 ± 4.0	40.1 ± 3.4	38.5 ± 4.9	39.2 ± 4.1
LES-PIP (cm)	3.1 ± 1.8	2.3 ± 1.5	2.7 ± 1.8	2.7 ± 1.7
LES length (cm)	3.3 ± 1.1	2.9 ± 1.5	3.6 ± 1.2	3.3 ± 1.3

* Mean ± 1 SD.
LES = lower esophageal sphincter; PIP = pressure inversion point; Esoph. length = esophageal length.

Table II
pH-Metric Results: Group Comparisons

	Nissen 18		Toupet 16		Lortat-Jacob 13	
	Pre	Post	Pre	Post	Pre	Post
Minaire's Score*						
severe	16	2	14	1	12	4
moderate	2	3	2	7	1	4
mild	0	5	0	2	0	2
none	0	8	0	6	0	3
Mean*	8.1 ± 1.2	2.1 ± 2.6	8.0 ± 1.5	2.7 ± 2.6	8.0 ± 1.2	4.9 ± 3.3
Mean net change in score per patients**	−5.9 ± 1.4		−5.2 ± 1.0		−3.2 ± 2.1	

* Mean ± 1 SD; ** Each patient is his own control; △ No statistical difference; △△ p < 0.05.

doscopy. Surgical revision was needed in two of these patients. Only one case of mild persistent dysphagia was seen (Nissen group). In the Nissen group, no surgical revision was needed, there was no inability to belch or vomit, and no persistent reflux esophagitis was observed.

pH-metry (Table II)

Of the 47 patients, GER was severe in 7, moderate in 14, mild or absent in 26. A comparison of the pre- and postoperative score for each group revealed that each procedure significantly decreased the mean pH-metric score. A comparison of the postoperative score among the three groups revealed a significant decrease in the pH-metric score when the Nissen or Toupet was compared to the Lortat-Jacob repair.

Manometry (Table III)

The Nissen repair significantly improved all manometry parameters. The Toupet repair improved LES length and the Lortat-Jacob repair improved TEL. Only Nissen repair significantly decreased (LES-PIP). In a comparison of the postoperative score between the three groups, the sphincter tonicity was significantly increased in Nissen repair compared to the other repairs.

Discussion

After a 2-year follow-up, the Nissen repair seems to be the most effective in our patients as evaluated by: (1) the best Minaire's score (Table II); (2) the only repair improving all manometric parameters; (3) the best LES tonicity (Table III); and (4) the best clinical and endoscopic improvement. These results were obtained with a low rate of morbidity and minimal side effects (one mild dysphagia). We believe that the use of an indwelling #50 F bougie as a routine and exclusion of motility disorders are the reason for our low rate of dysphagia and inability to belch or vomit.[6] Although disappearance of esophagitis was not retained as a criterion of judgment because esophagitis was not required for inclusion in this study, one-half of the patients had esophagitis at the onset of the study. Only the Nissen

Table III
Net Change Between Pre- and Postmanometry (each patient is his own control)

	Nissen	Toupet	Lortat-Jacobs
Patients	18	16	13
LES tonicity (cm H₂O)	+11.1 ± 8.9***	+2.4 ± 10.8	−1.5 ± 5.2
LES length (cm)	+1.4 ± 1.2**	+1.6 ± 1.5**	+0.8 ± 1.4
Pre-TEL/ Post-TEL (cm)	+3.8 ± 3.6**	+1.5 ± 4.1	+4.3 ± 3.4**
LES-PIP (cm)	−1.5 ± 2.1*	−1.0 ± 1.7	−0.9 ± 3.0

* $p < 0.05$; ** $p < 0.01$; *** $p < 0.001$ (compared to preoperative scores); △ No statistical difference; △△ $p < 0.05$; LES = lower esophageal sphincter; PIP = pressure inversion point; Pre-TEL/Post-TEL = pre- to postoperative total esophageal length difference.

group did not show esophagitis at 2 years of follow-up, again suggesting the superiority of the procedure. Minaire's score[5] has been chosen because (1) it is able to express GER in a semiquantitative manner and to take in account the height of GER thereby giving an indication of esophageal clearance; (2) it has been previously studied in symptomatic patients showing a sensitivity of 0.86 and a specificity of 1.0;[7] and (3) the alternative study, the 3-hour Kaye's technique, was not available at that time in all centers.

In our study, no clear difference was shown among the three procedures by clinical evaluation. Abnormal pH-metric scores (moderate or severe) were not always associated with clinical recurrence. This clearly highlights the need to assess the antireflux procedures by objective criteria, not only on symptomatology.[8]

Based upon manometry, the Nissen repair is the only one that significantly ameliorates mechanical factors by acting on LES tonicity (i.e.: TEL, LES length, [LES-PIP]). More than the other procedures, the Nissen technique significantly increases LES tonicity. This seems to be a permanent feature of Nissen technique.[9] The manometric superiority of the Nissen repair in this study can be explained by the following: (1) a return to a durable normal sphincter pressure due to the mechanical effect of the 360° wrap; (2) a better intra-abdominal fixation of the LES as confirmed by the different scores measured. DeMeester found similar results when comparing the Nissen to the Hill and Belsey repairs.[1] Thus, it seems that a gastric wrap is needed to be effective against reflux.[1,5,6,8] Indeed, the Lortat-Jacob repair, which is more a procedure for reducing and fixing a hiatal hernia, does not optimally improve GER. The Toupet repair, which is said to have fewer side effects than the Nissen, has a risk of long-term clinical recurrence.[10] Therefore, we would recommend the Nissen fundoplication as the procedure of choice given the entrance criteria used in this trial. Long-term follow-up is still necessary to evaluate the late or long-term results of the Nissen antireflux procedure.[11] However, any new surgical, antireflux prospective study should include the Nissen repair as the procedure of comparison.

References

1. DeMeester TR, Johnson LF, Kent AH: Evaluation of current operations for the prevention of gastro-esophageal reflux. Ann Surg 180:511, 1974.
2. Nissen R: Gastropexy and fundoplication in surgical treatment of hiatus hernia. Am J Dig Dis 6:654, 1961.
3. Toupet A: Technique d'oesophago-gastroplastie avec phrénogastropéxie appliquée dans la cure radicale des hernies hiatales et comme complément de l'opération de Heller dans les cardiospasmes. Mem Acad Chir 89:394, 1963.
4. Lortat-Jacob JL, Robert F: Les malpositions cardio-tubérositaires. Arch Mal Dig 42:750, 1953.
5. Minaire Y: Reflux gastro-oesophagien: Mesure et sens de la mesure. Gastoenterol Clin Bio 4:519, 1980.
6. DeMeester TR, Bonavina L, Aldertucci M: Nissen fundoplication for gastro-esophageal reflux: Evaluation of primary repair in 100 consecutive patients. Ann Surg 204–209, 1986.
7. Baptiste P, Segol P: Rentabilité diagnostique de l'exploration fonctionnelle de l'oesophage dans le diagnostic du reflux gastro-oesophagien. Gastoenterol Clin Bio 3:586, 1979.
8. Russel COH, Hill LD: Gastro-esophageal reflux. In Current Problems in Surgery, Ravitch MM (ed), Chicago-London, Year Book Medical Publishers Inc, 1983, p 204.
9. Goodall RJR, Temple JG: Effect of Nissen fundoplication on competence of the gastro-esophageal function. Gut 21:607, 1980.
10. Galmiche JP, Teniere P, Ducrotte P, et al: Traitement du reflux gastro-

oesophagien acide par hémi-fundoplicature posterieure: Résultats cliniques et pHmétriques. Gastoenterol Clin Bio 7:385, 1983.

11. Brand DL, Eastwood IR, Martin D, et al: Esophageal symptoms, manometry and histology before and after antireflux surgery: A long-term follow-up study. Gastroenterology 76:1393, 1979.

23

Does Fundoplication Improve Pulmonary Function?
Results of a Prospective Clinical Study

M. Ruth, B. Bake, N. Sandberg, L. Olbe, Lars Lundell

Introduction

Respiratory disorders are common (10–63%) among subjects suffering from gastroesphageal reflux disease (GERD).[1,2] In a survey of 636 subjects, Urschel and Paulson[3] found cough to be the most common (47%) followed by bronchitis (35%), asthma and pneumonitis (16%). The nature of the putative association between respiratory tract diseases and GERD is not settled. Acid stimulation of the distal esophagus may provoke a reflex-mediated bronchoconstriction or an increase of airway responsiveness,[4–6] while aspiration of gastric contents may cause not only acute inflammatory conditions, but also chronic respiratory disease.[7,8] On the other hand, others have suggested GERD to have little or no influence on respiratory disease.[9,10]

Surgical and medical treatment of patients with GERD and chronic respiratory disease including asthma has, however, been reported to improve symptoms and even ameliorate the respiratory condition.[11–13] The aim of the present study was to examine the effect of restoration of the antireflux barrier, achieved by a fundoplication, on respiratory symptoms, bronchial hyperreactivity, and spirometric

Little AG, Ferguson MK, Skinner DB: Diseases of the Esophagus, Vol. II: Benign Diseases. Futura Publishing Company, Inc., Mount Kisco, NY, © 1990.

Table I
Demographic Data

No. of subjects	47
Male to female ratio	25:22
Age (mean, range)	57 (28–74)
Smokers/nonsmokers (n)	10:37
Respiratory disease:	
asthma	7
chronic bronchitis	4
recurrent bronchitis	8
pneumonitis	16
pleuritis	1
tuberculosis	1
Respiratory symptoms	
cough	10
dyspnea	18
wheezing	10
No. with Barrett's esophagus	6
No. with esophageal stricture	1

values in patients with severe gastroesophageal reflux disease, but otherwise nonselected with regard to respiratory disorders.

Materials and Methods

Forty-seven consecutive patients (22 females) with a mean age of 57 (range, 28–74) years, with gastroesophageal reflux disease, refractory to medical treatment were studied (Table I). The GERD diagnosis was established by symptom evaluation, endoscopy, and 24-hour pH measurements. A history of respiratory disease and symptoms was assessed in conjunction with a spirometry and a metacholine provocation test, which were performed preoperatively and one year after a transabdominal fundoplication either according to Toupet or to Rosetti.

24-Hour pH Monitoring

Twenty-four-hour pH monitoring was performed before and 6 months after the operation, mainly as described by Johnson and DeMeester.[14] A pH-electrode (Synectics no. 0011) was positioned 5 cm above the lower esophageal sphincter as located by an esophageal manometric motility examination. The pH data, obtained every 4th second, were stored in a digital memory (Synectics Digitrapper model 6000) carried in a belt.

The patients were ambulatory throughout the recording and instructed to follow a normal pattern of living throughout the study period. The pH data and the information given in the diary were evaluated manually as well as by computer. A reflux episode was defined to start at a drop of pH below 4 and to end when pH rose above 5. The number of reflux episodes, the duration of the longest episode, the number of reflux episodes lasting more than 5 minutes, and reflux time in minutes as well as percentage of the recording time were analyzed as total values for the entire 24-hour study period and according to their occurrence in supine or upright positions.

Endoscopy

Esophagogastroduodenoscopy was performed with a flexible endoscope (Olympus model GIF P10 or XQ10) preoperatively, and at 3 and 12 months postoperatively. The endoscopic findings were classified as described by Sandmark et al.[15]

Spirometry

The spirometry measured the vital capacity (VC), the forced expiratory flow volume in 1 second (FEV_1), the $FEV_{1.0}/VC$ ratio (FEV%), the maximum midexpiratory flow rate (MMEF), and the alveolar ventilation by the single-breath N_2-test. Bronchial hyperreactivity was assessed by means of a metacholine provocation test.[16]

The metacholine provocation, which was performed in noninfected patients with a FEV_1 of >65% of predicted value, started with an inhalation of 2 mL saline to determine the baseline FEV_1 whereafter metacholine in rising concentrations was inhaled. An interval of 5 minutes was allowed between the inhalations. When FEV_1 decreased 20% or more, the provocation was terminated.

Statistics and Ethics

In the statistical evaluation the Student's two tailed *t*-test for paired observations and the Chi-square test was used. Informed con-

Table II
Pre- and Postoperative 24-Hour pH-Values in the Distal
Esophagus of 47 Subjects Treated with Fundoplication

pH Variable	Position	Preoperative		Postoperative		Comparison of Pre- and Post-Treatment Values
		mean	SE	mean	SE	
% Time pH <4	upright	22	3	3	1	0.001
	supine	18	3	2	1	0.001
	total	20	3	2	1	0.001
Time pH <4,	upright	189	22	24	6	0.001
min.	supine	92	17	10	7	0.001
	total	281	37	34	12	0.001
No. of reflux	upright	96	16	17	4	0.001
episodes	supine	16	2	2	1	0.001
(pH <4)	total	111	17	19	5	0.001
No. of reflux	upright	7	1	1	0	0.001
episodes	supine	4	1	0	0	0.001
lasting >5	total	10	1	1	0	0.001
min.						
Duration of	upright	36	7	7	2	0.001
longest	supine	38	8	9	6	0.001
reflux	total	54	10	13	6	0.001

sent was obtained from each patient and the study was approved by the local ethics committee.

Results

The antireflux procedure effectively controlled the gastroesophageal reflux disease, with no difference between the two operative techniques (Table II). Endoscopic grading of the esophageal mucosa pre- and postoperatively is presented in Figure 1. A profound improvement of reflux symptoms was experienced postoperatively in all patients.

A slight postoperative decrease was recorded for all spirometric values, a decrease reaching statistical significance for VC ($p<0.05$) and $FEV_{1.0}$ ($p<0.01$) (Table III). Airway hyperreactivity as assessed by the metacholine test was registered preoperatively in five patients (14%) of which two had asthma and two had respiratory symptoms.

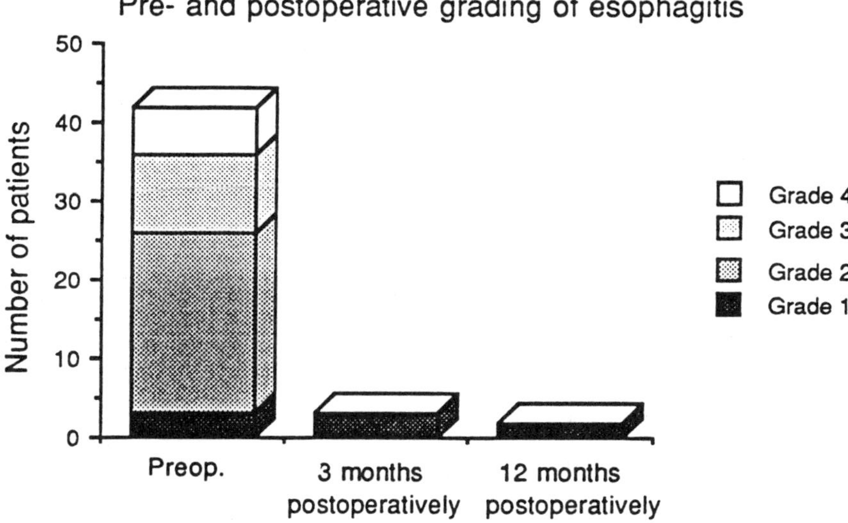

Figure 1: Endoscopic grading of the esophageal mucosa pre- and postoperatively.

Table III
Results of Spirometric Examination in 47 Subjects with GERD When Studied Preoperatively and One Year Postoperatively

	Preoperative		Postoperative		Comparison Between Pre- and Postop. Values
Airway Variable	mean	SE	mean	SE	p
VC (L)	4.1	0.1	4.0	0.1	0.0438
$FEV_{1.0}$ (L)	3.2	0.1	3.1	0.1	0.0069
FEV%	78.5	0.9	77.1	1.1	0.1538
MMEF (L)	3.1	0.2	2.9	0.2	0.4374
N_2-test ($\%N_2$/L)	1.3	0.1	1.0	0	0.5889

VC = vital capacity; $FEV_{1.0}$ = forced expiratory flow volume in one second; FEV% = $VC/FEV_{1.0}$; MMEF = maximum midexpiratory flow rate; N_2 test = slope of the alveolar plateau.

One year after the operation, only two (6%) patients reacted with a bronchospasm. The prevalence and severity of respiratory symptoms were not altered by the operation.

Patients with a history of chronic respiratory disease, asthma (n = 7) and chronic bronchitis (n = 4), as well as those with respiratory symptoms (n = 16) were also separately evaluated. Patients with respiratory symptoms had significantly lower pretreatment spirometry values ($FEV_{1.0}$, FEV%, and MMEF) than those with no history of respiratory disorders. A postoperative decrease was registered for all measured spirometric variables, reaching statistical significance for $FEV_{1.0}$ and VC as seen in Table IV. On the other hand, respiratory symptoms such as cough and dyspnea were significantly improved by the operation in the "symptom" group ($p < 0.05$).

Discussion

Respiratory symptoms and chronic respiratory disease are commonly encountered among patients with GERD and a causal relationship has been postulated. Medical antireflux therapy with alginic/antacid mixture, cisapride, and/or H_2-receptor antagonists has been alleged to improve respiratory symptoms.[11–13,17] The effect of therapy on respiratory tract function and/or hyperreactivity has, however, at best been of a moderate degree.[11,12] This discrepancy may be due to the incomplete control of the reflux of gastric contents into the esophagus, offered by the medical regimens so far used.[18] Surgery, however, is followed by a long-lasting and complete control of GERD and has been especially recommended in patients with airway disease and suspected aspiration.[19]

In the present study, we found a postoperative restrictive decrease in pulmonary function, an observation made also in patients with chronic respiratory disease or respiratory symptoms. These somewhat unexpected results may be due to a postoperative altered mobility of the diaphragm. The degree of change was, however, small (2–12%) and it deserves to be pointed out that a change of this magnitude is not likely to affect a healthy individual but might negatively influence a labile asthma.

Bronchial hyperreactivity was less frequently observed postoperatively and disappeared in two patients with a history of asthma. These results contrast to those of Sontag and co-workers,[20] who found no difference in the bronchial reactivity induced by metacholine in

Table IV
Preoperative and One Year Postoperative Spirometric Values in Subjects with Chronic Respiratory Disease (CRD) and Subjects with Respiratory Symptoms (RS)

Airway Variable	CRD (n = 7)		Difference Pre-Postop		Statistical Comparison	RS (n = 16)		Difference Pre-Postop		Statistical Comparison
	mean	SE	(L)	(%)	p	mean	SE	(L)	(%)	p
VC (L)	4.0	0.4	−0.3	−8	0.1177	3.9	0.2	−0.3	−7	0.0166
$FEV_{1.0}$ (L)	3.0	0.3	−0.2	−7	0.0205	2.9	0.1	−0.3	−10	0.029
FEV%	75.6	2.5	−0.3	0	0.1643	75.3	1.8	−0.7	−1	0.5657
MMEF (L)	3.2	0.3	−0.2	−6	0.2554	2.4	0.2	0	0	0.8834
N_2 ($\%N_2$/L)	1.7	0.3	−0.2	−12	0.433	1.6	0.2	−0.1	−6	0.1199

VC = vital capacity; $FEV_{1.0}$ = forced expiratory flow volume in one second; FEV% = VC/$FEV_{1.0}$; MMEF = maximum midexpiratory flow rate; N_2-test = slope of the alveolar plateau.

12 patients when tested preoperatively and 1 year postoperatively. These discrepancies are at present difficult to explain.

Several authors have reported favorable effects of surgical treatment both on respiratory symptoms and on the demand for medication.[3,19,21,22] The criteria for respiratory disease and treatment results, though, have in these studies often been a clinical evaluation only. Objective improvement of respiratory function after surgery has recently been demonstrated in adult asthmatics, but peak expiratory flow rate improved more than 10% in only three out of nine tested patients.[20] In the present prospective controlled study, a significant symptomatic improvement was experienced although no corresponding effects were seen in the objective functional parameters.

In conclusion, the present results would suggest that a general and close association between GERD and respiratory tract disease does not exist, at least when studied in an unselected population of patients with severe GERD.

References

1. Euler AR, Byrne WJ, Ament ME, Fonkalsrud EW, Strobel CT, Sheldon SG, Katz RM, Rachelefsky GS: Recurrent pulmonary disease in children: A complication of gastroesophageal reflux. Pediatrics 63:47, 1979.
2. Danus O, Casar C, Larrain A, Pope CE: Esophageal refllux: An unrecognized cause of recurrent obstructive bronchitis in children. J Pediatrics 89:220, 1976.
3. Urschel HC, Paulson DL: Gastroesophageal reflux and hiatal hernia. J Thorac Cardiovasc Surg 53:21, 1967.
4. Mansfield LE, Stein MR: Gastroesophageal reflux and asthma: A possible reflex mechanism. Ann Allergy 41:224, 1978.
5. Kjellén G, Tibbling L, Wranne B: Bronchial obstruction after oesophageal acid perfusion in asthmatics. Eur J Respir Dis 1:285, 1981.
6. Herve P, Denjean A, Jian R, Simonneau G, Duroux P: Intraesophageal perfusion of acid increases the bronchomotor response to metacholine and to isocapnic hyperventilation in asthmatic subjects. Am Rev Respir Dis 134:986, 1986.
7. Reich SB, Early WE, Ravin TH, Goodman M, Spector S, Stein MR: Evaluation of gastro-pulmonary aspiration by a radioactive technique: Concise communication. J Nucl Med 18:1079, 1977.
8. Boyle JT, Tuchman DN, Altschuler SM, Nixon TE, Pack AI, Cohen S: Mechanisms for the association of gastroesophageal reflux and bronchospasm. Am Rev Respir Dis 131:16, 1985.
9. Perpina M, Pellicier C, Marco V, Maldonado J, Ponce J: The significance of the reflux bronchoconstriction provoked by gastro-esophageal reflux in bronchial asthma. Eur J Resir Dis 66:91, 1985.

10. Ekström T: The importance of gastro-oesophageal reflux as a trigger factor in bronchial asthma. Linköping University Medical Dissertation, no. 278, Linköping, 1988.
11. Harper PC, Bergner A, Kaye MD: Antireflux treatment for asthma. Arch Intern Med 147:56, 1987.
12. Goodall RJR, Earis JE, Cooper DN, Bernstein A, Temple JG: Relationship between asthma and gastro-oesophageal reflux. Thorax 36:116, 1981.
13. Bengtsson U, Sandberg N, Bake B, Löwhagen O, Swedmyr N, Månsson I, Carlsson S: Gastro-oesophageal reflux and night time asthma. Lancet I:1501, 1985.
14. Johnson LF, DeMeester TR: Twenty-four hour pH monitoring of the distal esophagus. Am J Gastroenterol 62:325, 1974.
15. Sandmark S, Carlsson R, Fausa O, Lundell L: Omeprazole or ranitidine in the treatment of reflux esophagitis: Results of a double-blind, randomised, Scandinavian multicentre study. Scand J Gastroenterol 23(5):625, 1988.
16. Löwhagen O, Lindholm N: Short-term and long-term variation in bronchial response to histamine in asthmatic patients. Eur J Respir Dis 64:466, 1983.
17. Malfroot A, Vandenplas Y, Verlinden M, Piepsz A, Dab I: Gastroesophageal reflux and unexplained chronic respiratory disease in infants and children. Pediatr Pulmonol 3:208, 1987.
18. Ruth M, Enbom L, Lundell L, Lönroth H, Sandberg N, Sandmark S: The effect of omeprazole or ranitidine treatment on 24-hour esophageal acidity in patients with reflux esophagitis. Scand J Gastroenterol 23:1141, 1988.
19. Pellegrini CA, DeMeester TR, Johnson LF, Skinner DB: Gastroesophageal reflux and pulmonary aspiration: Incidence, functional abnormality, and results of surgical therapy. Surgery 86:110, 1979.
20. Sontag S, O'Connell S, Greenlee H, Schnell T, Chintam R, Nemchausky B, Chejfec G, Van Drunen M, Wanner J: Is gastroesophageal reflux a factor in some asthmatics? Am J Gastroenterol 82(2):119, 1987.
21. Overholt RH, Ashraf MM: Esophageal reflux as a trigger in asthma. NY State J Med 66:3030, 1966.
22. Lomasney TL: Hiatus hernia and the respiratory tract. Ann Thorac Surg 24(5):448, 1977.

24

Incidence and Clinical Relevance of Postfundoplication Vagal Nerve Damage

Joost M. L. M. Horbach, E. H. Jansen,
J. B. M. J. Jansen, H. G. Gooszen,
C. B. H. W. Lamers

Introduction

With the increasing success of medical treatment for reflux eso-phagitis, a distinct decline in the number of antireflux operations is reported. Not only is the number of operations performed decreasing, but with the success of H_2-receptor antagonists and especially ome-prazole, the results operation should attain in comparison with med-ical treatment are more critically evaluated. Success rates of operations should reach about 90% and morbidity should be negligible.

Vagal nerve damage is a well-known complication of antireflux surgery but the incidence is unknown since a sensitive and specific test to diagnose vagal nerve damage, with or without symptoms, has not been available until recently. The pancreatic polypeptide (PP) stimulation test seems to be such a sensitive and specific test. It is based on the knowledge that PP is secreted by the pancreas after

Little AG, Ferguson MK, Skinner DB: Diseases of the Esophagus, Vol. II: Benign Dis-eases. Futura Publishing Company, Inc., Mount Kisco, NY, © 1990.

stimulation of the vagal nerve by, for instance, insulin-induced hypoglycemia. After induction of hypoglycemia (blood sugar below 2.5 mMol/L), a rapid and distinct rise in plasma PP levels is observed. Truncal vagotomy and atropine almost completely abolish the PP response.[1,2] We have performed the PP stimulation test in different groups of patients to learn about the incidence of vagal nerve damage after fundoplication.

Patient Material

Three different patient groups were studied. The first group included nine patients with documented gastroesophageal reflux disease (five men, four women; median age 52, ranging from 21 to 77 years). Clinical symptoms were objictified with endoscopy and 24-hour pH monitoring. The second group included twenty-four patients who had undergone a Nissen repair for reflux esophagitis (14 men, 10 women; median age, 52, ranging from 29 to 87 years). The third group of six patients had undergone truncal vagotomy as part of different surgical procedures (one men, five women; median age 45, ranging from 28 to 75 years) and served as a control group for complete vagotomy. The patients with Nissen fundoplication and those with truncal vagotomy did not come to our attention because of postoperative symptoms but were randomly selected. In addition, 20 healthy volunteers were investigated to serve as a normal control group. All individuals were subjected to insulin-induced hypoglycemia after a 12-hour fast. Hypoglycemia was called "adequate" with plasma glucose levels below 2.5 mMol/L. Before and up to 90 minutes after hypoglycemia registration, blood samples were drawn for the determination of plasma PP levels. Plasma PP was determined by a sensitive and specific radioimmunoassay.[3] Test results (median and range) are described in basal PP concentration, in peak and in incremental (peak-basal concentration) PP response. Statistical analyses were done by the Wilcoxon test for unpaired observations and by the Chi-square test. The study was approved by the local ethics committees.

Results

As shown in Figure 1, basal plasma PP concentrations in the patients with Nissen fundoplication (24, 9–259 pM) were not signif-

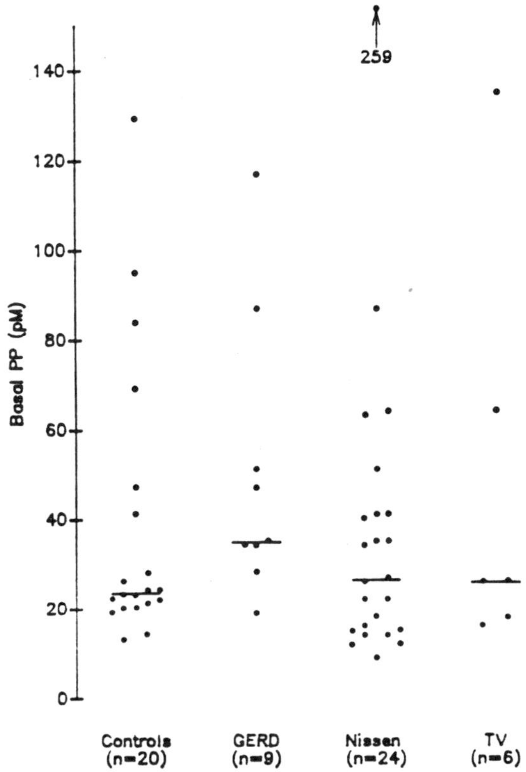

Figure 1: Basal plasma pancreatic polypeptide (PP) concentrations in 20 normal subjects, in 9 unoperated patients with gastroesophageal reflux disease (GERD), in 24 patients with previous Nissen fundoplication and in 6 patients with truncal vagotomy (TV). Reprinted from Scand J Gastroenterol with permission of the authors.

icantly different from the results in the patients with gastroesophageal reflux disease (35, 19–117 pM) and the normal subjects (24, 13–129 pM). In addition, basal plasma PP concentrations did not differ from those in the patients with previous truncal vagotomy (26, 16–135 pM).

Peak plasma PP concentrations in the patients with Nissen fundoplication (210, 10–1215 pM) were slightly ($p = 0.07$) lower than in normal control subjects (281, 135–750 pM, Fig. 2). Patients with gastroesophageal reflux disease had peak plasma PP responses (168, 137–940 pM) that were not significantly different from those in the normal subjects. As expected, patients with truncal vagotomy (44, 20–116

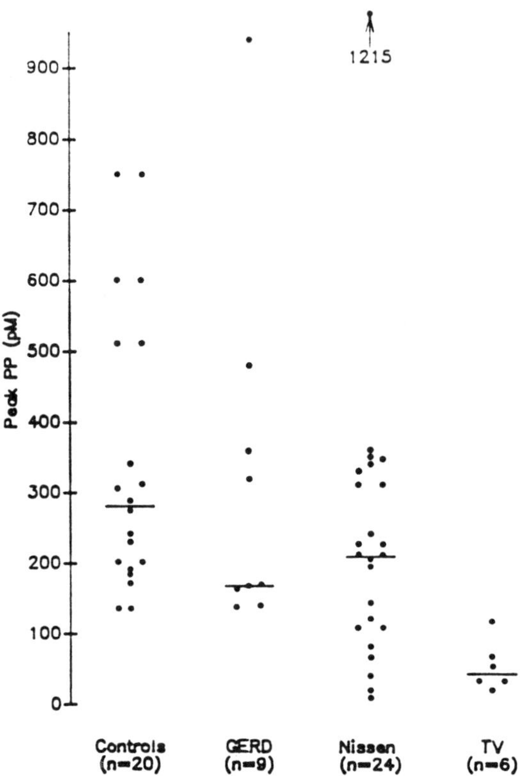

Figure 2: Peak plasma pancreatic polypeptide (PP) concentrations in response to insulin hypoglycemia in 20 normal subjects, in 9 unoperated patients with gastroesophageal reflux disease (GERD), in 24 patients with previous Nissen fundoplication, and in 6 patients with truncal vagotomy (TV). Reprinted from Scand J Gastroenterol with permission of the authors.

pM) had significantly (p<0.001) decreased peak plasma PP levels after insulin hypoglycemia. Abnormally low peak plasma PP concentrations were found in 8/24 (33%) of the patients with Nissen fundoplication (p<0.05), in all six (100%) with truncal vagotomy (p<0.001), and in none of the unoperated patients with gastroesophageal reflux disease.

As shown in Figure 3, plasma PP increments induced by insulin hypoglycemia were slightly lower (p = 0.08) in the patients with Nissen fundoplication (174, 0–956 pM) than in the normal subjects (209, 94–730 pM). Plasma PP increments in the unoperated patients with

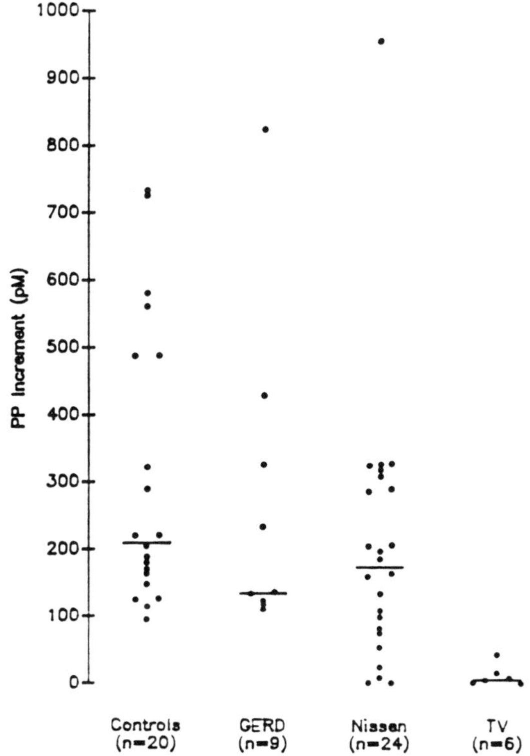

Figure 3: Plasma pancreatic polypeptide (PP) increments in response to insulin hypoglycemia in 20 normal subjects, in 9 unoperated patients with gastroesophageal reflux disease (GERD), in 24 patients with previous Nissen fundoplication, and in 6 patients with truncal vagotomy (TV). Reprinted from Scand J Gastroenterol with permission of the authors.

severe gastroesophageal reflux disease (134, 109–823 pM) were not different from normal, while the results in the patients with truncal vagotomy (6, 0–41 pM) were significantly ($p < 0.001$) decreased. Abnormally low plasma PP increments were found in 5/24 (21%) of patients with Nissen fundoplication ($p < 0.05$), in all six of those with truncal vagotomy ($p < 0.001$), but in none of the patients with gastroesophageal reflux disease.

From the data obtained in the control group, it was decided that an incremental PP response of over 100 pM should be called "normal." A PP response ranging from 40 to 100 pM was described as "intermediately disturbed" and a response of below 40 pM was considered to reflect complete vagotomy. After Nissen fundoplication, an intermediately disturbed PP response was observed in five patients (21%), and in four patients (17%) complete vagotomy must have taken place according to the above-mentioned criteria.

Discussion

The reason to conduct this study was in fact fourfold. We wanted to assess the incidence of vagal nerve damage, to gain more insight into postoperative morbidity and its potential cause(s), to get more data on the mode of action of antireflux surgery, and to re-assess the rationale of adding some type of vagotomy to the fundoplication.

The incidence of vagal nerve damage in the group of patients that were studied depends on the criteria used in interpretation of the PP data. Based on the data obtained in the group of patients who had undergone truncal vagotomy of some sort, with a mean incremental PP response of 6 pM ranging from 0 to 41 pM, we conclude that the Nissen fundoplication leads to complete vagotomy in 21% of patients. In 17%, a so-called "intermediately disturbed" PP response was observed. It is currently unknown what these data mean in terms of vagal nerve damage. We learned from experimental work[4] that cholinergic vagal innervation to the pancreas runs a long at least two different routes, i.e., along the anterior vagal trunk and along the posterior vagal trunk after connection with celiac and superior mesenteric ganglia. We hypothesize that in case of intermediately disturbed PP response, either the anterior or the posterior vagal nerve bundle is accidentally injured at operation. Further prospective studies, however, are needed to prove this hypothesis.

The question arises of whether the risk of vagal nerve damage is even higher in patients who have to undergo reoperation for recurrence of gastroesophageal reflux disease after previous fundoplication. Considering the difficulties that are encountered in reoperation, this is not unlikely, and our preliminary data in a group of 18 patients who were subjected to a PP stimulation test after reoperation support this contention. In five patients an intermediately disturbed PP peak response was found and eight had complete vagotomy. Since no preoperative data are available in this group, it is uncertain whether damage to the vagal nerve was inflicted during the first or the second operation (unpublished observations).

Regarding postoperative morbidity, we learned from our own clinical experience that epigastric fullness, sometimes referred to as the "gas bloat" syndrome, is observed in a distinct percentage of patients. Such symptoms may be the result of partial vagal nerve damage and are probably not necessarily an effect of a tight fundoplication. Symptoms of epigastric fullness or delayed gastric emptying do tend to improve with time and maybe neuropraxy at operation with restoration of function within 3 to 6 months can serve as an explanation for these temporary symptoms.

What do our PP data add to the knowledge of the mode of action of antireflux surgery? DeMeester has done important studies with mechanical models to define the criteria that antireflux surgery should fulfill to act as an adequate barrier to potential reflux.[5-7] The data of the effect of different types of operation on LES pressure are contradictory and it seems that elevation of LES pressure is not a prerequisite for successful antireflux surgery. From the PP response data we obtained, it can tentatively be concluded that success can be attained by a combination of fundoplication with an inadvertently performed partial or even truncal vagotomy even if the LES pressure is not raised by the fundoplication performed.

The role of additional vagotomy and highly selective vagotomy (HSV), in particular, has been criticized in the last decade because of lack of success of antacid administration on reflux esophagitis. With the impressive results of complete blockage of gastric acid secretion on reflux esophagitis and symptoms, renewed interest on reduction of acid secretion seems justified. HSV, however, only leads to a 60% or 70% reduction in acid secretion and is therefore inferior to omeprazole in regard to gastric acid inhibition.

Although these recent data suggest that the combination of fundoplication and HSV to treat reflux esophagitis may be worthwhile, the addition of HSV is by no means a reason to compromise the quality of the fundoplication.

In conclusion, accidental vagotomy seems to be far more common than reported in the literature so far. It has to be sorted out in prospective studies whether partial or complete vagal nerve damage adds to the efficacy of fundoplication or is a major cause of postoperative upper gastrointestinal symptoms.

ACKNOWLEDGMENT: The authors thank Ms. JFN Visser for typing the manuscript.

References

1. Taylor IL, Walsh JH, Carter D, Wood J, Grossman MI: Effect of atropine and bethanechol on bombesin-stimulated release of pancreatic polypeptide and gastrin in dogs. Gastroenterology 77:714–718, 1979.
2. Jonung M, Jonung T, Chen MH, Murphy RF, Joffe SN: Effect of extragastric vagotomy on pancreatic polypeptide in dogs. Digestion 29:103–106, 1984.
3. Lamers CBHW, Kiemel JM, Van Leer E, Van Lensen R, Peetoom J: Mechanisms of elevated serum: Pancreatic polypeptide concentrations in chronic renal failure. J Clin Endocrinol Metab 55:922–926, 1982.
4. Guicherit OR, Gooszen HG, Jansen JBMJ, Van der Burg MPM, Frölich M, Lamers CBHW: Effects of extrinsic denervation and duodenal transection on pancreatic polypeptide response patterns from the right lobe of the canine pancreas: A model for complete pancreatic denervation. Digestion 40(2):83–84, 1988.
5. DeMeester TR, Wernly JA, Bryant GH, et al: Clinical and in vitro analysis of gastroesophageal competence: A study of the principles of antireflux surgery. Am J Surg 137:39, 1979.
6. O'Sullivan GC, DeMeester TR, Joelsson BE, et al: The interaction of the lower esophageal sphincter pressure and length of sphincter in the abdomen as determinants of gastroesophageal competence. Am J Surg 143:40, 1982.
7. Bonavin L, Evander A, DeMeester TR, et al: Length of the distal esophageal sphincter and competency of the cardia. Am J Surg 151:25, 1986.

25

Delayed Vagotomy in Total Duodenal Bypass

Michel J. Noirclerc, A. Caamano, L. Durif, P. Alziar, P. Campan, B. Dupin

Total duodenal bypass consisting of antrectomy with Roux-en-Y anastomosis (ARYA) is gaining in popularity for the treatment of complicated esophageal reflux. Although this procedure compares favorably with fundoplication or resection,[1-3] with regard to reflux control, it leads to unwanted iatrogenic complications, namely stomal ulcer (SU) and gastric emptying disorders (GED).

Vagotomy has been implicated in this problem. While it prevents SU, it is probably a major cause of GED. The incidence of SU, which is easy to treat, is not greater than GED, which is difficult to control. In most cases in our series, vagotomy was not usually performed at the same time as ARYA. The results suggest that delaying vagotomy may be a good policy to adopt.

Materials and Methods

Between 1977 and 1987, 21 ARYA procedures were performed by the same surgical group. Indications are listed in Table I. In 14 cases, ARYA was the primary treatment. The operative technique was as follows (Fig. 1, 2, and 3A,B): conservative antrectomy closing the pylorus with staples; creation of a 60-cm Roux-en-Y loop; side-to-side

Little AG, Ferguson MK, Skinner DB: Diseases of the Esophagus, Vol. II: Benign Diseases. Futura Publishing Company, Inc., Mount Kisco, NY, © 1990.

Table I
Antrectomy with Roux-en-Y Anastomosis: 21 Cases

Alkaline GER–Brachyesophagus–Scleroderma	7
Postop GER	3
Peptic Stenosis	2
GER + Causal Antral Stenosis (Primary 14, Secondary 7)	9

GER = gastric emptying disorders

---

or side-to-end gastrojejunal anastomosis at the lowest point of the stomach. Vagotomy was performed in only four cases (once by the abdominal route and three times by the thoracic route).

Results

Immediate

No patient died as a result of the operation. No transit disorders were noted in the 17 patients who did not undergo vagotomy. On the other hand, acute gastric dilatation requiring reoperation occurred in two of the four patients who underwent vagotomy.

Late

SU occurred in three patients who did not undergo vagotomy. In these cases, transthoracic vagotomy was performed between 3 months and 1 year after ARYA. One patient who underwent immediate vagotomy presented with persistent GED requiring reoperation.

Follow-Up

At 1 year after surgery, 19 patients were re-examined. Of these, four had undergone vagotomy and 15 had not. All were classified Visick I or II.

Comments

Concomitant vagotomy with ARYA is widely recommended to prevent SU.[4] In some cases, however, vagotomy is difficult and haz-

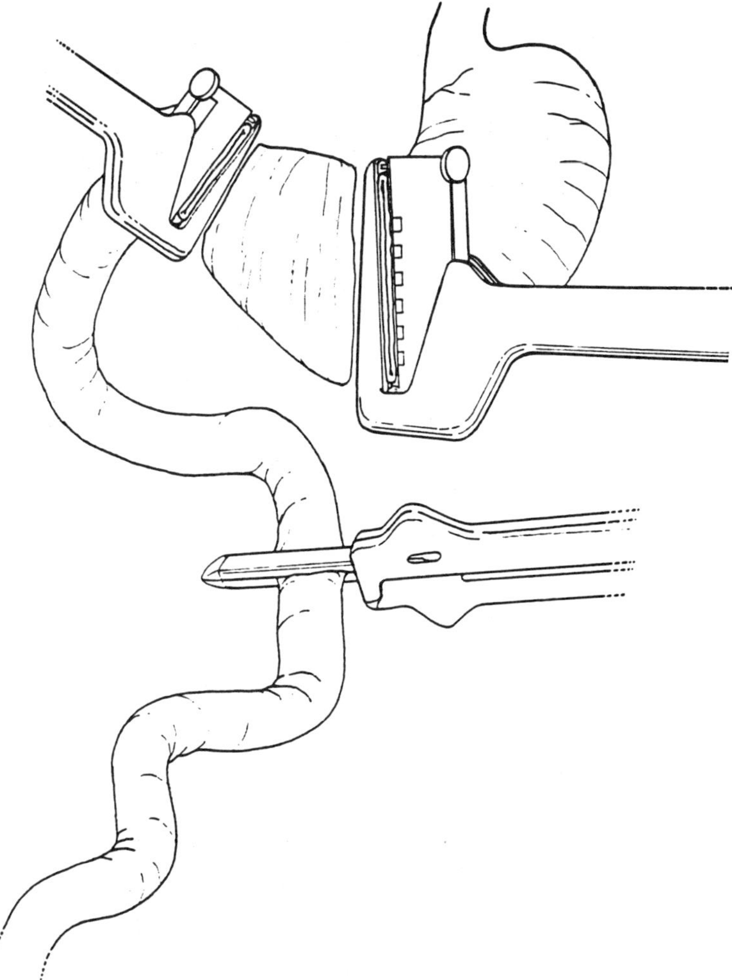

Figure 1: Cross-sectional views of the antrum and jejunum.

ardous to perform. For safety reasons, the thoracic route should be used for patients who have undergone previous hiatus surgery. This considerably lengthens the duration of surgery. In fact, perusal of the literature reveals that SU is far from being a systematic complication in patients who did not undergo vagotomy[2,3,5,6] (Table II). Furthermore, in most cases SU can be successfully treated using antisecretory

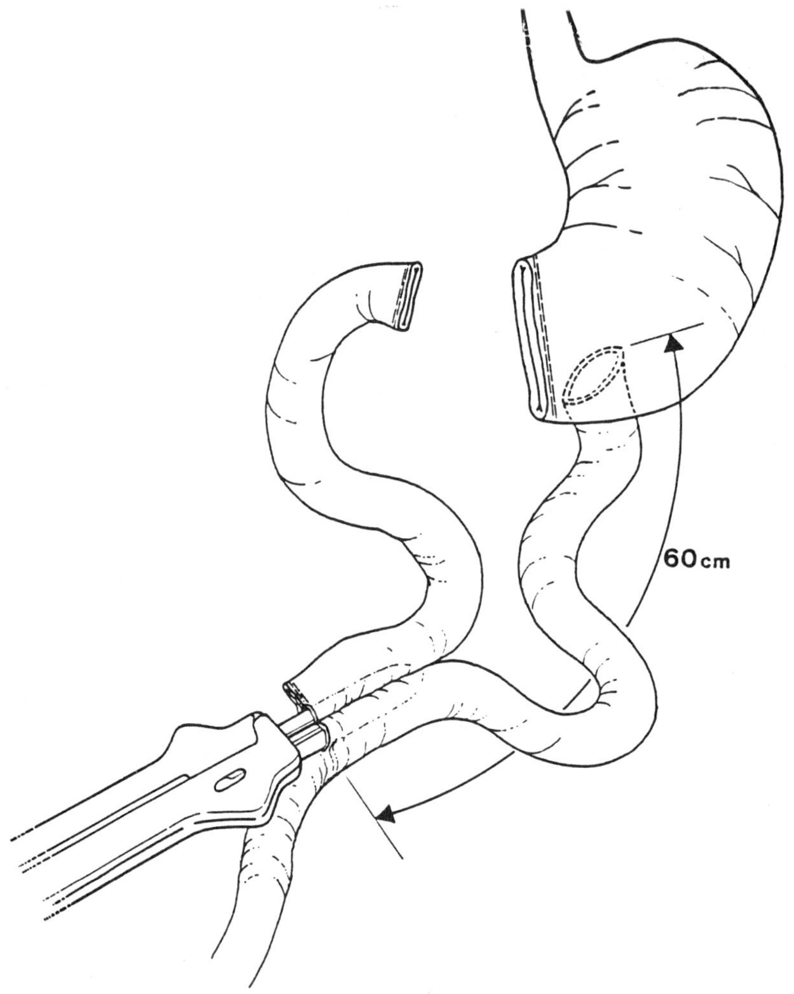

Figure 2: Roux-en-Y loop.

agents and antacids.[2] If therapy fails, transthoracic vagotomy can be used as a simple and definitive solution to the problem.

GED is a more frequent complication[3,5-8] (Table III). In some cases it is due to acute postoperative gastric dilatation[9] or to chronic dysfunction. With prolonged parenteral nutrition and aspiration, these problems usually reverse spontaneously within 2 to 4 weeks.

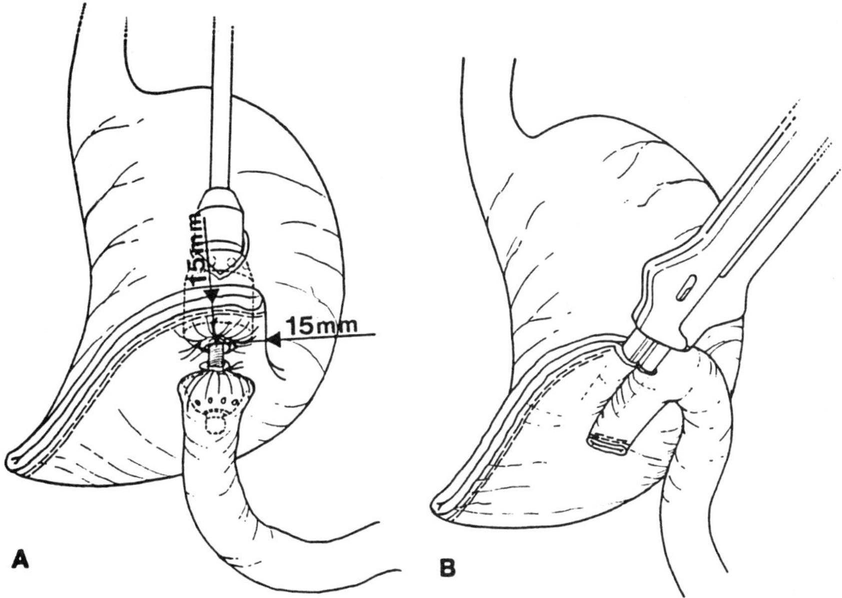

Figure 3A,B: Side-to-side or end anastomosis of the jejunum to the lowest point of the stomach.

In some cases, however, these problems lead to a severe condition not susceptible to drug therapy and require radical gastric resection.[10]

The mechanism underlying GED in these cases is poorly understood. Besides misfashioning in the creation of the anastomosis (one case in our series), another possibility is the Roux-en-Y loop dismotility. It has often been implicated either because of the bypass in relation to the duodenal "pacemaker"[11–13] or because of its excessive

Table II
Antrectomy with Roux-en-Y Anastomosis (ARYA)
Anastomotic Ulcer: Incidence (ARYA Without Vagotomy)

Viard	Lyon Chir	1988	1/6
Perniceni	Br J Surg	1988	3/7
Washer	Ann R Coll Surg Engl	1986	4/24
Britton	Br J Surg	1987	0/12
Noirclerc		1989	3/17

Table III
Antrectomy with Roux-en-Y Anastomosis Gastric Emptying Disorders: Incidence

				Reoperations
Perniceni	Br J Surg	1988	5/59 (9%)	1
Boulez	Lyon Chir	1988	3/17 (18%)	1
Viard	Lyon Chir	1988	5/23 (22%)	2
Gustavsson	Am J Surg	1988	49/163 (30%)	?
Britton	Br J Surg	1987	32/48 (67%)	?
Noirclerc		1989	3/21 (14%)	3

length.[8] However, the fact that good results can be obtained by re-gastrectomy without modification of the Roux-en-Y loop contradicts this hypothesis.

The role of vagotomy is controversial. Experimental findings differ according to the methodology used.[11,15–17] Clinical and scintigraphic studies show stasis to originate in the stomach.[14] It can be speculated that leaving the vagus nerves intact preserves gastric motility especially since the volume of remaining stomach is larger. GED was not observed in any of our patients after conservative antrectomy without vagotomy. In our opinion, performing a more extensive gastrectomy is an excessive alternative to vagotomy.[5,18]

Conclusion

Total duodenal bypass for complicated esophageal reflux raises a problem with regard to vagotomy. Vagotomy exposes the patient to the risk of severe and intractable postoperative GED. Not performing vagotomy exposes the patient to the risk of SU which is often susceptible to medication and always curable by transthoracic vagotomy.

In view of the findings described here, we propose the following policy:

- achieve total duodenal bypass by conservative antrectomy without vagotomy;
- systematically administer anti-H_2 and antacids postoperatively;

- carry out endoscopic inspections after the first, second, and third months;
- perform transthoracic vagotomy after the third month in case of persistent stomal ulcer.

References

1. Washer GF, Gear MWL, Dowling BL, Gillison EW, Royston CMS, Spencer J: Randomized prospective trial of Roux-en-Y duodenal diversion versus fundoplication for severe reflux oesophagitis. Br J Surg 71:181–184, 1984.
2. Washer GF, Gear MWL, Dowling BL, Gillison EW, Royston CMS, Spencer J: Duodenal diversion with vagotomy and antrectomy for severe or recurrent reflux and esophagitis stricture: An alternative to the operation of the hiatus. Ann R Coll Surg Engl 68:222–226, 1986.
3. Perniceni T, Gayet B, Fekete F: Total duodenal diversion in the treatment of complicated peptic oesophagitis. Br J Surg 75:1108–1111, 1988.
4. Fekete F, Hugentobler JP, Breil P: Place de la diversion duodenale totale dans le traitement de l'oesophagite peptique. In: Actualities chirurgicales, Masson Edit., Paris, 1983, p 82–89.
5. Viard H, Fraisse J, Bernard A, Haas O: La diversion duodenale dans le traitement de l'oesophagite peptique. Lyon Chir 84:405–406, 1988.
6. Britton JP, Johnston D, Ward C, Axon ATR, Barker MCJ: Gastric emptying and clinical outcome after Roux-en-Y diversion. Br J Surg 74:900–904, 1987.
7. Boulez J, Beaune B, Chabal J: Bilan de la diversion duodenale totale dans le traitement du reflux oesophagien. Lyon Chir 84:411–413, 1988.
8. Gustavsson S, Ilstrup DM, Morrison P, Kelly KA: Roux-Y stasis syndrome after gastrectomy. Am J Surg 155:490–494, 1988.
9. Jebira A, Benamor N, Ayachi K, Benyounes MA, Gargouri MA, Fourati M: La diversion duodenale totale (a propos de 4 cas). Med Chir Dig 15:559–562, 1986.
10. Vogel SB, Woodward ER: The surgical treatment of chronic gastric atony following Roux-Y diversion for alkaline reflux gastritis. Ann Surg 209:756–763, 1989.
11. Vogel SB, Brock Vair D, Woodward ER: Alterations in gastro intestinal emptying of 99m-technetium-labeled solids following sequential antrectomy, truncal vagotomy and Roux-Y gastroenterostomy. Ann Surg 198:506–515, 1983.
12. Mathias JM, Fernandez A, Sninsky CA, Clench MH, Davis RH: Nausea, vomiting and abdominal pain after Roux-en-Y anastomosis: Motility of the jejunal limb. Gastroenterology 88:101–107, 1985.
13. Perino LE, Adcock KA, Goff JS: Gastro intestinal symptoms, motility and transit after the Roux-en-Y operation. Am J Gastroenterol 83:380–385, 1988.
14. Hinder RA, Esser J, DeMeester TR: Management of gastric emptying disorders following the Roux-en-Y procedure. Surgery 104:765–772, 1988.

15. Hocking MP, Vogel SB, Falasca CA, Woodward ER: Delayed gastric emptying of liquids and solids following Roux-en-Y billiary diversion. Ann Surg 194:494–501, 1981.
16. Hocking MP, Brunson ME, Vogel SB: Effect of various prokinetic agents on post Roux-en-Y gastric emptying experimental and clinical observations. Dig Dis Sci 33:1282–1287, 1988.
17. Yamagishi T, Debas HT: Control of gastric emptying: Interaction of the vagus and pyloric antrum. Ann Surg 187:91–94, 1978.
18. Hollender LF, Meyer CH, Marrie A, Keller D, Zeyer B, Goldschmidt P: La place de la fundo-jejunostomie sur anse exclue en y dans les echecs therapeutiques chirurgicaux du reflux gastro-oesophagien. Chirurgie 107:139–145, 1981.

III.

Barrett's Esophagus:
Editors' Overview

Chapter 26 provides results from a long-term and careful analysis of a large group of patients with Barrett's esophagus diagnosed at the Mayo Clinic between 1972 and 1988. The data show that the length of columnar mucosa in these patients tends to remain stable over many years, whether or not endoscopic esophagitis is present. In other words, neither upward progression nor downward regression are usually seen. The author interprets this study to suggest that the columnar epithelium is acquired from gastroesophageal reflux but remains stable after initial development. An alternative hypothesis is that Barrett's esophagus, when it is defined as a significant extension of columnar mucosa upwards in the esophagus, may be of congenital origin.

Chapter 27 addresses the difficult problem of long-term follow-up and surveillance of patients with Barrett's mucosa, a premalignant condition. This study suggests that analysis of nucleolar organizer region proteins, loops of DNA encoded for RNA, can be used to differentiate between dysplasia associated with carcinoma and dysplasia that is not associated with carcinoma. If this type of analysis truly provides the ability to differentiate malignant from nonmalignant dysplasia, it would be of tremendous aid in follow-up of these patients.

26

A Follow-Up Study of Barrett's Esophagus:
Does the Length of Columnar Mucosa Progress or Regress?

Alan J. Cameron

Introduction

In Barrett's esophagus, the normal squamous epithelial lining of the lower esophagus is replaced by columnar mucosa. This condition is thought to be acquired, and is associated with severe gastroesophageal reflux.[1] Patients with Barrett's esophagus often have esophagitis, inflammation, and ulceration seen immediately above the columnar-lined segment.[2] It has been proposed that reflux esophagitis causes destruction of the squamous mucosa and that, in the presence of continuing reflux, the ulcerated area may be re-epithelialized by cells that differentiate to form the columnar mucosa of Barrett's esophagus.[3] In a few reported cases, the level of the junction between squamous and columnar mucosa has been found to ascend the esophagus over a period of years.[4–6] Naef et al.[7] therefore suggested that "the pathogenesis could be clearly defined by following the progressive replacement of the squamous mucosa by columnar epithelium."

The aim of the present study was to find whether, in the presence of continuing esophagitis, the length of columnar mucosa in Barrett's

Little AG, Ferguson MK, Skinner DB: Diseases of the Esophagus, Vol. II: Benign Diseases. Futura Publishing Company, Inc., Mount Kisco, NY, © 1990.

BARRETT'S ESOPHAGUS
Length of Follow-Up

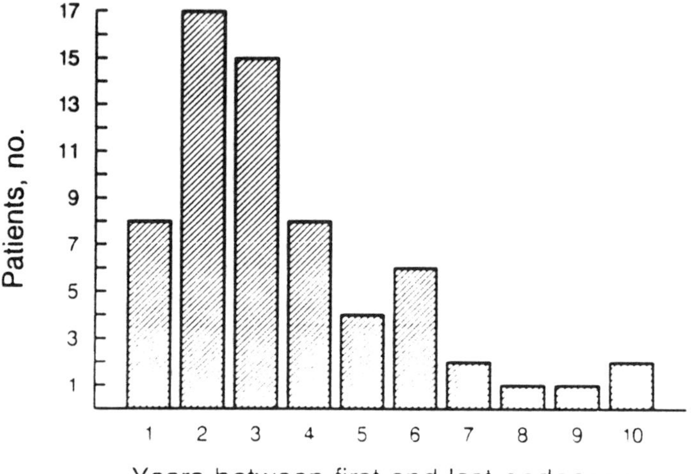

Figure 1: See text.

esophagus did indeed progress. Also, because of the known association of Barrett's esophagus with adenocarcinoma, evidence of regression of columnar mucosa when esophagitis was not present was sought.

Methods

Mayo Clinic records were searched for cases of Barrett's esophagus diagnosed between 1972 and 1988. The diagnosis was accepted if the squamous-columnar junction was seen at endoscopy 3 cm or more above the lower end of the esophagus, together with biopsy proof of columnar mucosa in the lower esophagus. Cases were included in the present report if they had at least two endoscopic examinations, one year or more apart, the length of columnar mucosa being recorded on each examination. Esophagitis was defined as any type of inflammation, erosions, or ulceration noted on endoscopy at the junction of squamous and columnar epithelium. This definition excluded localized ulcers surrounded by columnar mucosa. Patients

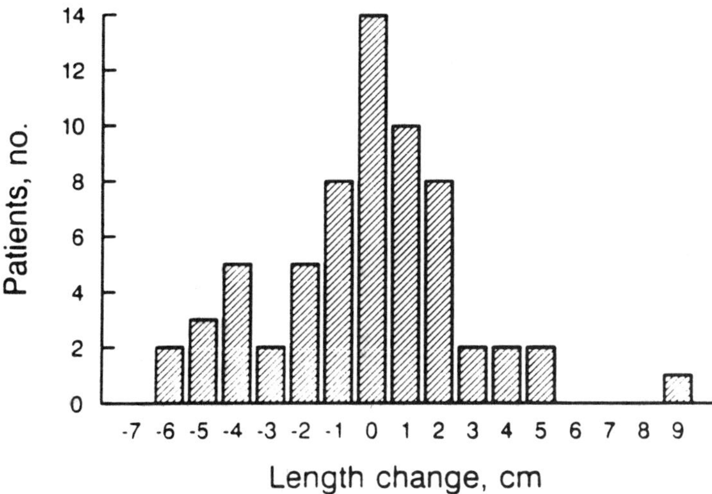

Figure 2: See text.

were usually managed with dietary and postural advice, antacids, and H_2-receptor antagonists; omeprazole was not given. Patients having antireflux surgery were excluded from this report.

Results

A total of 64 patients fulfilled the entry criteria for this study (46 men and 18 women). The mean interval between the first and last endoscopic examinations was 3.5 years (Fig. 1).

The changes in recorded length of columnar mucosa between the first and final examinations are shown in Figure 2. The length appeared to increase in 25 patients, to decrease in 25 patients, and to remain unchanged in 14 patients. However, small changes in recorded length may be due to observer error; in 70% of patients the difference in length was 2 cm or less.

In 14 of these patients, endoscopic evidence of esophagitis was

BARRETT'S ESOPHAGUS
Change in Length of Columnar Mucosa: Patients With Persisting Esophagitis

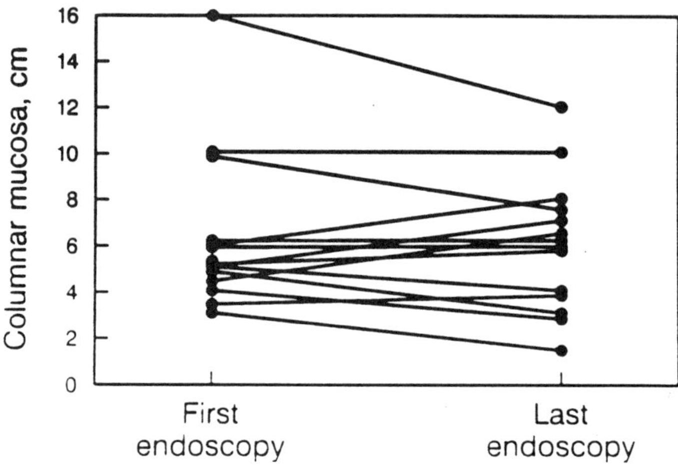

Figure 3: See text.

seen on the first and on the final endoscopic examinations and on any intermediate examinations that were performed. Their mean age was 62.1 years and the mean interval between first and last examinations was 2.9 years. Continuing inflammation was not associated with any trend toward upward extension of the Barrett's esophagus, the mean initial length of columnar mucosa being 6.4 cm and mean final length being 6.0 cm (Fig. 3).

Table I
Barrett's Esophagus: Length of Columnar Mucosa in Different Age Groups

Patients age, years	40–49	50–59	60–69	70–79	80–89
n	9	10	33	9	3
Mean length, cm	8.2	7.4	7.3	6.2	6.0

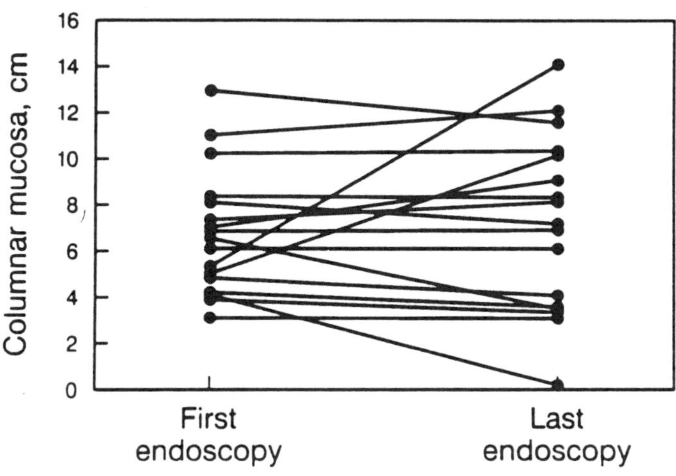

Figure 4: See text.

In 17 patients there was no sign of esophagitis on any endoscopic examination. Their mean age was 62.3 years and the mean interval between first and last endoscopies was 2.6 years. No trend towards regression of columnar mucosa was seen, the mean initial length being 6.7 cm and mean final length being 7.0 cm (Fig. 4).

These findings indicate that the length of columnar mucosa remained stable over a few years, but the possibility remains that changes evolve gradually over a longer time span. If this is so, and Barrett's esophagus is an acquired disorder, then the length of columnar mucosa might be expected to increase with age. This was found not to be the case (Table I), there being instead a slight trend towards shorter lengths of columnar mucosa in older patients. This trend does not necessarily indicate regression of columnar mucosa; an alternative explanation is reduced apparent length of the esophagus due to enlargement of diaphragmatic hernias and the development of kyphosis in the elderly.

Discussion

The information presented is not consistent with the belief that columnar mucosa gradually extends upwards, replacing damaged squamous epithelium. It seems more likely that the development of Barrett's esophagus is a fairly rapid event, with relative stability of the length of columnar mucosa in subsequent years, whether esophagitis continues or not. A possible sequence of events that is consistent with this new data is as follows. Esophageal reflux might damage the squamous mucosa at the gastroesophageal junction. A length of several centimeters of squamous mucosa might then become detached. Because continuing acid reflux prevents squamous regeneration, the denuded area is then covered by newly formed columnar mucosa, which persists.

References

1. Iascone C, DeMeester TR, Little AG, Skinner DB: Barrett's esophagus: Functional assessment, proposed pathogenesis, and surgical therapy. Arch Surg 118:543, 1983.
2. Naef AP, Savary M: Conservative operations for peptic esophagitis with stenosis in columnar-lined lower esophagus. Ann Thorac Surg 13:543, 1972.
3. Spechler SJ, Goyal RK: Barrett's esophagus. N Engl J Med 315:362, 1986.
4. Goldman MC, Beckman RC: Barrett syndrome: Case report with discussion about concepts of pathogenesis. Gastroenterology 39:104, 1960.
5. Mossberg SM: The columnar-lined esophagus (Barrett's syndrome): An acquired condition? Gastroenterology 50:671, 1966.
6. Borrie J, Goldwater L: Columnar-lined esophagus. Assessment of etiology and treatment: A 22-year experience. J Thorac Cardiovasc Surg 71:825, 01976.
7. Naef AP, Savary M, Ozzello L: Columnar-lined lower esophagus: An acquired lesion with malignant predisposition: Report on 140 cases of Barrett's esophagus with 12 adenocarcinomas. J Thorac Cardiovasc Surg 70:826, 1975.

27

Nucleolar Organizer Regions in Endoscopic Surveillance of Barrett's Esophagus

R.C. Stuart, N. Nolan, T.F. Gorey, P. Gillen, P.J. Byrne, E. Jones, T.P.J. Hennessy

Introduction

"Barrett's esophagus" is an acquired metaplastic change of the normal squamous epithelium of the esophagus to columnar epithelium, first recognized in 1950.[1] The columnar epithelium shows differentiation towards specialized and nonspecialized gastric epithelium and also small intestinal epithelium.[2] Most researchers now accept that Barrett's esophagus results from chronic gastroesophageal reflux.[3] The association of adenocarcinoma with Barrett's metaplasia has been noted and the risk of developing carcinoma has been estimated to be about forty times greater than for the normal population.[4] As a result, endoscopic surveillance has been recommended by some workers,[5] but the value and cost-effectiveness have been questioned.[4]

Epithelial dysplasia of varying degrees is commonly found in Barrett's esophagus and frequently in epithelium adjacent to adenocarcinoma. Hence, a dysplasia-carcinoma sequence is postulated, analogous to that in the colon;[6] however, the natural history of this progression is unknown. While there are definite criteria[5-7] for each grade of dysplasia, their application to a given case may be interpreted

Little AG, Ferguson MK, Skinner DB: Diseases of the Esophagus, Vol. II: Benign Diseases. Futura Publishing Company, Inc., Mount Kisco, NY, © 1990.

differently by separate observers, particularly between adjacent grades of dysplasia (e.g., mild and moderate).

Nucleolar organizer regions (NORs) are loops of DNA encoded for ribosomal RNA production. The associated proteins are argyrophilic and as such can be easily demonstrated on formalin-fixed, paraffin-embedded tissue.[8] Several studies have demonstrated significant differences in scores obtained from benign and malignant tissues.[9–13] Other workers and studies have been less enthusiastic as "borderline" lesions were not so clearly demarcated by the method.[14–16] It has been established, however, that NORs are related to cellular activity and proliferation.[17]

The aim of this study was to examine tissue sections from patients with Barrett's esophagus and to examine the correlation of the NOR score with histologic grades of carcinoma, dysplasia, and metaplastic mucosa in order to determine the prognostic significance of the NOR score.

Materials and Methods

Thirty-five patients with biopsy-proven Barrett's esophagus were selected from the files in our hospital (Fig. 1A). The biopsies were taken during endoscopy from macroscopically abnormal, intraesophageal mucosa. Fourteen patients had associated adenocarcinoma. Two patients had been followed up for over 4 years, four patients for 3 years, and six patients for 2 years (one of whom subsequently developed adenocarcinoma). Two were followed for 1 year each and the remainder were single biopsies or the patients presented with adenocarcinoma and were found to have Barrett's mucosa. The hematoxylin and eosin stained sections were assessed for the presence and grade of dysplasia. Dysplasia was determined as "mild" (Fig. 2A). if the nuclear-cytoplasmic ratio was slightly increased, with stratification of the nuclei within the epithelium. "Moderate" dysplasia was attributed to epithelium showing marked stratification, with loss of polarity, mitotic figures, and increased nuclear-cytoplasmic ratio. "Severe" dysplasia (Fig. 3A) was applied where the above criteria were more markedly present with the addition of architectural changes, i.e., glandular crowding and proliferation. The adenocarcinomas were classified into well, moderate, and poorly differentiated groups.

Further sections were then cut from each corresponding block at

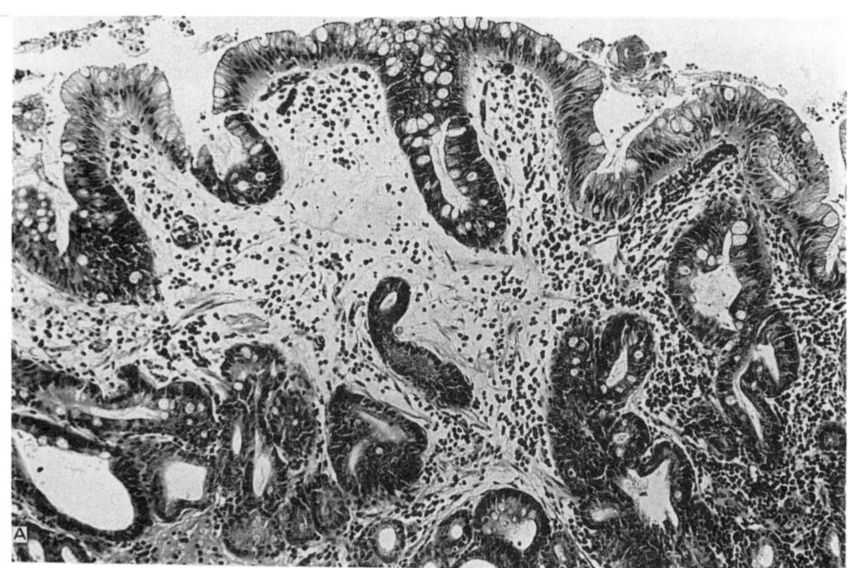

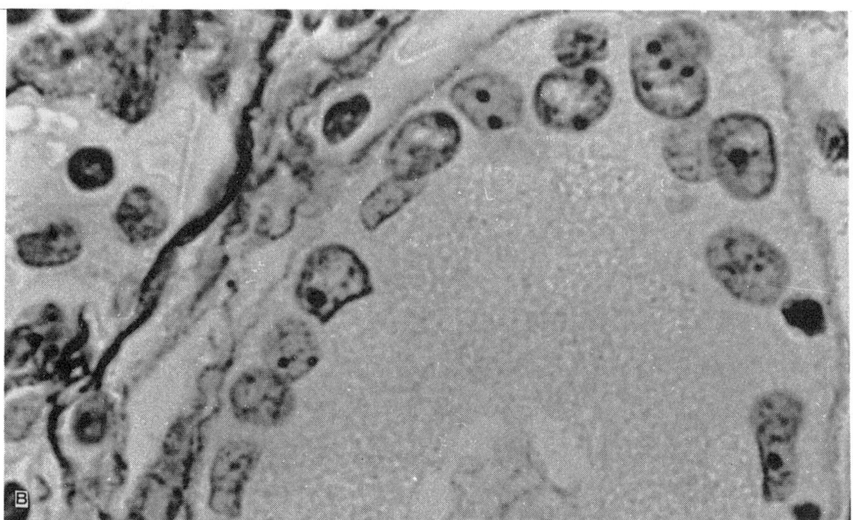

Figure 1: (A) Columnar-lined esophagus including goblet-cell i.e., small intestine differentiation of Barrett's mucosa. (B) AgNOR staining of this metaplastic, nondysplastic tissue demonstrating nuclei, each containing a range of dots corresponding to a score of 2 and 6.

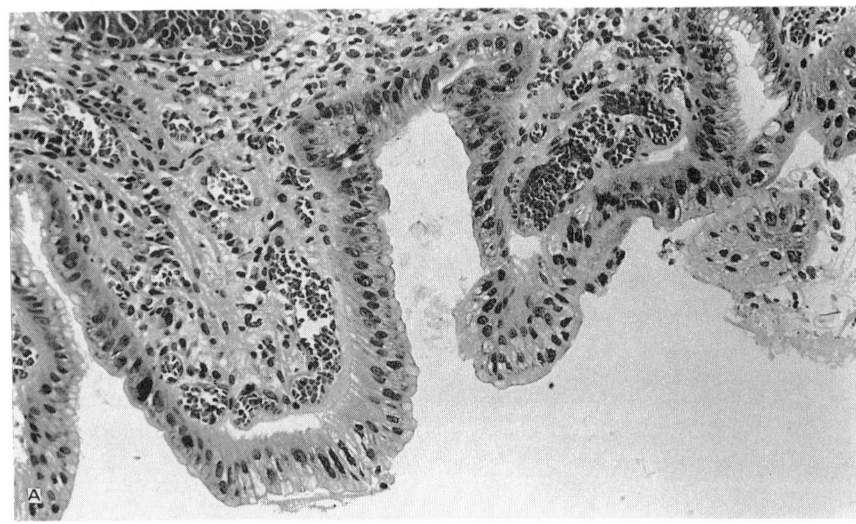

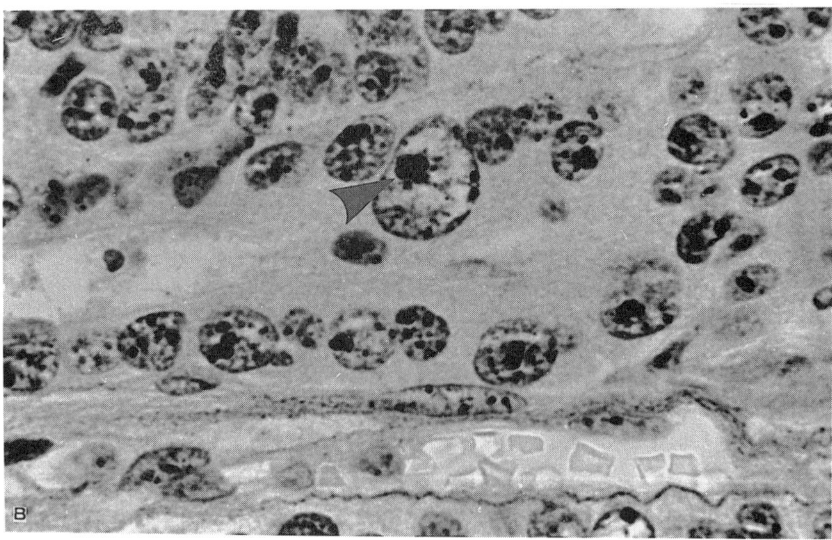

Figure 2: (A) Barrett's mucosa with stratified nuclei, increased nuclear cytoplasmic ratio, and hyperchromatic nuclei. This is mildly dysplastic epithelium. (B): AgNOR stain demonstrating larger dots in all nuclei, some single ones (arrow), meriting a score of 7.

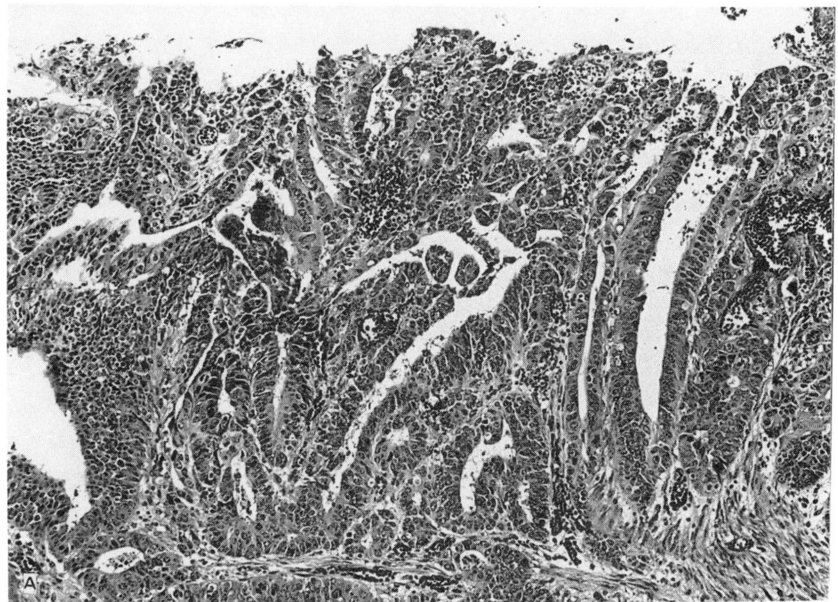

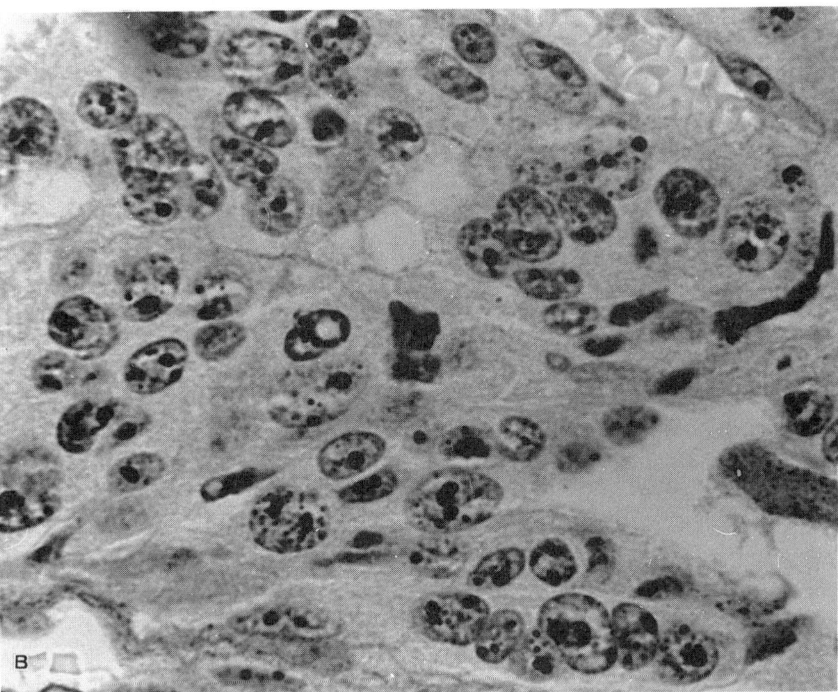

Figure 3: (A) Severely dysplastic Barrett's mucosa showing architectural distortion with glandular proliferation and crowding.
(B): Correspondingly high AgNOR score in which the nuclei contain large aggregates plus multiple small dots.

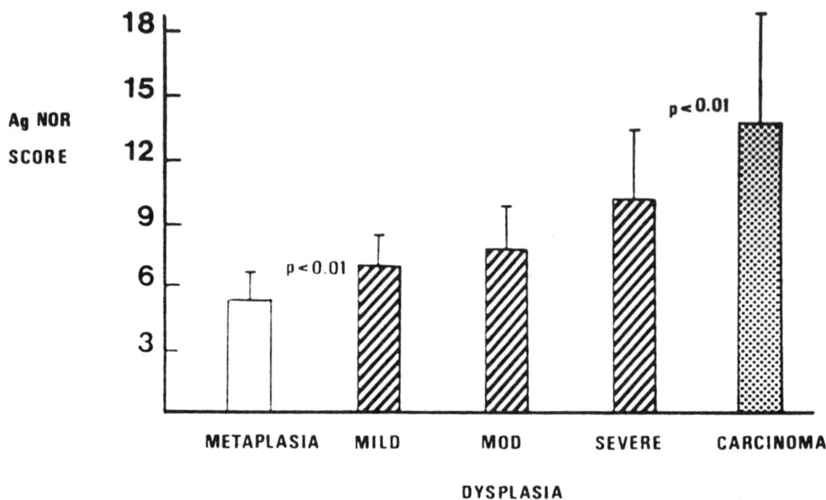

Figure 4: AgNOR score showing progressive increase for metaplastic Barrett's mucosa through grades of dysplasia to carcinoma.

3 microns and stained for NORs in a solution of 2% gelatin in 1% silver formic acid and 50% silver nitrate for 50 minutes at room temperature as previously described.[8] Methyl green counterstain was applied. NORs were then visible within the nuclei as black dots under oil immersion objective (xlOO) as single dots or clumped aggregates. The "clumps" were allocated a score of 3, 5, or 7 depending on how many single (allocated score of 1) dots could either be discerned, or estimated to be, within the clump (Figs. 1B, 2B, 3B). Two researchers (NN and RCS) individually assessed each section. One hundred nuclei were counted within a predesignated area on the slide (judged representative, but the slide was then "coded" to reduce observer bias). These were epithelial nuclei; care was taken to exclude endothelial or inflammatory cell nuclei. A mean score was obtained for each section; the scores from each observer were pooled, and the mean for each case calculated. Subsequently, the scores were matched with the two histologic grades and analyzed statistically (chi-square test).

Results

The AgNOR score obtained for each group is illustrated in Figure 4. When the overall group was examined, there was a significant progressive increase in the score obtained for metaplastic Barrett's mucosa through all grades of dysplasia to carcinoma. The score for metaplastic tissue 5.3 ± 1.2 was significantly lower than all other groups (p<O.01); the score for the carcinoma group 13.9 ± 5.1 was significantly higher than the other groups (p<0.01). Within the dysplastic tissue, the score for severe dysplasia was higher than the scores for both mild and moderate dysplasia p<0.01 (Fig. 4). The patients were then divided into cases with and without associated carcinoma. Representatives of each group were present. The AgNOR score was significantly higher for cases with associated carcinoma than for those without P<0.01 (Fig. 5). One patient was followed over a period of 3 years showing histologic grades of dysplasia ranging from mild to moderate to severe, without associated carcinoma. In this case also the AgNOR score for severe dysplasia was 6.8, i.e., lower than that seen in severe dysplasia associated with carcinoma.

Discussion

Barrett's mucosa has been evaluated as a pre-neoplastic condition for many years. The type of mucin present within the nongoblet-cell epithelium was investigated as a possible prognostic indicator of malignancy since sulfomucin was frequently associated with adenocarcinoma.[19] However, it was later shown that this was a poor prognostic factor.[20] Adenocarcinoma of the esophagus is almost always associated with dysplastic Barrett's mucosa adjacent to it.[2] Light microscopic parameters of dysplasia, as seen on hematoxylin and eosin stained sections, are principal factors applied to assess a given biopsy. It is known that while the dysplasia-carcinoma sequence is of importance, not all cases of dysplastic Barrett's mucosa evolve to malignancy; all cases, however, are regularly surveyed. Nucleolar organizer regions are loops of DNA which transcribe for ribosomal RNA and can be found in both activated and inactive forms in the nucleolar and extranucleolar nuclear compartments, respectively. The proteins associated with the NORs are the portion that can be detected by silver staining (argyrophilia), hence known as "AgNORs." The AgNORs are then visible as black dots either clustered or dispersed. It is suggested that dispersal of the AgNOR staining is associated with more malignant tissue. A single cluster of AgNOR is thought to represent the nucleolus, although multiple clusters may in fact be small nucleoli. The AgNOR stain is related to the amount of protein

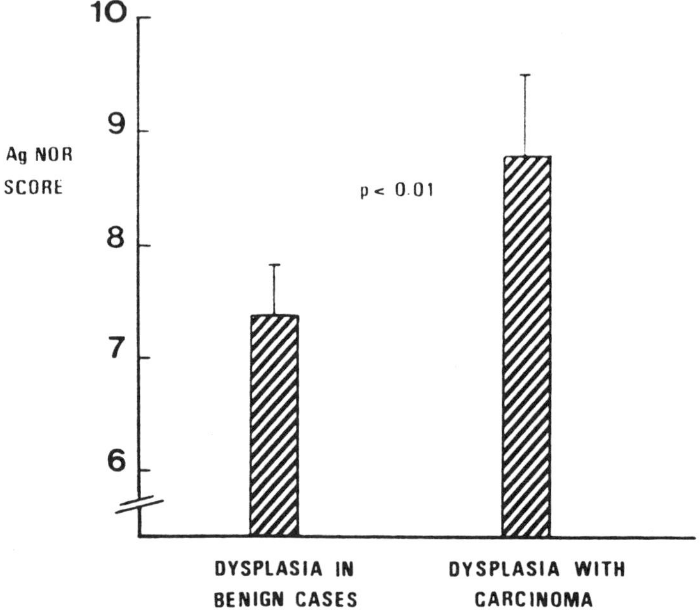

Figure 5: AgNOR score comparing dysplastic change with and without associated carcinoma.

synthesis that the nucleus is undertaking and reflects cellular proliferation; the greater the amount of activity (i.e., the more NORs seen), the more rapidly the cell is dividing and the more malignant the tissue.

AgNOR estimation has provided clear differences between benign and malignant tissue in cases of benign nevi versus malignant melanoma,[10] mesothelial pleural lesions,[11] and breast neoplasms;[13] in cases of virally induced proliferation[15] (squamous papilloma of the larynx versus verrucous carcinoma versus invasive squamous cell carcinoma), the differences were not so clear-cut and probably reflect gene amplification within the virally infected tissue. Similarly, Spitz nevi and malignant melanoma were indistinct.[14]

The AgNOR staining technique is relatively simple to perform; however, it should be said that the counting is laborious, time-consuming, and also subjective. We scored aggregates of NORs within nuclei as 3, 5, or 7 depending on size whereas others have coded only 1 per dot, irrespective of size.[14] This may account for our high score in the metaplastic-only group relative to ''benign'' scores in other studies. However, while the absolute values may vary, within our own study, the scoring system remained constant and thus we can compare and contrast the scores from different groups. Other workers have observed that on a routine basis the difference in score between benign and malignant tissue is very obvious and only a few cells need to be counted. This would hold true at both extremes in our study but is of doubtful validity between mild and moderate dysplasia (Fig. 4).

Our study was carried out on a small number of cases, with a short follow-up period. The results, however, show that the AgNOR score in dyplastic Barrett's mucosa associated with carcinoma is higher in all grades than the score for dysplastic Barrett's mucosa without malignancy. This may reflect an earlier stage in the evolution of the disease when cellular activity is lower. It may on the other hand suggest that there are two distinct groups of patients, one high-scoring, which will develop carcinoma. If this is confirmed in further studies, the dilemma of how best to treat patients with severe dysplasia[20] in Barrett's esophagus may be resolved, or at least aided by the AgNOR technique.

Summary

The malignant potential of Barrett's esophagus is undisputed although the degree of risk to the individual patient is undetermined. As a result, endoscopic surveillance of patients with Barrett's esophagus is advocated. Carcinoma may develop as a progression from benign metaplastic columnar epithelium through degrees of dysplasia. However, the distinction between grades of dysplasia is subjective and the prognostic significance of each stage is unclear. Nucleolar organizer region proteins, which are loops of DNA (rDNA) encoded for ribosomal RNA, have been utilized to detect differences between benign and malignant tissue using an argyrophilic reaction on formalin fixed, paraffin-embedded tissue. We have studied the role of NORs in Barrett's disease using 83 sections from 35 patients in the following groups: (1) metaplasia (n = 25, NOR score = 5.3); (2) dysplasia (mild: n = 19, NOR score 7.0; moderate: n = 17, NOR score = 7.97; severe: n = 8, NOR score = 10.2); and (3) adenocarcinoma (n = 14, NOR score = 13.9). The NOR score correlated well with the histologic grading of dysplasia, and was also significantly higher in patients with dysplasia associated with carcinoma than in patients with dysplasia in benign Barrett's esophagus (p<0.01). This may provide a means of quantifying progression and risk in serial follow-up.

References

1. Barrett NR: Chronic peptic ulcer of the esophagus and "oesophagitis." Br J Surg 38:175, 1950.
2. Thompson J, Enterline H: Pathology of the Esophagus, New York, Springer Verlag, 1984, p 109.
3. Sjogren RN, Johnson LF: Barrett's esophagus: A review. Am J Med 74:313, 1983.
4. Spechler SJ, Robbins AH, Rubins HB, et al: Adenocarcinoma and Barrett's esophagus: An overated risk? Gastroenterology 87:927, 1984.
5. Smith RRL, Boitnott JK, Hamilton SR, Rogers EL: The spectrum of carcinoma arising in Barrett's esophagus: A clinico- pathologic study of 26 patients. Am J Surg Pathol 8:563, 1984.
6. Riddel RH, Goldman H, Ranshaff DF, et al: Dysplasia in inflammatory bowel disease: Standardized classification with provisional clinical applications: Hum Pathol 14:931, 1981.
7. Thompson JJ, Zinser KR, Enterline HT: Barrett's metaplasia and adenocarcinoma of the esophagus and gastroesophageal junction. Hum Pathol 14:42, 1983.
8. Crocker J, Nar P: Nucleolar organizer regions in lymphomas. J Pathol 151:111, 1987.
9. Morgan DW, Crocker J, Watts A, Shenoi PK: Salivary gland tumors studied by means of AgNOR technique. Histopathology 13:553, 1988.
10. Crocker J, Skilbeck N: Nucleolar organizer regions in cutaneous melanotic lesions: A quantitative study. J Clin Pathol 40:885, 1987.
11. Ayres JG, Crocker J, Skilbeck NQ: Differentiation of malignant from normal reactive mesothelial cells using the AgNOR technique. Thorax 44:366, 1988.
12. Crocker J, Ayres JG, McGovern J: Nucleolar oranizer regions in small cell carcinoma of the bronchus. Thorax 42(12):972, 1987.
13. Smith R, Crocker J: Evaluation of nucleolar organizer region-associated proteins in breast malignancies. Histopathology 12:113, 1988.
14. Howat AJ, Giri DD, Cotton DWK, Slater DN: Nucleolar organizer regions in Spitz nevi and malignant melanomas. Cancer 63:474, 1989.
15. Bryan RL, Allcock RA, Crocker J, Shenoi PM: Nucleolar organizer regions in squamous tumors of the pharynx and larynx. J Clin Pathol 89(2):218, 1989.
16. Fallowfield ME, Cook MG: The value of nucleolar organizer regions in the differential diagnosis of borderline melanocytic lesions. Histopathology 14:299, 1989.
17. Hall PA, Crocker J, Watts A, Stansfeld AG: Comparison of nucleolar organizer region staining and Ki-67 immunostaining in non-Hodgkin's lymphomas. Histopathology 12(4):373, 1988.
18. Jass JR: Mucin histochemistry of the columnar epithelium of the esophagus: A retrospective study. J Clin Pathol 34:866, 1981.

19. Jauregui HO, Davessan K, Hale JH, et al: Mucin histochemistry of intestinal metaplasia in Barrett's esophagus. Mod Pathol 1:188, 1988.
20. Mitros FA: Inflammatory and neoplastic diseases of the esophagus. In: Contempory Issues in Surgical Pathology: Pathology of the Esophagus, Stomach and Duodenum, New York, Churchill Livingstone, 1984, p 19.

IV.

Stricture:
Editors' Overview

Peptic or reflux-induced esophageal strictures constitute a challenging and somewhat controversial therapeutic dilemma. Controversy stems from the surgical instinct that these patients require antireflux surgery and the gastroenterology community's knowledge that many patients can be treated successfully with a combination of antacid therapy and esophageal dilation. Chapter 28 provides important information which allows prediction of a patient's response to dilation. It is shown that patients with long (more than 2 cm) and tight (less than 9 mm in diameter) strictures respond poorly to dilation. It is also clear that successful antireflux surgery will reduce the need for dilation and in fact eliminate it in the majority of patients. These are important data which allow the appropriate selection and timing of therapy for patients with reflux strictures.

The remaining two chapters in this section should be read together and compared. They report alternative techniques for treatment of a very challenging problem, that of upper esophageal and pharyngeal caustic strictures. The authors of both chapters report utilization of long colon segments to replace the injured esophagus but one team outlines a thoughtful, multistage approach while the other group recommends a one-stage approach. Both techniques have pros and cons which should be weighed by the reader.

28

Reflux-Induced Esophageal Strictures:
Factors Influencing Long-Term Results of Dilation

Luigi Bonavina, Lorenzo Norberto,
Antonio Cusumano, Marco Baessato,
Giovanni L. Pappagallo, Valentino Fontebasso,
Stefano Merigliano, Alberto Ruol, Alberto Peracchia

Introduction

Esophageal strictures represent the end-stage of chronic reflux esophagitis. Despite the multiple surgical options available for treatment, the ideal management of these patients is not well defined at present.

During the past two decades there has been a trend away from resectional procedures, since it has become apparent that most strictures can be successfully dilated and that dilation combined with standard antireflux repair can restore comfortable swallowing in the majority of the patients.[1-5] However, this form of treatment is not always applicable, especially in elderly patients who often have concomitant heart and lung disease and are not eligible for surgery.[6]

Although dilation is considered an effective short-term therapy, the rate of stricture recurrence and the results of dilation plus medical treatment in the long-term management of these patients are still

Little AG, Ferguson MK, Skinner DB: Diseases of the Esophagus, Vol. II: Benign Diseases. Futura Publishing Company, Inc., Mount Kisco, NY, © 1990.

unknown. We attempted to evaluate the clinical course of reflux-induced esophageal strictures by identifying factors influencing the long-term outcome of dilation in a series of patients.

Materials and Methods

From January 1980 to December 1987, 106 consecutive patients with reflux-induced esophageal strictures were referred to our institution. There were 75 males and 31 females, with a median age of 59 years (range 14–86). The median time from the onset of symptoms was 12 months (range 1–180). All patients had radiological evidence of distal esophageal stricture; a hiatal hernia was present in 89 cases (84%). None of the patients had previously undergone esophageal or gastric surgery.

All patients underwent fiberoptic endoscopy using a pediatric instrument (Olympus GIF-XP, 7.9 mm diameter). Dilation was performed using the Savary-Gilliard bougies with positioning of the flexible guidewire under endoscopic control.[7] The diagnosis of malignancy was excluded by performing vital staining with multiple biopsies and brush cytology of the area of esophageal narrowing.[8] Associated findings on endoscopy were grade II or III esophagitis in 48 patients (45.3%), and Barrett's esophagus in 16 (15%).

In nearly all cases, the endoscopic procedures were performed on an outpatient basis by two staff physicians, using mild intravenous sedation and local anesthesia. An average of three bougienages per session were performed.

An initial trial of dilation (median 4; range 1–6) was carried out during the first 3 to 4 weeks of treatment. Twenty patients (19%), who showed early recurrence of dysphagia and drop of the esophageal caliber to less than 10 mm within one month, were considered nonresponders to conservative treatment and are excluded from the present study.

The remaining 86 patients (81%) who initially responded to dilation entered the follow-up study and were treated with a standard dose of H_2-antagonists (cimetidine or ranitidine). Esophageal function studies, i.e., manometry and 24-hour pH monitoring, were performed after the initial dilations in 47 of the 86 patients according to standard techniques.[9] During the follow-up period, all patients returned to the clinic for repeat endoscopy; dilation was performed when dysphagia was present or the esophageal caliber was less than 10 mm.

Twenty-two selected patients (26% of the 86) received surgical treatment within the first year of follow-up. An antireflux repair was performed in 20 patients (16 Toupet, 2 Collis-Nissen, 1 Nissen, 1 Dor) and a Roux-en-Y gastrojejunostomy in one. The last patient required esophageal resection to relieve a disabling, early recurring dysphagia.

The time free of dysphagia after dilation was calculated according to the Kaplan-Meier method. Differences between curves were analyzed by the log-rank and Wilcoxon tests (univariate analysis). A stepwise selection (maximum partial likelihood ratio and the Cox's proportional hazard method) were performed to identify factors able to independently predict the need of further dilation.[10]

Results

There was no mortality related to the endoscopic procedures. The overall morbidity rate was 2.3% and consisted of two perforations which were treated conservatively.

The 86 patients who initially responded to dilation were followed 6 months or more (median 17 months). The estimated time free of dysphagia was 14 months. Sixteen patients (18.6%) remained free of dysphagia after the initial dilations. Thirteen patients (15.1%) needed only a single dilation after the initial treatment. Fifty-seven of the 86 patients (66.3%) required further dilation to maintain an adequate caliber of the esophageal lumen. Of these 57 patients, 48 (84.2%) underwent redilation within the first year of follow-up.

Esophageal manometry showed a mean lower esophageal sphincter pressure of 10.9 ± 3.5 mmHg, which is significantly lower than control values obtained in our laboratory from a group of 25 asymptomatic volunteer subjects (23.3 ± 7.2 mmHg, p<.001). Ten patients had a motility disorder of the esophageal body; in five, the pattern was that typical of scleroderma, and in the remaining cases a nonspecific motor abnormality was detected. Prolonged pH monitoring of the distal esophagus revealed abnormal esophageal acid exposure in 36 of the 47 studied patients.

Surgery reduced the need of further dilation. This trend is reflected by the diminished number of dilations per time during the postoperative period (Fig. 1). A statistically significant increase of LES pressure was observed after fundoplication (Fig. 2). No remarkable changes in the motility of the esophageal body were noted. Eighteen patients (81.8%) had a successful surgical outcome. Of these, seven

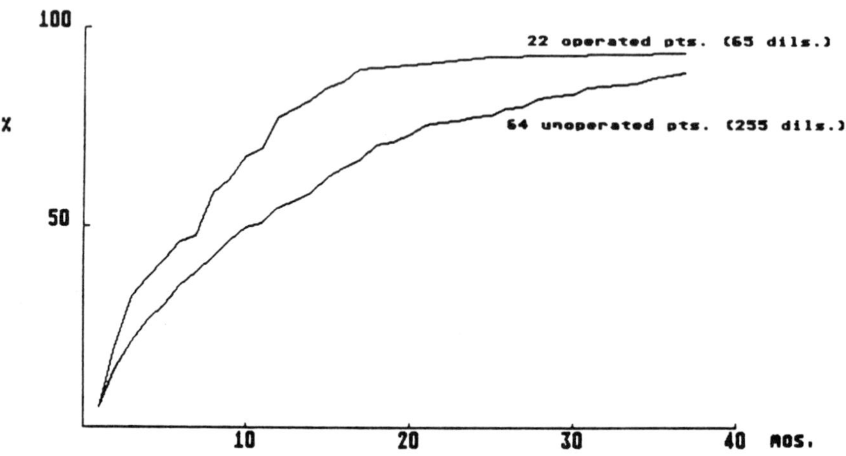

Figure 1: Cumulative probability of esophageal dilation in the patient population according to treatment.

required postoperative dilation. However, only two patients were further dilated after the first year of follow-up. There were four surgical failures (18.2%); three of these patients, one of whom had scleroderma, required esophageal resection for relief of dysphagia; a Roux-en-Y gastrojejunostomy was performed in another patient due to persistent reflux.

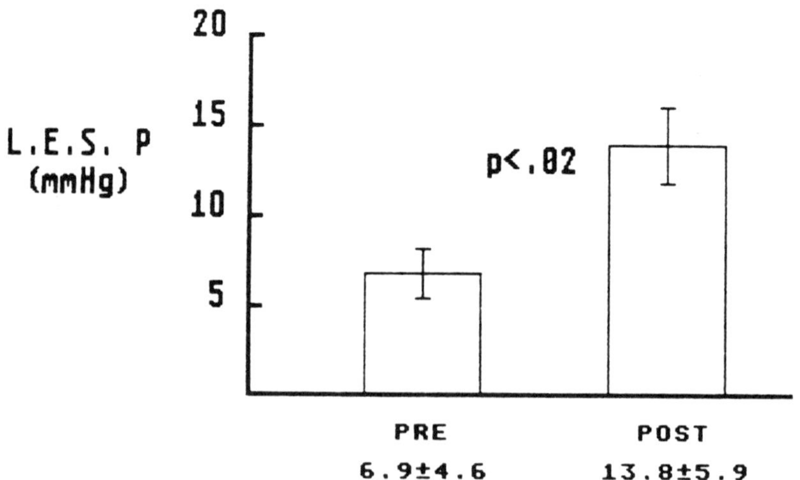

Figure 2: Effect of fundoplication on lower esophageal sphincter pressure.

Table I
Factors Predicting Dysphagia after Initial Dilation
(Univariate Analysis)

Factor	*Log-Rank*	*Wilcoxon*
Length (2 cm)	p = 0.019	p = 0.012
Diameter (9 mm)	p = 0.005	p = 0.015
No. of Initial Dilations (4)	p = 0.040	p = 0.153 (N.S.)

The univariate analysis of the factors predicting dysphagia after initial dilation (Table I) showed that a length of the stricture of less than 2 cm (Fig. 3) and a diameter of 9 mm or more (Fig. 4) could predict a greater duration of the symptom-free interval. The multivariate analysis showed that length and diameter of the stricture are independent prognostic factors (Fig. 5). This holds true even when the 22 operated patients are excluded from the analysis.

Discussion

Although it is current clinical practice to palliate reflux-induced esophageal strictures by means of dilation, the long-term results of

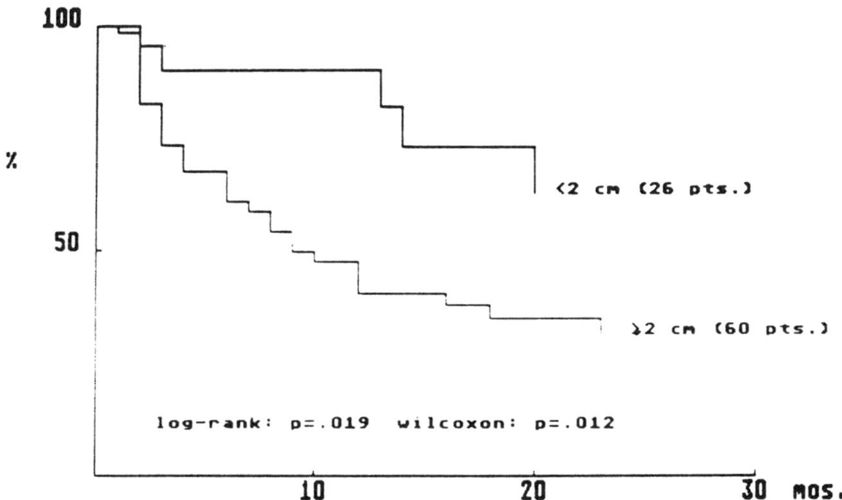

Figure 3: Influence of initial length of the stricture on the time free of dysphagia after dilation (Kaplan-Meier).

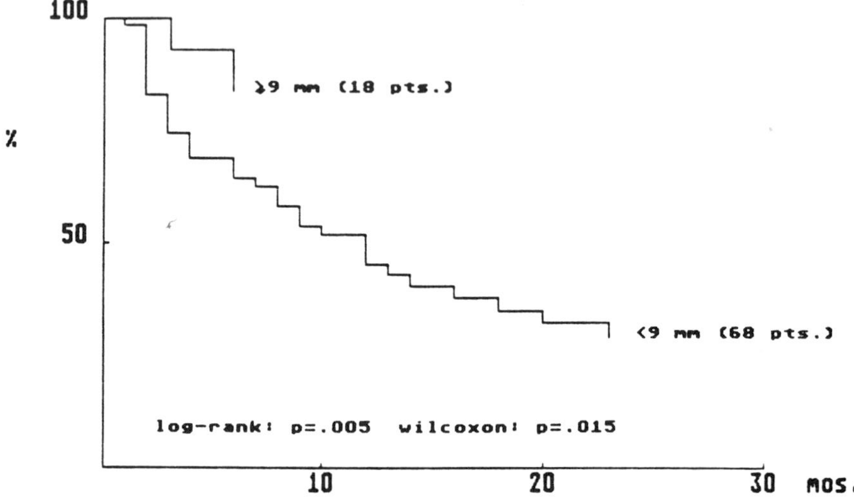

Figure 4: Influence of initial diameter of the stricture on the time free of dysphagia after dilation (Kaplan-Meier).

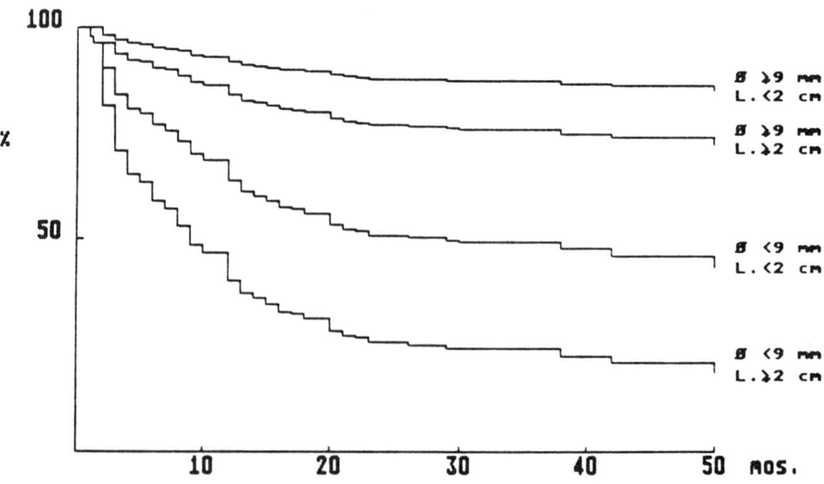

Figure 5: Expected time free of dysphagia based on initial length and diameter of the stricture (Cox's proportional hazard model).

such a conservative approach are conflicting.[11–15] The response to dilation is often described as bimodal in that some patients receive virtually permanent relief of dysphagia, whereas others follow an unpredictable course.

We found that dilation plus pharmacological control of reflux is an appropriate initial treatment for peptic esophageal strictures. The radial and longitudinal stretching produced by bougienage can improve compliance of the esophageal wall and reduce axial tension.[16] The use of the Savary-Gilliard dilators allows a very gentle and progressive dilation with minimal mucosal trauma and, as a consequence, carries an acceptably low risk of complications.[17]

The primary goal of our work was to identify parameters useful to predict the long-term outcome of patients with reflux-induced esophageal strictures undergoing conservative treatment. The present study shows that the best results of dilation can be expected in patients with a stricture length of less than 2 cm and a diameter of the esophageal lumen greater than 9 mm. In fact, 90% of these patients are estimated to be symptom-free at 2 years. An initial diameter of less than 9 mm decreases to 50% or less the probability of being symptom-free at 2 years (Fig. 5).

Another finding of this study is that antireflux surgery favorably influences the natural history of the disease by reducing the need of subsequent dilations. The choice of the most appropriate surgical technique in patients with reflux-induced strictures is still a matter of controversy. Undoubtedly, the lower success rate than that usually achieved in uncomplicated reflux disease is due to a combination of difficulty in restoring competency to the cardia, especially in the presence of esophageal shortening, and the fact that underlying motility disorders may cause esophageal dysfunction after fundoplication.

We believe that an antireflux operation should be undertaken early in the course of the disease to avoid progression of the fibrosis through the esophageal wall and further functional damage secondary to repetitive dilations. Resection of the stricture should be considered only in patients unresponsive to dilation. Recent studies have demonstrated that when a severe motility disorder of the esophageal body is detected, esophageal resection represents the treatment of choice in these patients.[18]

In conclusion, esophageal dilation represents only a palliative procedure in reflux-induced strictures, but results are acceptable in selected patients, i.e., those whose stricture length is less than 2 cm and/or diameter exceeds 9 mm. Also it may be the only therapeutic option available in patients who are not surgical candidates. In the ideal patient, early antireflux surgery is strongly recommended to prevent progression of the disease and to provide a better quality of life.

References

1. Hayward J: The treatment of fibrous stricture of the esophagus associated with hiatal hernia. Thorax 16:45, 1961.
2. Hill LD, Gelfand M, Bauermeister D: Simplified management of reflux esophagitis with stricture. Ann Surg 172:638, 1970.
3. Larrain A, Csendes A, Pope CE: Surgical correction of reflux: An effective therapy for esophageal strictures. Gastroenterology 69:578, 1975.
4. Siewert R: Surgical therapy of peptic stenoses. In: Medical and Surgical Problems of the Esophagus, Stipa S, Belsey RH (eds). New York, Academic Press, 1980, p 146.
5. Salo JA, Kulju KA, Kalima T: Fibre-endoscopic dilatation of peptic esophageal strictures. Acta Chir Scand 153:365, 1987.
6. Watson A: Reflux stricture of the esophagus. Br J Surg 74:443, 1987.
7. Monnier Ph, Hsieh V, Savary M: Endoscopic treatment of esophageal stenosis using Savary-Gilliard bougies: Technical innovations. Acta Endosc 15:119, 1985.
8. Norberto L, Cusumano A, Bonavina L, et al: Endoscopic vital staining in the diagnosis of esophageal cancer. In: Diseases of the Esophagus, Siewert JR, Holscher AH (eds), Berlin, Springer Verlag, 1988, p 135.
9. Bonavina L, Evander A, DeMeester TR, et al: Length of the distal esophageal sphincter and competency of the cardia. Am J Surg 151:25, 1986.
10. Buyse ME, Staquet MJ, Silvester RJ: Cancer clinical trials: Method and practice. Oxford Medical Publications, 1988.
11. Ogilvie AL, Ferguson R, Atkinson M: Outlook with conservative treatment of peptic esophageal stricture. Gut 21:23, 1980.
12. Glick ME: Clinical course of esophageal stricture managed by bougienage. Dig Dis Sci 27:884, 1982.
13. Wesdorp IC, Bartelsman JF, Den Hartog FC, et al: Results of conservative treatment of benign esophageal strictures: A follow-up study in 100 patients. Gastroenterology 82:487, 1982.
14. Patterson DJ, Graham DY, Smith JL, et al: Natural history of benign esophageal strictures treated by dilatation. Gastroenterology 85:346, 1983.
15. Tytgat GN: Dilation therapy of benign esophageal stenoses. World J Surg 13:142, 1989.
16. Little AG, Naunheim KS, Ferguson MK, Skinner DB: Surgical management of esophageal strictures. Ann Thorac Surg 45:144, 1988.
17. Dumon JF, Meric B, Sivak MV, Fleischer D: A new method of esophageal dilation using Savary-Gilliard bougies. Gastrointest Endosc 31:379, 1985.
18. Zaninotto G, DeMeester TR, Bremner CG, et al: Esophageal function in patients with reflux-induced strictures and its relevance to surgical treatment. Ann Thorac Surg 47:362, 1989.

29

Surgical Treatment of Caustic Strictures of the Hypopharynx and Cervical Esophagus

Romeo Bardini, Massimo Asolati, Luigi Bonavina, Maurizio Pavanello, Ermanno Tiso, Alberto Peracchia

Introduction

The reported incidence of caustic hypopharyngeal strictures varies from 0.7% to 6% of caustic ingestions.[1,2] Reconstructive surgery in these patients is challenging, since it is necessary to restore digestive continuity and preserve function of the larynx to avoid aspiration.

We reviewed our experience in patients with severe caustic stricture of the hypopharynx to formulate criteria of surgical therapy.

Patients and Methods

From 1968 to 1989, 148 patients with caustic lesions of the esophagus have been referred to our institution. Overall, 38 patients (25.6%) had severe hypopharyngeal strictures. Six of them, who presented with associated laryngeal lesions, required surgical therapy. There were four females and two males, mean age 29 years, range 9 to 43.

The mean time elapsed from the ingestion of the corrosive agent was 23 months (range 8 months to 6 years). Five patients ingested

Little AG, Ferguson MK, Skinner DB: Diseases of the Esophagus, Vol. II: Benign Diseases. Futura Publishing Company, Inc., Mount Kisco, NY, © 1990.

acid and one ingested an alkaline solution. The five adults had attempted suicide, while in the 9-year-old patient, the severe burns had been caused by accidental swallowing of a solution of acetic acid.

In all but one patient, surgical reconstruction of the esophagus was carried out in three stages. Stage I consists of performing an external pharyngostomy on the least damaged pyriform sinus. This results in stretching the pharynx laterally and inferior to the laryngeal inlet. The pharyngeal stoma allows daily digital calibration and provides an excellent training to the patient for rehabilitation of the deglutitory mechanism.

Stage II consists of a pharyngocoloplasty with "open" cervical anastomosis, i.e., a visceral suture limited to the lateral and posterior walls with the remaining circumference of the viscera sutured to the skin.

Stage III of the procedure is performed 3 weeks later, and consists of restoring digestive continuity by rotating the contiguous skin in order to form the anterior wall of the anastomosis.[3] This technique of delayed reconstruction avoids internal pressure on the anastomosis and allows visual evaluation of the mucosa of the transposed viscera through the stoma.

Case Histories

Case 1

M.M., female, age 39. This patient had previously undergone laryngoplasty, tracheostomy, and gastrostomy. We performed a pharyngostomy and, subsequently, a one-stage pharyngocoloplasty. A severe anastomotic stricture developed, which required multiple dilations and eventually led to reoperation. However, the clinical outcome has never been satisfactory. The experience with this patient convinced us of the importance of a three-stage reconstruction.

Case 2

S.H., female, age 9. She had tracheostomy and gastrostomy performed elsewhere for an established hypopharyngeal stricture. We used the three-stage technique: pharyngostomy and pharyngocoloplasty with open anastomosis.

Case 3

S.M., female, age 25. She had pharyngostomy, laryngofissure, and tracheostomy performed 4 years before. Subsequently, a pharyngo-jejunoplasty had been attempted. The postoperative course was complicated by necrosis of the jejunal loop which required a gastrostomy and a cervical jejunal stoma. We performed a new pharyngostomy; subsequently, we dismantled the jejunoplasty and used the left colon to restore digestive continuity. An open pharyngocolic anastomosis was performed.

Case 4

C.L., male, age 29. This psychotic drug-addicted individual had previously undergone total esophagogastrectomy, jejunostomy, and cervical esophagostomy because of extensive esophageal and gastric necrosis. We performed a pharyngostomy, and, later, a pharyngo-coloplasty with open anastomosis. The stoma was closed 20 days later, and a tracheostomy was performed.

Case 5

S.A., male, age 30. He had undergone an emergency total eso-phagogastrectomy with splenectomy, jejunostomy, cervical esopha-gostomy, and tracheostomy; later, a retrosternal hypopharyngocol-oplasty had been performed but the hospital course was complicated by dehiscence of the anastomosis. Multiple attempts at surgical repair had been unsuccessful, and the patient was left with a pharyngeal fistula and fibrosis of the colonic loop above the jugulum. Through a median sternotomy, we were able to mobilize the colonic loop and bring it up to the pharynx where an open anastomosis was performed.

Case 6

S.G., female, age 43. This patient had previously undergone repair of a duodenal perforation and a feeding jejunostomy. Because of the presence of devastating lesions involving the epiglottis and the la-ryngeal aditus, we performed a pharyngostomy and a superior transverse laryngectomy. Subsequently, a pharyngocoloplasty with an open anastomosis was performed.

Results

There was no mortality related to the surgical procedures. Morbidity consisted of a pleural empyema in the patient whose retrosternal jejunoplasty was dismantled without opening the chest. Oral feeding proved satisfactory in all patients, and no significant episodes of aspiration were recorded. The tracheostoma was closed within 2 months of the operation in the five patients who underwent the three-stage procedure. Mean follow-up is 44 months (range 6–120 months). The patient described in case 1 died of suicide 48 months after surgery.

Discussion

Reconstruction of digestive continuity in patients with strictures following corrosive burns of the hypopharynx is difficult. The goal of surgery is to restore comfortable swallowing while preserving good phonatory function and preventing aspiration. Standard surgical procedures have proven unsatisfactory when the larynx has been preserved, and this may be due to pharyngeal wall fibrosis, anastomotic stricture, or to the location of the anastomosis at the level of the laryngeal inlet.[4] However, there are little data on this subject in the current literature, and only a few significant contributions have been reported.[5–8]

We agree with Celerier[8] that the initial assessment of the upper digestive tract and larynx should be performed about a month after the ingestion of the corrosive, i.e., when the patient is out of the acute phase of disease. Such evaluation should be repeated monthly until the lesions are stabilized, and this assessment is critical for planning appropriate surgical treatment. Of course, massive oropharyngeal lesions associated with lip and tongue retraction represent a contraindication of reconstructive surgery.

In our opinion, it is advisable to wait at least 10–12 months before undertaking surgical reconstruction of the esophagus, since the scarring process is usually slower than in the stomach.[9] We believe that the first surgical step should consist of a pharyngostomy on the least damaged pyriform sinus; this approach allows daily calibration of the stoma and rehabilitation of the deglutitory mechanism. The patient is trained to swallow properly, and will maintain this ability after the esophageal reconstruction. In addition, pharyngeal stretching and lateralization allow the future anastomosis to be located below the laryngeal inlet, thereby avoiding aspiration. When the hypopharynx is obliterated, a superior transverse laryngectomy is mandatory to reduce the declivity of the laryngeal inlet and prevent aspiration.

Once relative stabilization of the lesions has been obtained, the patient should undergo reconstructive surgery. Colon bypass has been advocated for hypopharyngeal and cervical esophageal replacement since 1950.[10,11] The left colon is, in our opinion, the most suitable segment for restoration of digestive continuity, either through a substernal route or through the posterior mediastinum should esophagectomy be performed. The technique of pharyngocoloplasty with open anastomosis allows visual control of the colonic mucosa and has the advantage of avoiding potential leaks.[3,12] Delayed reconstruction can be accomplished about 3 weeks later, is simple, and restores an adequate lumen without risk of subsequent anastomotic stricture.

References

1. Cardona J, Daly J: Current management of corrosive esophagitis: An evaluation of results in 239 cases. Ann Otol Laryngol 80:521, 1971.
2. Schild J: Caustic ingestion in adult patients. Laryngoscope 95:1199, 1985.
3. Bardini R, Bonavina L, Asolati M, et al: Surgical treatment of cervical anastomotic leaks following esophageal reconstruction. Int Surg 72:163, 1987.
4. Gupta S: Total obliteration of esophagus and hypopharynx due to corrosives: A new technique of reconstruction. J Thorac Cardiovasc Surg 60:264, 1970.
5. Thomas A, Dedo H: Pharyngogastrostomy for treatment of severe caustic stricture of the pharynx and esophagus. J Thorac Cardiovasc Surg 73:817, 1977.
6. Tran Ba Huy P, Assens P, Mislawski R, et al: L'oesopharyngoplastie par transposition d'un greffon ileo-colique droit dans le traitement des sequelles des stenoses caustiques de l'oesophage et de l'hypopharynx. Ann Otol Laryngol 99:489, 1982.
7. Cecconello I, Zilberstein B, Pollara W, et al: Pharyngocoloplasty for the treatment of caustic stricture of the esophagus and pharynx. In: Esophageal Disorders: Pathophysiology and Therapy, DeMeester TR, Skinner DB (eds), New York, Raven Press, 1985, p 271.
8. Tran Ba Huy P, Celerier M: Management of severe caustic stenosis of the hypopharynx and esophagus by ileocolic transposition via suprahyoid or transepiglottic approach. Ann Surg 207:439, 1988.

9. Peracchia A, Bardini R, Bonavina L, et al: Lesioni da caustici dell'esofago: Esperienza su 143 casi osservati. Chirurgia 2:1, 1989.
10. Brain R, Reading P: Colon transplantation into the pharynx and cervical esophagus. Br J Surg 53:933, 1966.
11. Belsey R: Corrosive strictures of the esophagus. In: Esophageal Disorders: Pathophysiology and Therapy, DeMeester TR, Skinner DB (eds), New York, Raven Press, 1985, p 261.
12. Peracchia A, Bardini R, Asolati M, et al: Esophagovisceral anastomotic leak: Prevention, diagnosis, and treatment. In: Diseases of the Esophagus, Siewert JR, Holscher AH (eds), Berlin, Springer Verlag, 1988, p 484.

30

Pharyngoesophageal Postcorrosive Stricture Treated by One-Stage Retrosternal "Bypass" Coloplasty

Zoran Gerzic, Jelena Knezevic, Miroslav Milicevic

Introduction

Severe postcorrosive esophageal stricture will develop in 5–20% of patients sustaining corrosive damage to the esophagus even with adequate postinjury emergency management.[1-4] The prognosis of a corrosive injury to the esophagus is determined at the time of ingestion, and the dominant factors influencing outcome are type, concentration, and quantity of ingested corrosive agent as well as the degree and depth of destruction to the esophageal wall.[5] The type of initial management does not affect outcome in patients with extensive lesions. A small number of patients will have strictures of adjacent structures as well, including the pharynx, epiglottis, hypopharynx, larynx, and sometimes the entire esophagus and stomach, resulting in impairment of respiration, swallowing, and phonation. In patients with severe damage, due to progressive scarring of the injured esophagus, endoscopic dilation is futile. The only possible way to avoid the misery of life-long gastrostomy and to restore swallowing is by total reconstruction of the esophagus.

Little AG, Ferguson MK, Skinner DB: Diseases of the Esophagus, Vol. II: Benign Diseases. Futura Publishing Company, Inc., Mount Kisco, NY, © 1990.

A Historical Review of Pharyngoesophageal Reconstruction

Roux, in 1907,[6] performed the first successful antethoracic esophagojejunoplasty reconstructive procedure. Lexer[7] added a cutanoplasty to the original esophagojejunoplasty procedure in 1911 in an attempt to avoid frequent jejunal necrosis. The combined procedure significantly lowered mortality, but long-term results were not satisfactory. At the same time, Kelling[8] employed the colon and in 1920, Kirschner[9] used the stomach for reconstruction of the esophagus. There is no ideal reconstructive procedure, although many modifications and new procedures have been introduced.

Procedures and techniques for subtotal esophageal reconstruction have improved during the past decades. Functional results are good and some centers have accumulated considerable experience.

Many procedures for total esophagoplasty have been developed and used in the past, but predominantly for reconstruction following laryngeal resection[10–12] for hypopharyngeal carcinoma. Such procedures have been very infrequently used in attempts to bypass combined postcorrosive lesions to the pharynx and larynx.[13–17]

Reconstructive surgery for combined, high strictures of the esophagus and pharynx is technically very difficult. Postoperative complications are frequent (leakage, stenosis of the anastomoses) and since the number of operated patients is small, evaluation and comparison of the different procedures, especially in view of long-term functional results, is uncertain.

Our Method of Reconstruction

The rationale for the procedure we employ stems from our 5-year experience in the management of postcorrosive esophageal stricture by reconstruction using the right colon (with the terminal ileum) or the left (transversosplenic) colon segment (Fig. 1). We have been using colon transplants in the management of high, combined, postcorrosive strictures of the pharynx and esophagus since 1971.

Postcorrosive stricture is a benign disease, so that the requirements for a reconstructive procedure are strict and well defined: (1) long-lasting, good, functional results, (2) acceptable postoperative mortality, (3) low postoperative morbidity, (4) good cosmetic results, and (5) one-stage procedure. Colon transplants have distinct advan-

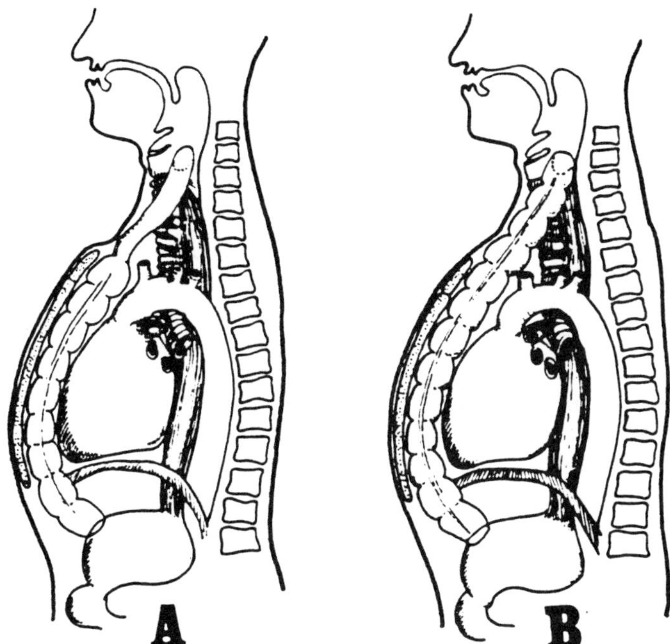

Figure 1: Appearance after pharyngoesophageal "bypass" reconstruction with (A) right colon with long segment of terminal ileum, and (B) left colon (transversosplenic) segment.

tages in comparison to the stomach for esophageal replacement, since a sufficient length of the colon segment is generally easily obtainable and regurgitation is prevented, due to active peristalsis of the ileum and the valve of Bauchini. It is difficult, sometimes impossible, to bring the stomach all the way up to the pharynx. In such attempts, transplant necrosis presents a serious threat, especially if the patient sustained corrosive injury to the stomach or had a feeding gastrostomy. Furthermore, it seems logical to preserve the stomach whenever possible.

All operations were done with endotracheal anesthesia. Intubation of the patient can be difficult in the presence of extensive supraglottic scarring, so it might be necessary to perform reconstructive surgery of the pharynx[13] or laser surgery to obtain a suitable lumen. Technique of "bypass" total pharyngoesophagocoloplasty is very similar to routine retrosternal esophagocoloplasty.

The approach is through an upper midline incision and a long

Table I
Corrosive Agents and Level of Stricture

	Supraglottic	Hypopharyngeal	High Cervical	Total
Liquid lye	5	8	3	16
Concentrated acid	2	11	5	18
Total	*7*	*19*	*8*	*34*

left cervical incision (from the suprasternal notch to the angle of the mandibula). Either the right colon, with a long segment of ileum (15–25 cm), or the transversosplenic segment of the left colon is mobilized in the usual manner. Obtaining a segment of sufficient length to reach the angle of the jaw is usually not a problem. The continuity of the intra-abdominal gastrointestinal tract is achieved by end-to-end anastomosis. Cologastric anastomosis is performed close to the lesser curvature of the stomach.

At this point the cervical esophagus is dissected along the anterior border of the sternocleidomastoid muscle, from the angle of the jaw to the suprasternal notch. In patients with hypopharyngeal and high cervical strictures, the posterolateral wall of the pharynx and hypopharynx is approached after ligation of the superior thyroid artery. The carotid sheath is retracted laterally. The omohyoid muscle is divided. The prevertebral space is entered by blunt dissection and the entire mass (larynx, pharynx, and esophagus) is mobilized and rotated to the right in order to expose the posterolateral wall of the pharynx. An instrument (peanut, blunt probe, etc.) is passed through the mouth to demonstrate the position of the stricture.

A retrosternal tunnel of sufficient width is created and the transplant positioned through it. It is essential to pass the transplant carefully without twisting the vascular pedicle. The sternohyoid, sternothyroid, and omohyoid muscles are divided.

The site of the anastomosis at the level of the pharynx and hypopharynx depends on the location and extent of the stricture. In the presence of a low hypopharyngeal or high cervical stricture, a longitudinal incision is created through the main body of the right inferior constrictor muscle of the pharynx. This incision can be extended caudally through the cricopharyngeal muscle. In the presence of a high supraglottic stricture, in order to place the anastomosis at the oropharyngeal level, it is necessary to divide the stylopharyngeal muscle and resect the greater horn of the hyoid bone. The superior laryngeal nerve may be sacrificed. The pharyngeal wall is usually thick and scarred. The mucosa at the site of the anastomosis should be unaltered. The end-to-side or side-to-side anastomosis is done in a one-layer technique (interrupted or running sutures), using Vicryl 3-0 or 4-0 and it should be at least 2.5 cm long. A penrose drain is always used to drain the site of the anastomosis.

Patients

During the period ranging from January 1,1964 to January 1, 1989, a total of 176 esophagocoloplasties were performed for undilatable postcorrosive stricture of the esophagus at The Center for Esophageal Surgery, Institute for Digestive Diseases of the University Clinical Center, Belgrade, Yugoslavia. Thirty-four (19.31%) of the patients had combined, extensive stricture of the esophagus involving the hypopharynx, the pharynx, and the entire esopagus. The majority of patients (80%) had attempted suicide by swallowing corrosive liquids. The extent and upper level of the stricture varied. All patients were classified into three groups according to the uppermost level of the stricture (Table I).

The diagnosis of the stricture was established by X-ray (barium swallow) examination and rigid endoscopy for hypopharyngeal and high cervical lesions. X-ray investigation was of no value for supraglottic pharyngeal strictures.

The interval from corrosive injury to reconstruction ranged from 6 months to 37 years. Surgical procedures prior to reconstruction were: gastrostomy (27 patients), jejunostomy (4 patients), pharyngostomy (2 patients), tracheostomy (8 patients), and laser resection of laryngeal stricture and supraglottic fibrous tissue (4 patients). Retrosternal "bypass" ileocoloplasty was performed in 16 patients and coloplasty in the remaining 18 patients. In seven patients with stricture of the gastric antrum, corrective surgery had been performed during the reconstructive procedure.

Results

Three patients (8.9%) died in the early postoperative period (necrosis of the transplant, pulmonary embolism, and major leakage of

Table II
Follow-Up of Operated Patients

Level of Stricture	No. Pts.	Time of Closure of Gastrostomy	Swallowing			Lost to Follow-Up
			Good	Fair	Poor	
Pharynx	7	7 mo. to 1 year	5	1	1	
Hypopharynx	16	14 days to 2 mo.	12	1		3
High cervical	8	14 days	7			1
Total	31		24	2	1	4

pts. = patients; mo. = months

the cervical anastomosis). Early postoperative complications were infrequent. A small cervical leak occurred in four patients and healed spontaneously. Compression of the transplant at the upper thoracic outlet occurred in another three patients requiring partial resection of the clavicle and manubrium of the sternum. One patient sustained injury to the left laryngeal nerve which did not affect swallowing.

The most frequent late complication was stricture of the cervical anastomosis encountered in six patients. Reoperation was necessary in four patients while the remaining two were managed by transoral digital dilatation. All six patients are doing well. One patient developed a peptic ulcer close to the distal end of the colon transplant above the cologastro anastomosis. The patient was treated by partial gastrectomy, Billroth I reconstruction, and selective vagotomy and is doing well 14 years after reoperation.

From the functional point of view, good swallowing could not be achieved in the early postoperative period in all patients. All patients treated for supraglottic strictures required several months or even a whole year of exercise in order to achieve exclusive oral alimentation. Long-term follow-up results (1 to 18 years postoperatively) are presented in Table II.

The most important criteria for evaluating patients postoperatively were: pattern of swallowing of both solids and liquids, gain in body weight, and presence of aspiration and regurgitation.

Normal swallowing was achieved in the majority of patients (77.41%), although patients with supraglottic reconstruction demanded an exercise period ranging from a couple of months to a whole year. Repeated yearly check-ups (X-ray examination, barium

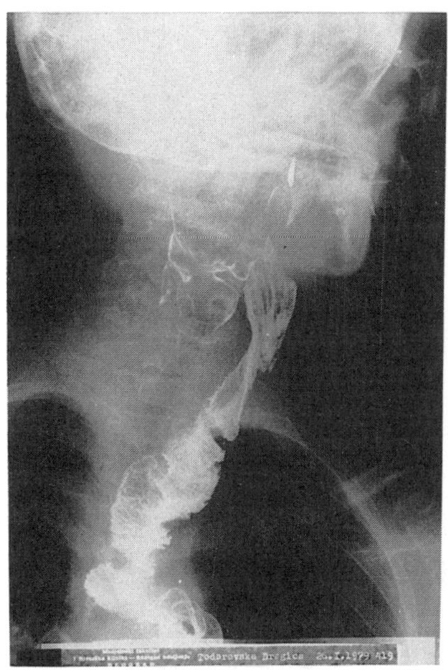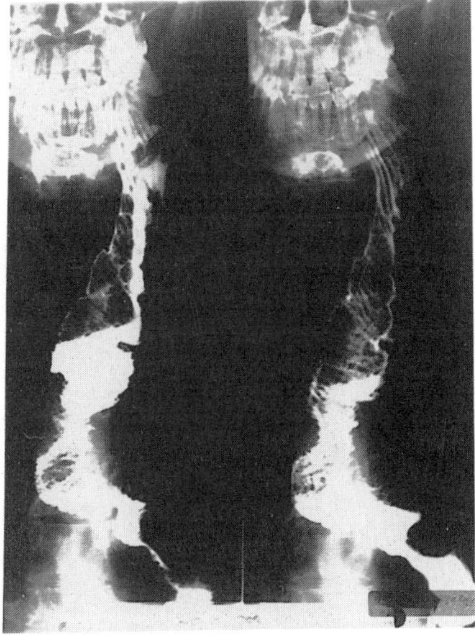

Figure 2A: Postoperative barium swallow in two patients 3 and 5 years after reconstruction demonstrating barium passage through the esophageal replacement (right colon and terminal ileum) without regurgitation or aspiration into the trachea.

swallow) demonstrated good patency of the cervical anastomosis and good function of the colon transplant (Fig. 2).

Presently only one patient, treated for supraglottic stricture, still has a gastrostomy, because swallowing of liquids causes aspiration. Two other patients complained of frequent aspiration, but with time, the frequency of complaints decreased although aspiration never disappeared entirely. Some patients needed psychiatric monitoring and treatment due to varying degrees of psychiatric disability. Four patients were lost to follow-up.

Discussion

Experience with reconstructive surgery in patients with established, extensive pharyngoesophageal stricture is limited, since these patients are rare. Published data are scarce and experience is based on small series. The exact site of the stricture is not described in most

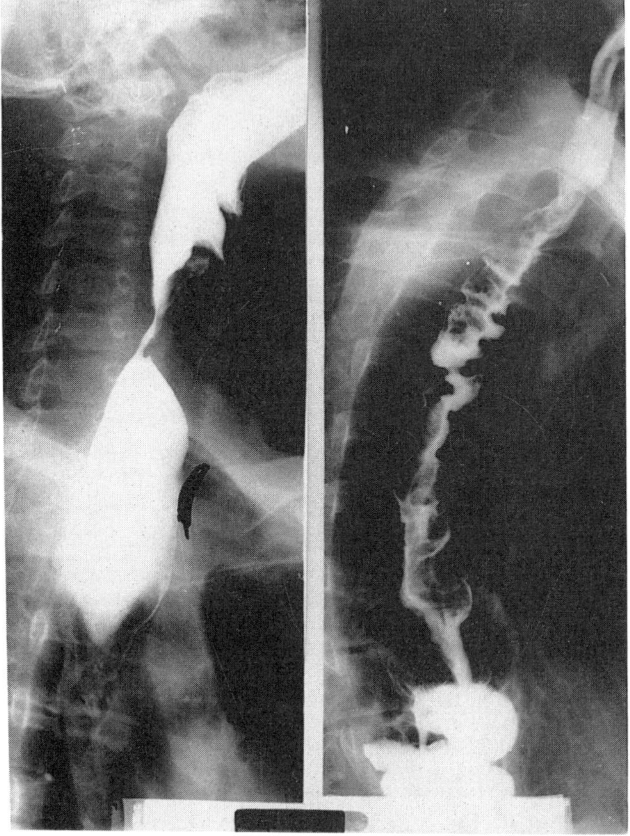

Figure 2B: Preoperative barium swallow examination in a patient with multiple strictures (hypopharyngeal and esophageal). One month postoperative barium swallow shows good passage through left colon transmediastinal replacement after esophagectomy without thoracotomy.

series so they are of little comparative value. Careful endoscopic evaluation is essential for the exact localization of the caustic lesions.

When the hypopharynx is completely obstructed, different approaches are proposed. The posterior pharyngeal[15–17] and the transepiglottic[18] approaches are the most common. Some authors perform pharyngocoloplasty as two- or three-stage procedures.[13,19] We prefer the posterolateral pharyngeal approach for anastomosis with the colon as an one-stage procedure. Esophagectomy should not be a routine procedure since most patients have a high, complete stricture of the esophagus.[14,18] If esophagectomy needs to be performed, we prefer transhiatal esophagectomy without thoracotomy.

All authors have observed several frequent complications in patients with such high anastomosis. One of the most frequent and troublesome postoperative complications is aspiration during swallowing. The second is stricture of the anastomosis, which can prove to be undilatable.[18] In order to prevent stricture of the anastomosis, extensive resection of the scarred pharyngeal wall prior to anastomosis has been advocated.[15,17]

Since 1950, colon bypass has been the most widely used method of esophageal replacement. Petrov et al.[14] and Ogura et al.[13] used colon transplants for postcorrosive pharyngoesophageal stricture with good results. Recently, some authors have stressed advantages of the stomach in such patients,[15–17] but their experience is limited to only a few patients. Transposition of the stomach to replace the hypopharynx as cervical esophagus has been used most often in treatment of cervical esophageal, laryngeal, and hypopharyngeal carcinoma.[12] In patients with benign strictures, where life expectancy is long, we prefer colon transplants, as do most authors with relevant experience.[13,18] There are two reasons for choosing the colon: first, the colon has a better blood supply, and second, the stomach is frequently unusable due to initial caustic damage or previous feeding gastrostomy.

Postoperative functional results depend on the extent and level of stricture. Reconstruction for supraglottic stricture is most difficult and the functional results are uncertain. There is a significant difference in function between anastomosis at the pharyngeal or esophageal level. In pharyngeal anastomosis, the upper esophageal sphincter function does not exist and aspiration during swallowing can be a problem. It seems that better functional results are attained with right colon and terminal ileum segments, probably due to active peristalsis of the ileum and the valve of Bauchini. Substantial data are lacking and further investigations are necessary. In our opinion, incision of the posterolateral wall of the pharynx should be in a vertical direction and at least 2.5 cm long. Definitive assessment of functional results should be postponed, since some patients witnessed significant improvement in swallowing during periods ranging from a few months to more than a year postoperatively.

References

1. Oakes DD, Sherk JP, Mark JBD: Lye ingestion. J Thorac Cardiovasc Surg 83:194, 1982.
2. Haller JA Jr, Andrews HC, et al: Pathophysiology and management of acute corrosive burns of the esophagus. J Pediatr Surg 6:578, 1971.
3. Borja MR, Ransdell HT Jr, et al: Lye injuries of the esophagus. J Thorac Cardiovasc Surg 57:533, 1969.
4. Bikhazi HB, Thompson ER, Shumrich DA: Caustive ingestion: Current status. Arch Otolaryngol 89:770, 1969.
5. Triggiani E, Belsey R: Esophageal trauma. Incidence, diagnosis and management. Thorax 32:241, 1977.
6. Roux C: L'esophago-jejuno-gastroanastomoses, nouvelle operation pour retrecissement infranchissable de l'esophage. Semin Med 4:37, 1907.
7. Lexer E: Vollstandigier Ersatz der Speiserohre. Munich Med Wschr 58:1548, 1911.
8. Kelling G: Oesophagoplastic mit Hilfe des Quiercolon. Zentralb F Chir 38:9, 1911.
9. Kirschner M: Ein neues Verfaren der oesophagoplastik. Arch Klin Chir 114:553, 1920.
10. Wookey H: The surgical treatment of carcinoma of the pharynx and upper esophagus. Surg Gynecol Obstet 75:499, 1942.
11. Seidenberg B, Hurwitz ES: Immediate reconstruction of the cervical esophagus by a revascularised isolated jejunal segment. Surg Forum 9:413, 1958.
12. Ong GB, Lee TC: Pharyngogastric anastomosis after pharyngectomy for carcinoma of the hypopharynx and cervical esophagus. Br J Surg 48:193, 1960.
13. Ogura JH, Roper CL, Burford TH: Complete functional restitution of the food passage in extensive stenosing burns of the esophagus. J Thorac Cardiovasc Surg 42:340, 1961.
14. Petrov BA, Sitnik AP: Totalnaja kisecnaja ezofagoplastika pri rubcovik suzenija pisevoda u glotki. Hirurgija 11:14, 1962.
15. Gupta S: Total obliteration of the esophagus and hypopharynx due to corrosives. J Thorac Cardiovasc Surg 2:264, 1970.
16. Thomas AN, Dedo HH, et al: Pharyngoesophageal caustic stricture. Am J Surg 132:195, 1976.
17. Ti TK: Oesophageal resection with pharyngogastrostomy for corrosive stricture of the pharynx and esophagus. Br J Surg 27:798, 1980.
18. Ba Huy PT, Celerier M: Management of severe caustic stenosis of the hypopharynx and esophagus by ileocolic transposition via suprahioid or transepiglotic approach. Ann Surg 207:439, 1988.
19. Peracchia A, Bardini R: Pharyngoplasty in three or two stages after damages caused by caustics. VIII GEEMO Meeting, Leuven, 1988, Proceedings.

V.

Esophageal Perforation:
Editors' Overview

Chapters 31 and 32 review an experience with a total of 20 patients treated with emergency esophagectomy for perforations complicating benign disease. This primarily addresses patients with esophageal perforations for whom the decision for resection is based upon the presence of such severe esophageal disease that long-term, satisfactory function is unlikely, and/or the presence of mediastinitis and sepsis. Both reports document that resection with reconstruction of gastrointestinal continuity with an esophagogastrostomy located in the neck is a satisfactory undertaking as it completely eliminates the possibility of continuing mediastinal or pleural sepsis. Long-term gastrointestinal function is satisfactory. The two groups differ in their preferred technique for esophagectomy but, as results are equivalent, it would appear that the primary point is that there is a role for this aggressive procedure in order that some patients can not only survive but survive with good results. The technique of esophagectomy should be based upon the surgeon's experience and preference.

31

Emergency Subtotal Esophagectomy

Hugoe R. Matthews, I.M. Mitchell, J.A. McGuigan

Introduction

Esophageal conditions that are bad enough to require resection as an emergency are not common. When they do occur, however, they pose very difficult problems of management for a number of reasons: patients are often elderly, decrepit, and in severe shock, the diagnosis of the nature and extent of the injury and the presence or absence of associated disease such as tumor or stricture may be incomplete and there may be involvement of the mediastinum, and abdominal or both pleural cavities by contamination.

The permutations that arise from these factors mean that individual cases vary widely and there is correspondingly a wide spectrum of possibilities as to the best surgical treatment. For the same reason comparative studies are difficult and none have so far been reported with homogeneous populations. Since 1981, therefore, we have attempted to unify the management of these cases by performing one-stage resection and reconstruction with esophagogastric anastomosis in the neck as the standard operation for emergency esophageal resection whenever possible. The purpose of this paper is to present our results and discuss the merits of this approach in the treatment of surgical esophageal emergencies.[1]

Little AG, Ferguson MK, Skinner DB: Diseases of the Esophagus, Vol. II: Benign Diseases. Futura Publishing Company, Inc., Mount Kisco, NY, © 1990.

Patients and Methods

From 1981 to 1987, a total of 318 esophageal resections were performed for standard indications, including both benign and malignant disease. Of these operations, nine (2.8%) were done as an emergency on patients ranging from 27 to 71 years (mean 54 years), of whom six were male. Intrathoracic perforation communicating with the pleural space was the indication in six patients. Five of these had endoscopic perforation (four from outside hospitals, one from our own) and all of these had an associated carcinoma, though this was not diagnosed until operation in two patients. The sixth patient had undergone an intrathoracic Nissen fundoplication for short esophagus and reflux stricture 3 months previously at another hospital and was admitted in profound shock with spontaneous necrosis and perforation of the gastric fundus into the left chest. In several of these cases, there was a delay in diagnosis and transfer to our unit so that three of the patients were not operated on until more than 24 hours after the perforation, the others being operated on at 8, 12, and 14 hours, respectively; mean interval from perforation to operation was 18 hours for all six patients.

Two other patients were resected for severe hemorrhage. One of these had esophageal varices and portal hypertension from chronic active hepatitis B and was continuing to bleed despite multiple sclerotherapy and a Sengstaken tube. The other patient had a bleeding Barrett's ulcer in a columnar-lined esophagus with hiatal hernia and reflux and was operated on after the transfusion of 13 units of blood.

The ninth patient had a hiatal hernia and reflux with an esophageal ulcer penetrating into the mediastinum. Three days after esophagoscopy and dilatation, he developed acute pain and shock and operation revealed an acute sterile mediastinitis with gross edema but no perforation. It was postulated that dilatation may have aggravated his reflux with resultant mediastinal inflammation.

Perioperative Management

Operation was performed as soon as possible in all patients after initial resuscitation but was not delayed even if normal circulation could not be restored. Chest drains were inserted before operation in all patients with collections of fluid or air and intravenous antibiotics given to all those with intrathoracic leaks. Emergency contrast studies were obtained in five patients, but not in two patients who were too ill and in the two bleeding patients who had already had recent studies. Endoscopy was not used in any patient.

Operation consisted of subtotal esophagectomy in all patients in two parts, through a left thoracolaparotomy in the 6th intercostal space and an oblique left neck incision, since the esophagogastrostomy is our standard practice for the elective resection of esophageal carcinoma.[2] Two patients had complicating factors in the form of a benign gastric ulcer in one case and an enlarged thyroid in the other, but neither of these interfered with the successful completion of the operation. The only patient to have any stomach resected was the one with a gastric perforation, where the area of necrosis adjacent to the cardia was resected with a cuff of stomach.

Postoperative regimes were kept as simple as possible. Nasogastric tubes were not used routinely but the patient with gastric perforation had a small Foley catheter inserted across the neck as a temporary gastrostomy to decompress the severely inflamed stomach. Artificial ventilation was used only if spontaneous respiration was unsatisfactory. Oral fluids were commenced on the second postoperative day, progressing to soft diet by the time of discharge from the hospital. Postoperative antibiotics were used only in those patients with intrathoracic sepsis at the time of operation.

Results

Eight patients made a satisfactory recovery and were discharged from the hospital at intervals ranging from 10 to 27 days (mean 18 days). One patient (11% of the whole group and 17% of the perforated group) died on the third postoperative day from irreversible shock. This patient had required inotropic support even before operation and never regained an adequate circulation. Autopsy confirmed death from circulatory failure with the alimentary reconstruction intact.

Two patients required ventilation postoperatively and one other developed sputum retention requiring minitracheotomy. One patient was found to have a localized anastomotic leak on routine postoperative barium studies but was asymptomatic and required no treatment. No other postoperative complications occurred.

Of the five patients with perforated carcinoma, four survived to be discharged from the hospital. Of these, one died at 4 years 9 months from a second primary tumor in the pelvis and one died at

9 months from recurrence of his esophageal carcinoma. The other two are alive at 2 years 7 months and 9 months, respectively.

The four patients with nonmalignant disease all survived and were discharged from the hospital but one died at 2 months from an aggressive primary hepatoma that was not identified at the time of operation. The remaining three are all alive and well at 9 months to 2 years from operation. One patient required a single anastomotic dilatation but no other surgical revision or attention has been necessary for any of the survivors.

Discussion

The first emergency esophageal resection with immediate reconstruction was reported by Satkinsky and Kron in 1952[3] and it has since come to be accepted that this is an effective and satisfactory form of treatment when the operative findings are favorable and the patient's condition permits.[4] All the reported anastomoses, however, have been performed inside the chest.

Our experience suggests that the neck offers a more attractive option as a site for anastomosis. Larsson and Petterson[5] have stressed the importance of a high anastomosis in diminishing late postoperative reflux but access to the apex of the chest on either side can be difficult and anastomosis is certainly technically easier in the neck. Additional advantages of this site are that the short esophageal stump has a good blood supply, the anastomosis is made in a clean field, and if postoperative leaks do occur, they are less likely to lead to the death of the patient. Lymphatic clearance in patients with carcinoma is clearly better than with intrathoracic anastomosis and lesions at any level of the intrathoracic esophagus can be dealt with.

Our results would certainly seem to indicate that this two-part left-sided subtotal esophagectomy is a satisfactory emergency operation. No technical difficulty was encountered in getting the fundus of the stomach up to the neck in any patient and the postoperative mortality of 11% for the whole group is as good as our figures for the elective resection of esophageal carcinoma,[2] despite the fact that most of the patients in this series were critically ill. The long-term results have also been satisfactory in terms of the reconstruction with no patient having any major long-term complications or requiring any further surgical revision of the alimentary tract. Some patients with esophageal emergencies requiring resection may be too ill for immediate reconstruction and should have a gastrostomy and terminal esophagostomy with later reconstruction, but in suitable cases we would suggest that the neck should be the first choice for the site of anastomosis in patients who are suitable for resection and reconstruction at a single stage.

References

1. Matthews HR, Mitchell IM, McGuigan JA: Emergency subtotal esophagectomy. Br J Surg 76, 1989 (in press).
2. Matthews HR, Steel A: Left-sided subtotal esophagectomy for carcinoma. Br J Surg 74:1115, 1987.
3. Satkinsky VP, Kron SD: One-stage esophagectomy in presence of mediastinitis. Arch Surg 64:124, 1952.
4. Kerr WF: Emergency esophagectomy. Thorax 23:204, 1968.
5. Larsson S, Petterson G: Advisability of concomitant immediate surgery for perforation and underlying disease of the esophagus. Scand J Thorac Cardiovasc Surg 18:275, 1984.

32

One-Stage Esophagectomy and Reconstruction for Esophageal Perforation in Benign Disease

Mark B. Orringer

Introduction

Disruption of the intrathoracic esophagus has long been among the most serious of challenges faced by the esophageal surgeon. The physiological consequences of mediastinal contamination by oral bacteria, saliva, and refluxed gastric contents are generally fatal without surgical intervention. As treatment is delayed, the mortality from this injury increases, to 40–60% after 24 hours.[1-3] While the need for surgical intervention in the majority of these patients is almost uniformly acknowledged, opinion as to the operative approach and method of treatment varies widely. The decision-making process is influenced by multiple factors: the patient's age and general condition, associated systemic illness, the degree of esophageal inflammation at the site of the tear, the extent of pleural contamination, and the duration of time between the injury and its diagnosis .Drainage or attempted repair that results in another esophageal leak commit the patient to a prolonged, often complicated hospital course. Esophageal diversion re-

Little AG, Ferguson MK, Skinner DB: Diseases of the Esophagus, Vol. II: Benign Diseases. Futura Publishing Company, Inc., Mount Kisco, NY, © 1990.

sults in the need for a subsequent operation to restore the ability to swallow and complicates reconstructive procedures. This chapter reviews an experience with 11 patients with benign esophageal disease and an intrathoracic esophageal disruption treated by esophagectomy and immediate reconstruction with a cervical esophagogastrostomy.

Patients

During the past 15 years, 50 patients with perforations of the intrathoracic esophagus have been treated by the University of Michigan Thoracic Surgery Service. Twenty-seven patients (54%) were treated either by primary repair (22) or drainage (5). This latter group had either minimal intrinsic esophageal disease or endoscopic, postoperative, or postemetic perforations that were diagnosed early and were favorable for repair. One patient with an endoscopically perforated carcinoma underwent esophagectomy and primary esophagogastrostomy. Twenty-two additional patients (44%) with perforations unassociated with esophageal cancer have been treated by esophagectomy: one-half with a proximal cervical or anterior thoracic esophagostomy and one-half with esophageal resection and immediate reconstruction. This latter group of 11 patients is the subject of this chapter.

Among the 11 patients with intrathoracic esophageal perforations unassociated with cancer were eight women and three men ranging in age from 31 to 88 years (average 68 years). The oldest patients were 78, 79, 86, and 88 years (Table I). The etiology of the esophageal perforations included esophageal dilation in six (mercury-weighted in four, balloon in two), esophagoscopy in one, emesis in two, penetrating Barrett's ulcer in one, and swallowed dental prosthesis in one. Ten of the 11 patients had pre-existing esophageal disease, the presence of which influenced the decision for resection: reflux strictures (seven), monilial esophagitis (one), esophageal spasm associated with a pulsion diverticulum (one), and megaesophagus of achalasia (one).

The esophageal resections were performed within 4 hours to 20 days (average 4 days) after the diagnosis of the perforation. Four patients were operated upon within 6 hours of their injury, two from 6–12 hours, one at 18 hours, and four patients were operated upon after 3, 7, 14, and 20 days, respectively. In four patients undergoing

Table I
Esophagectomy for Esophageal Disruption: Single Stage Resection and Reconstruction

Patient no.	Age	Sex	Etiology of Disruption	Intrinsic Esophageal Disease	Interval-Leak to Esophagectomy	Operation	Complications	Hospitalization After Esophagectomy (Days)
1	69	M	Emesis	Reflux Stricture	<12 Hrs	THE/ Cerv E-G	Continued Sepsis, Death—3 Wks P.O.	—
2	86	M	Barret's Ulcer	Reflux Stricture	20 Days	THE/ Cerv E-G	Resp. Insufficiency, Sudden Death 9 Days P.O.	—
3	31	M	Endoscopy	Monilial Esophagitis	7 Days	THE/ Cerv E-G	Anastomotic Leak, Sepsis, Death 2 Mos. P.O.	—
4	65	F	Maloney Dilation	Scleroderma Reflux Stricture	<12 Hrs	THE/ Cerv E-G	Aspiration, Resp. Insufficiency	120
5	60	F	Balloon Dilation	Megaesophagus Achalasia	THE/<6 Hrs	Cerv E-G	None	12
6	78	F	Maloney Dilation	Reflux Stricture	<4 Hrs	THE/ Cerv E-G	None	15
7	88	M	Maloney Dilation	Reflux Stricture	<4 Hrs	THE/ Cerv E-G	None	15
8	79	F	Maloney Dilation	Reflux Stricture	72 Hrs	THE/ Cerv E-G	None	10
9	69	F	Balloon Dilation	Spasm, Pulsion Diverticulum	<6 Hrs	THE/ Cerv E-G	None	10
10	69	F	Emesis	Reflux Stricture	14 Days	THE/ Cerv E-G	None	12
11	59	F	Swallowed Dental Prosthesis	None	18 Hrs	TTE/ Cerv E-G	None	10

THE = Transhiatal esophagectomy without thoracotomy; CERV E-G = Cervical esophagogastrostomy; TTE = Transthoracic esophagectomy.
Reproduced (in part) with permission from Orringer MB and Stirling MC: Esophagectomy for esophageal disruption. Ann Thorac Surg (in press).

rigid esophagoscopy and dilation under general anesthesia, there was immediate concern that a perforation may have occurred during the instrumentation. The flexible esophagoscope was introduced, air was insufflated into the esophagus, and a portable chest roentgenogram was obtained. With the finding of mediastinal air on the chest film and the diagnosis of a perforation confirmed, the patient was allowed to awaken from anesthesia, and an emergency water-soluble contrast esophagogram was obtained to localize the site of the tear prior to surgical intervention. The presence of distal esophageal obstruction (reflux stricture), intrinsic esophageal disease (monilial esophagitis, diffuse spasm with pulsion diverticulum), or severe local mediastinal inflammation were regarded as factors that would so jeopardize the healing of an attempted repair that resection was a more reliable option.

In all but one patient in whom a swallowed dental prosthesis had lodged in the esophagus and caused a local perforation, the esophagectomy was performed transhiatally without a thoracotomy, and copious irrigation of the mediastinum was carried out. After removal of the esophagus, a sump catheter was inserted into the low posterior mediastinum through the diaphragmatic hiatus, and through a rubber catheter placed in the superior mediastinum through the cervical incision, 3–6 liters of saline solution were flushed into and aspirated from the mediastinum. The stomach was then mobilized through the posterior mediastinum in the original esophageal bed, and a cervical esophagogastric anastomosis was performed as described previously.[4,5] No mediastinal drain was used after the esophagectomy, although in each case, a chest tube was placed because of entry in one pleural cavity during the esophagectomy. The patient with the dental prosthesis impacted in the esophagus had undergone a prior esophagoscopy in an attempt to remove it. Sharp metallic barbs on the prosthesis resulted in multiple lacerations making repair impossible. A transthoracic approach was used for the esophagectomy, and a cervical esophagogastrectomy performed.

In the four patients with chronic disruptions 3, 7, 14, and 20 days after their injuries, the perforations were contained within the mediastinum and did not communicate with either pleural cavity. Two of these patients were edentulous and had little systemic evidence of infection. Each of the seven patients with perforations of less than 24 hours' duration required chest tube insertion because of an associated pneumothorax, but none had gross contamination of the pleural cavity or an empyema requiring a decortication. All had required vigorous intravenous rehydration and were receiving broad-spectrum antibiotic therapy at the time of their esophagectomy. A pyloromyotomy and feeding jejunostomy were used routinely in every patient.

Results

Despite the gravity of the situation, every patient tolerated the esophagectomy and esophageal replacement well. Measured intraoperative blood loss averaged 750 ml (range 100–1900 ml). These patients required intensive care monitoring for 72 hours after esophagectomy for treatment of intravascular fluid volume shifts and transient bacteremia. There were three hospital deaths (27% mortality), none related to the esophagectomy per se. One death occurred in an 86-year-old woman with a chronic contained perforated Barrett's ulcer and reflux stricture. She had been treated with anticoagulants 6 months earlier for deep venous thrombosis. After her esophagectomy, she required prolonged ventilatory assistance for respiratory insufficiency, and she died suddenly on the ninth postoperative day, either of a pulmonary embolus or a primary cardiac event (infarction or arrhythmia).

The other two deaths occurred in immunosuppressed patients with chronic renal failure, one of whom had undergone a renal transplant and was taking steroids and Imuran. His esophagus was perforated during endoscopic assessment of monilial esophagitis. He developed an anastomotic leak after his esophagectomy and remained septic throughout his hospital course, eventually dying 2 months later.

The third patients also had chronic renal failure and was on peritoneal dialysis when he developed a postemetic perforation. He remained septic after his esophagectomy and died 3 weeks later. One patient developed a left subphrenic abscess that was drained 6 weeks after the esophagectomy, 1 month after the patient's discharge from the hospital.

Another patient with scleroderma involvement of the esophagus and lungs required prolonged mechanical ventilation and a tracheostomy for respiratory insufficiency and was hospitalized for 4 months. She died 1 month later in a nursing facility of pneumonia. The remaining seven patients were discharged from the hospital 10–

15 days (average 12 days) after their esophagectomy. They have been followed from 6 to 84 months (average 30 months), and have been well and able to eat comfortably, with varying degrees of mild early satiety, regurgitation, and postvagotomy diarrhea.

Discussion

This report does not endorse a uniform policy of esophageal resection for every perforation. When a perforation is diagnosed within the first few hours after the injury has occurred, particularly in an otherwise normal or minimally diseased esophagus, closure of the tear and buttressing of the suture-line with intercostal muscle, pleura, pericardium, or omentum[6–8] is appropriate. Our decision to resect the perforated esophagus is influenced primarily by three factors: (1) the presence of intrinsic esophageal disease that will continue to impede comfortable swallowing even if repair of the injury is successful; (2) an estimate of the likelihood that the repair will heal primarily and the patient's ability to tolerate recurrent mediastinitis if it does not; and (3) an evaluation of the patient's overall condition. In general, the more ill the patient from mediastinitis and sepsis, the less tolerant we are of accepting a tenuous esophageal repair. A patient recovering from an initial bout of mediastinitis from an esophageal perforation may not be able to tolerate recurrent infection from breakdown of the repair. While an esophagectomy in a critically ill patient with mediastinitis is a major undertaking that inflicts an additional physiological insult initially, this approach completely eliminates the source of the sepsis, i.e., the perforation, and therefore provides the patient the best chance for survival.

In our opinion, repair of a perforation in a significantly diseased esophagus is unwise. A 23% mortality rate for perforations occurring in an intrinsically diseased esophagus, compared with 4% for perforations in an otherwise normal esophagus, has been reported by Michel et al.[3] An existing reflux stricture combined with fibrosis that follows healing of an esophageal perforation closure insures only increased dysphagia for the patient. A megaesophagus of achalasia that is perforated will not function well even if the injury heals.

Patient 9 (see Table I), who sustained a perforation of the esophagogastric junction during balloon dilation, had a large midesophageal pulsion diverticulum and associated esophageal spasm. Repair of the perforation alone would have left untreated the underlying motor disturbance. Resection of the diverticulum, esophagomyotomy, and repair of the perforation would have resulted in two esophageal suture lines in a recently contaminated mediastinum. Esophagectomy was felt to be the safest option that would also restore comfortable swallowing to this patient. The functional results of esophageal resection and replacement with stomach anastomosed to the cervical esophagus are sufficiently reliable[9] that we now favor this approach when a perforation in a clearly abnormal esophagus is encountered.

Nonoperative management of perforations of the thoracic esophagus that are confined to the mediastinum and unassociated with empyema or sepsis has been advocated.[10,11] Most argue, however, that the risk of a subsequent mediastinal abscess and empyema in such patients is too great to leave the leak uncontrolled.[2,3] Other options have been described, including T-tube drainage to establish an esophagopleural cutaneous fistula,[12] use of an indwelling esophageal prosthesis to occlude the fistula,[13] or occlusion of the fistula with a pleural or omental flap.[7] Unless these methods are successful in controlling the leak, the patient is relegated to a prolonged hospitalization, continued sepsis, and possibly death. We generally avoid esophageal exclusion procedures[15,16] which only complicate subsequent reconstruction and interrupt or result in an incision in the relatively normal cervical esophagus.

Treatment of an esophageal perforation that is not associated with significant mediastinal and pleural contamination is far less complicated than when such bacterial and chemical inflammation is present. Therefore, the sooner a perforation occurring as a result of esophageal instrumentation can be diagnosed, the better. We routinely insufflate air into the esophagus through a flexible fiberoptic esophagoscope whenever we have serious concern that a tear has occurred. This results in mediastinal emphysema on a chest radiograph and signals the need for a contrast study to localize the site of the perforation prior to surgical intervention. When extensive pleural contamination has not occurred in association with an esophageal perforation for which an esophagectomy is planned, the transhiatal route without thoracotomy is an excellent option. This approach opens the mediastinum widely and allows vigorous irrigation through the neck and abdominal incisions. If the patient is too ill to tolerate immediate esophageal reconstruction, a cervical or upper thoracic esophagostomy can be constructed and a feeding tube inserted. Alternatively, mobilization of the stomach into the posterior mediastinum in the original esophageal bed fills the potential space left by the resected esophagus with a viable, well-vascularized organ that helps to control the infection. The cervical anastomosis, placed outside the field of contamination, is no more at risk for a leak than under standard conditions. Experience and surgical judgment are critical to the successful management of these patients. But the more dependable and predictable results of esophagectomy and cervical esophagogastrostomy for selected patients with perforation of the thoracic esophagus often make this approach safer than less "radical" attempts at drainage, exclusion, or diversion.

References

1. Sandrasagra FA, English TAH, Milstein BB: The management and prognosis of esophageal perforation. Br J Surg 65:629, 1978.
2. Skinner DB, Little AG, DeMeester TR: Management of esophageal perforation. Am J Surg 139:760, 1980.
3. Michel L, Grillo HC, Malt RC: Operative and nonoperative management of esophageal perforation. Ann Surg 194:57, 1981.
4. Orringer MB, Sloan H: Esophagectomy without thoracotomy. J Thorac Cardiovasc Surg 76:643, 1978.
5. Orringer MB, Stirling MC: Cervical esophagogastric anastomosis for benign disease: Functional results. J Thorac Cardiovasc Surg 96:887, 1988.
6. Orringer MB: Complications of esophageal surgery and trauma. In: Complications in Surgery and Trauma, Greenfield LJ (ed), Philadelphia, J.B. Lippincott Co., 1984, p 260.
7. Mathisen DJ, Grillo HC, Vlahakes GJ, et al: The omentum in the management of complicated cardiothoracic problems. J Thorac Cardiovasc Surg 95:677, 1988.
8. Grillo HC, Wilkins EW Jr, Michel L, et al: Esophageal perforation: the syndrome and its management. In: Esophageal Disorders: Pathophysiology and Therapy, DeMeester, TR, Skinner DB (eds), New York, Raven Press, 1985, p 493.
9. Orringer MB: Transhiatal esophagectomy for benign disease. J Thorac Cardiovasc Surg 90:649, 1985.
10. Cameron JL, Kieffer RF, Hendrix TR, et al: Selective nonoperative management of contained intrathoracic esophageal perforations. Ann Thorac Surg 27:404, 1979.
11. Sarr MG, Penberton JH, Payne WS: Management of instrumental perforations of the esophagus. J Thorac Cardiovasc Surg 84:211, 1982.
12. Abbott OA, Mansour KA, Logan WD Jr, et al: Atraumatic so-called "spontaneous" rupture of the esophagus: A review of 47 personal cases with comments on a new method of surgical therapy. J Thorac Cardiovasc Surg 59:67, 1970.

13. Berger RL, Donato AT: Treatment of esophageal disruption by intubation: A new method of management. Ann Thorac Surg 13:27, 1972.
14. Grillo HC, Wilkins EW Jr: Esophageal repair following late diagnosis of intrathoracic perforations. Ann Thorac Surg 20:387, 1975.
15. Johnson J, Schwegman CW, Kirby CK: Esophageal exclusion for persistent fistula following spontaneous rupture of the esophagus. J Thorac Cardiovasc Surg 32:827, 1956.
16. Urschel HC, Razzuk MA, Wood RE, et al: Improved management of esophageal perforation: Exclusion and diversion in continuity. Ann Surg 179:587, 1974.

VI

Motility Disorders:
Editors' Overview

Chapter 33 outlines the surgical options in the management of achalasia. The authors feel that relatively early achalasia, prior to extensive esophageal dilation, can be managed by myotomy plus fundoplication. This is a reasonable view which is shared by many surgeons. The authors advocate a more radical approach to patients who have an extremely dilated esophagus and recommend esophagectomy and reconstruction using the stomach for this group. The editors feel this latter option is appropriate for some patients but is probably only required for an extremely small subset of patients. Chapter 34 is an important patient series which shows that properly performed esophageal dilation is the appropriate initial treatment for most achalasia patients, although there is a suggestion that younger patients are more likely to fail dilation and should be considered for early operation. These authors also state their preference for adding an antireflux procedure to the myotomy but admit that this is an unresolved issue.

The next two chapters focus on the upper esophageal sphincter. Chapter 35 reports an experience utilizing a sleeve manometry technique for study of the upper sphincter and finds that this method detects a higher pressure gradient remaining at the end of sphincter relaxation than does conventional manometry. The suggestion is made that sleeve manometry may become a very important tool in the diagnosis of upper esophageal sphincter disorders. Chapter 36 reports an experience with 100 patients with a Zenker's, or pharyngoesophageal, diverticulum. In addition to showing that myotomy plus diverticulopexy provides excellent results, the authors also document that there are clear pathological changes identifiable in the cricopharyngeal muscle in these patients. The combination of clinical and manometric data and these morphologic changes suggests that this diverticulum is one expression of a generalized neurogenic disorder.

Chapter 37 is consistent with other reports in the literature, all of which document the etiologic relationship between esophageal motor disorders and esophageal diverticula. This chapter illustrates the heterogeneity of these motor abnormalities but emphasizes their importance and, therefore, the necessity of an esophagomyotomy when surgical treatment is required. Chapter 38 presents information regarding a relatively new technique for investigation of esophageal motor abnormalities, the radionuclide esophageal transit study. The esophageal transit study seems to be a useful, noninvasive test for screening of patients which can be used to quantitate esophageal emptying patterns.

The pathophysiologic connection between abnormal esophageal contractions and chest pain has remained obscure. Despite the suggestion that a hypertensive lower esophageal sphincter may be important in the genesis of this pain, Chapter 39 shows that a hypertensive sphincter occurs only in a minority of patients and that dysphagia, when present, is usually due to an associated motility disorder of the esophageal body.

33

Surgery of Achalasia of the Esophagus

Henrique W. Pinotti, Ivan Cecconello,
Bruno Zilberstein, Ary Nasi

Introduction

We have adopted a classification in order to arrive at a more adequate management of achalasia or megaesophagus during its different stages. It is based on functional behavior, evaluated by manometric and radiological studies of the organ. It is as follows:

(1)*Early:* undilated esophagus or esophageal dilation less than 10 cm;

(2)*Advanced:* dilation of over 10 cm and elongation of the esophagus usually with loss of its rectilinear orientation. Manometric studies show weak contractions or an atonic esophagus.

Treatment should be chosen on an individual basis, considering the overall clinical situation prior to surgery, in addition to the proposed classification. The early cases are submitted to conservative operation. The goal is to overcome the obstacle at the level of the cardia so food can pass to the stomach. For advanced forms, we prefer to resect the esophagus.

Surgical Treatment of Early Megaesophagus

Even though peristalsis is absent in early forms of megaesophagus, the esophageal muscle is still capable of good contractility. In

Little AG, Ferguson MK, Skinner DB: Diseases of the Esophagus, Vol. II: Benign Diseases. Futura Publishing Company, Inc., Mount Kisco, NY, © 1990.

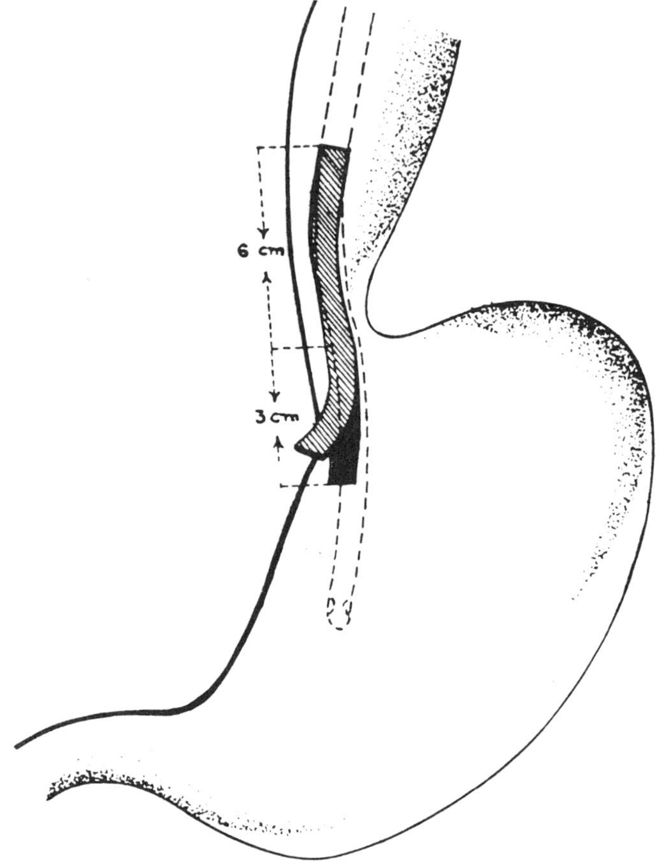

Figure 1: Cardiomyectomy.

these cases, when the barrier represented by the inferior sphincter of the esophagus is overcome, we observe immediate resolution of dysphagia and radiologically we see reduction in diameter of the organ with decrease of stasis. For this reason, the operation for this type of megaesophagus should be nonresectional and of low risk.

Surgical Technique

Laparotomy via a median supraumbilical incision is used for the procedure. The anterior surface of the distal esophagus and proximal

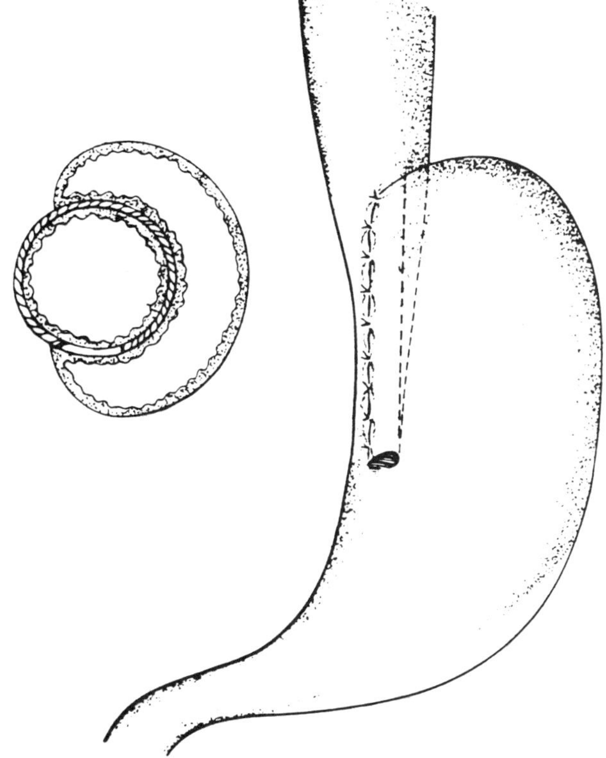

Figure 2: Diagram of the final appearance of the operation after fundoplication. The inset depicts the transverse section of the valve showing how;
the myectomy is covered by the serosa of the gastric fundus.

stomach are used for the extramucosal cardiomyectomy. A strip of
muscle 0.5 to 1 cm wide extending from 3 cm below to 6 cm above
the gastroesophageal junction is resected (Fig. 1). After mobilization
of the gastric fundus, a partial fundoplication is done. For this purpose, the gastric fundus is sutured to the posterior aspect of the
esophagus and to the anterior surface along the left and right margins
of the myectomy[1,2] (Fig. 2).

Results

Seven hundred and thirty six patients with early megaesophagus
were submitted to cardiomyectomy with fundoplication in our department (1969–1989).

The intraoperative complications included injury to the spleen in 27 cases (3.7%) and perforation of the mucosa in 30 cases (4.1%). We have managed to reduce these complications by displacing the spleen by placing packs in the splenic bed drawing it near to the stomach and avoiding tension when the gastric fundus is freed. A catheter 10 cm in diameter placed in the esophagus before myectomy greatly facilitates the procedure and significantly decreases the rate of perforation of the mucosa. If this occurs, the mucosa is sutured with 4-0 nylon and the region is covered with the gastric fundus.

There were no deaths in this series of 736 patients. Out of this total, excellent results were obtained in 83.88% of the cases (absence of dysphagia or reflux); good results were obtained in 11.64% (occasional short episodes of dysphagia and/or retrosternal burning). Poor results were obtained in 4.48% of the cases due to persistent dysphagia and/or retrosternal heartburn.

Surgical Management of the Advanced Form

In this stage, the organ no longer contracts, and the operation of choice is resection. The technique we use is transmediastinal esophagectomy without thoracotomy and re-establishment of continuity by esophagogastrostomy.[3–5]

Surgical Technique

Two surgical teams work simultaneously in the abdominal and cervical regions. The access to the esophagus is via a supraumbilical median incision. The diaphragm is opened, going from the anterior surface of the muscle of the hiatal ring toward the xiphoid process, cutting the aponeurotic part of the diaphragm (Fig. 3).[5] Scissors are used to free the esophagus, and then proceeding cranially, it is detached from the pulmonary vessels. This procedure is facilitated by using long glass type retractors, carefully retracting the pericardium to the front and both pleura to the sides (Fig. 4). The esophagus is also dissected in a cranio-caudal direction via a transverse cutaneous incision in the neck, 6 to 8 cm long and 2 cm above the clavicle. The esophagus is dissected between ligatures in the cervical region at the level previously chosen for its anastomosis to the stomach.

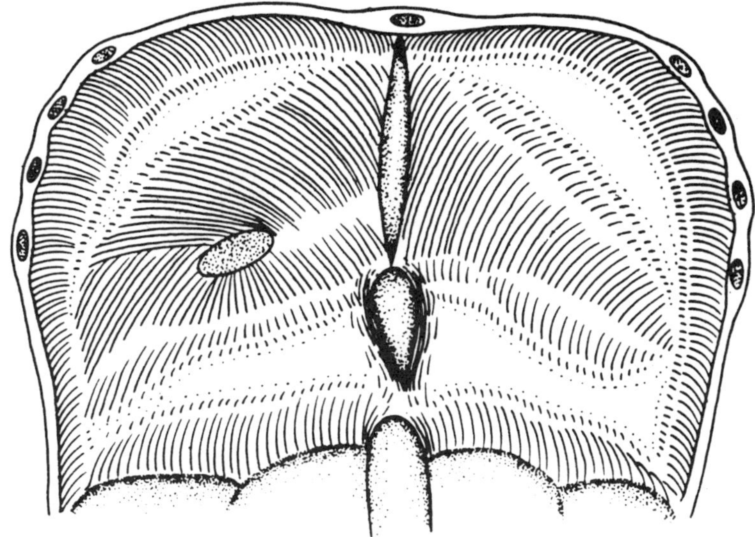

Figure 3: Phrenotomy.

Continuity is re-established directly by the stomach. The arcade of the greater curvature is maintained via the right gastroepiploic vessels and the lesser curvature by the right gastric vessels. Extramucosal pyloromyectomy is carried out. The stomach is brought via the mediastinal tunnel into the cervical region where the esophagogastric anastomosis is performed in two layers. They are internal or mucosal and external between the gastric seromuscular layer and the adventitia of the esophagus (Fig. 5). Two jejunostomies are then executed: one proximal to aspirate gastric secretions and the other distal for enteral feeding.

Results

One hundred and eighteen patients with advanced megaesophagus were operated on by this technique. Complications included: pleural effusion, 26 cases (22.0%); pneumonia, nine cases (7.6%); pyloromyectomy fistula, two cases (1.7%); hemorrhage of the mediastinal bed, two cases (1.7%); and tracheal injury, one case (0.8%). Operative mortality was 3.4% (four patients). Two deaths occurred from hemorrhage and two from sepsis.

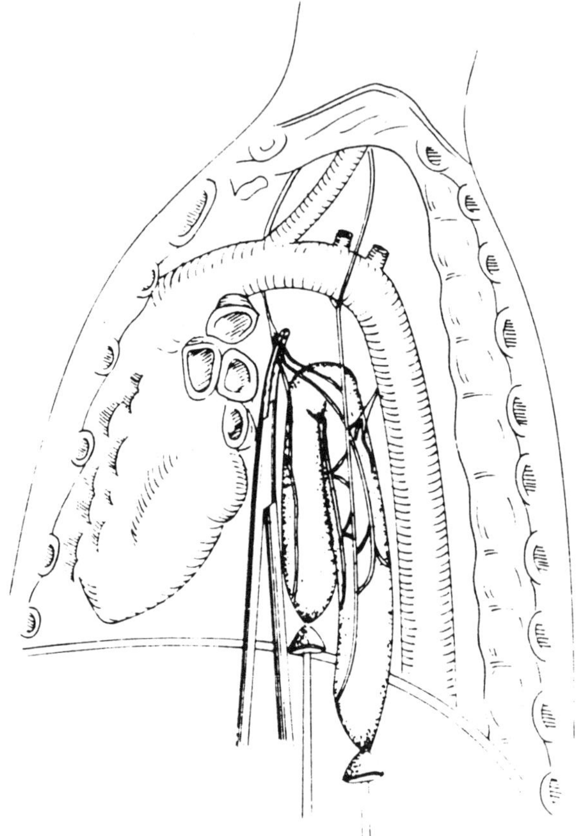

Figure 4: Esophageal resection.

Sixty-four patients with achalasia submitted to gastroplasty were followed up for 6 months to 12 years. The most frequent complaint was regurgitation in 16 (15.7%) patients. This occurred mainly at night in six patients (10.9%), requiring them to sleep slightly elevated. In spite of this, there was no case of aspiration bronchopneumonia. Slight dysphagia was observed in four (6.2%); all had a slight stenosis of the anastomosis resulting from postoperative fistula. Heartburn was present in four (6.2%). Diarrhea occurred in 11 (15.9%) and dumping in five (4.7%), which tended to diminish with time. Regarding body weight, 55 (86.0%) of the 64 patients gained weight, five (7.8%) showed no significant change, and four (6.2%) lost weight after gastroplasty.

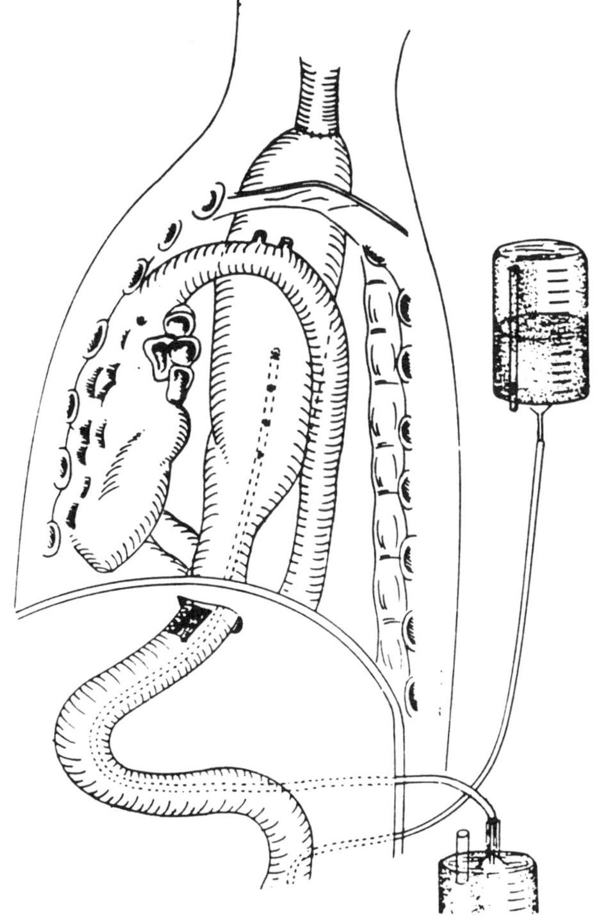

Figure 5: Gastroplasty.

Management of Special Circumstances

In early forms where the esophagogastric junction is extremely altered due to prior manipulations, we performed the operation proposed by Merendino and Dillard[6] by phrenolaparotomy without thoracotomy. In thirty-nine cases, we observed the following complications: atelectasis, four cases (10.2%); pleural empyema, one case (2.6%); fistula of the esophagojejunal anastomosis, one case (2.6%); necrosis of mobilized jejunum, one case (2.6%); and acute renal insufficiency, one case (2.6%). Mortality in this group was 7.6% (three cases).

As has been shown, depending on the case, management of megaesophagus may involve different therapeutic approaches and surgical procedures with different risks. Therefore, for successful management, it is crucial to choose the correct procedure in accordance with the phase of the disease and the patient's clinical condition.

References

1. Pinotti HW, Gama-Rodrigues JJ, Ellengoben G: Nova bases para o tratamento cirúrgico do megaesôfago: Esofagocardiomiotomia e esofagofundogastropexia. AMB Rev Assoc Med Bras 20:331–335, 1974.
2. Pinotti HW, Sakai P, Ishioka S: Cardiomyotomy and fundoplication for esophageal achalasia. Jpn J Surg 13:399–403, 1988.
3. Pinotti HW: Esofagectomia subtotal, por túnel transmediastinal sem toracotomia. Revista da Associacão Médica Brasileira 23:395–398, 1977.
4. Pinotti HW, Zilberstein B, Pollara WM, Raia A: Esophagectomy without thoracotomy. Surg Gynecol Obstet 152:344–346, 1981.
5. Pinotti HW: Acesso extrapleural ao esôfago por frenolaparotomia. AMB Rev Assoc Med Bras 22:57–61, 1976.
6. Merendino M, Dillard DH: The concept of sphincter substitution by an interposed jejunal segment for anatomic and physiologic abnormalities at the esophago-gastric junction, with special reference to reflux esophagitis and esophageal varices. 142:486–509, 1955.

34

Pneumatic Dilation and Cardiomyotomy with Modified Thal Fundoplasty in the Treatment of Achalasia of the Esophagus

Jouko Isolauri, Hubertus Feussner,
Arnulf H. Hölscher, and Jörg Reudiger Siewert

Introduction

Loss of peristaltic activity of the tubular esophagus and defective relaxation of the lower esophageal sphincter to swallowing stimuli are the characteristic features of achalasia.[1,2] Treatment is directed to relief of the symptoms by means of weakening the abnormal lower esophageal sphincter. Pneumatic dilation and modified Heller's myotomy are the most effective means of therapy.[1,3–6] Controversy, however, exists as to whether pneumatic dilation or esophagomyotomy is the preferable form of therapy and whether an antireflux procedure should be added to esophagomyotomy when operation is the treatment of choice.[1,2–9]

The present study was undertaken to assess the results of the treatment of patients with achalasia using pneumatic dilation as initial

Little AG, Ferguson MK, Skinner DB: Diseases of the Esophagus, Vol. II: Benign Diseases. Futura Publishing Company, Inc., Mount Kisco, NY, © 1990.

therapy and modified Heller's myotomy with Thal fundoplasty when dilation failed to relieve the symptoms.

Patients and Methods

Between July 1982 and May 1988, 63 patients without previous therapy for achalasia were treated at the Department of Surgery of the Technical University of Munich. The median duration of the symptoms before the diagnosis was 24 (range 1–684) months. Dysphagia and regurgitation were the most frequent symptoms.

The diagnosis was established by esophagogram, esophagoscopy with histological examination of the biopsy specimens, and by manometry. Thirty-five patients had 24-hour pH measurement before the treatment.

A water perfusion system was used for station pull-through and rapid pull-through manometry. A triple-lumen catheter (internal diameter of each single channel 1.0 mm, outer diameter 1.2 mm) was connected with three Statham P-23b transducers. This system was perfused by a low-compliance pneumohydraulic pump (Arndorfer medical specialities, USA) which generates a flow of 0.5 ml/minute. The analogue data were transferred to the central recording unit (Hellige, FRG), printed out on an a four-channel pen-writer, and, in parallel, sent to an A/D converter. The digital data entered via an eight-bit data base computing system (Anacomp 220, Kontron FRG). Evaluation of tubular motility was performed automatically (computer-aided) whereas the lower and upper sphincters (LES and UES) were interpreted manually. Station pull-through manometry was done in 1-cm steps; rapid pull-through velocity was 1 cm/second.

The system used in long-term pH monitoring was an Autronic CM 18 pH with a sampling rate of 0.2 Hz (360 Kbyte of RAM) and a glass electrode (with built-in reference) (F. Ingold, Frankfurt, FRG). A pH drop below 4 was considered as a reflux, and a percentage of pH<4 more than 3% of the whole recording time was taken as pathological.

The mean LES pressure before the treatment was 15.6 (SD ± 9.6) mmHg. Pathological acid reflux (pH<4) was observed in 4/35 patients with pretreatment 24-hour pH monitoring. The esophagocardiac junction could be passed during endoscopy in each case. Signs of grade I–II esophagitis were observed in six esophagoscopies. Two of these patients had pathological acid reflux in 24-hour pH measurement. Despite overnight fasting, food remnants were seen in the esophagus in 24 cases. Esophageal dilation more than 6 cm visualized radiographically was classified as severe. Five (18%) of the patients had a severely dilated esophagus before the treatment.

Pneumatic dilation was the first choice of treatment and, if failed, modified Heller's myotomy with Thal's fundoplasty was performed. The dilation was performed without anesthesia or premedication. The Rusk pneumatic dilator was positioned at the level of cardia under fluoroscopic control. The balloon was inflated to 300 mmHg for 3 minutes, deflated and removed. Endoscopy was repeated after the procedure to exclude perforation of the esophagus. In most cases, some bleeding was seen in the cardia. A plain chest radiograph was obtained after the procedure to exclude mediastinal emphysema. The day after the procedure, before starting oral intake, the patients were subjected to gastrografin swallow.

When two or three dilations failed to relieve the symptoms, the patients were subjected to operation. A modified Heller's myotomy,[10,11] extending 4–5 cm proximal to the esophagus and 1 cm distal to the stomach from the esophagogastric junction was performed. A fundic patch (Thal fundoplasty) was added in all patients.[13] The procedure was performed by the transabdominal route.

After the initial treatment in this clinic, the patients were reexamined regularly. The reexamination included interview, esophagoscopy, manometry, and 24-hour pH measurement. Those who refused reexamination were interviewed by telephone or by letter.

The results are presented in means (median) and 1SD (ranges). To compare these, Student's two-tailed independent *t*-test was used when appropriate. To compare the proportions, a chi-square test was applied.

Results

Forty-nine patients underwent one dilation, 12 patients underwent two, and two patients had three or more dilations. The results were excellent or good in 48 cases (76%). The result of the therapy was considered to be excellent if the patient was completely asymptomatic. The patient classified as having good results had occasional dysphagia. The patients with fair results experienced improvement of the symptoms but continued to have occasional to frequent episodes of dysphagia and regurgitation. Patients with poor results experienced no improvement, worsening of the condition, or the development of new symptoms. There were two esophageal perforations (3%). These were observed immediately after the dilation and were operated on by suturing the ruptured mucosa after myotomy and performing Thal fundoplasty. Both patients survived without other complications.

Twelve patients (19%) did not benefit from dilation(s). Both patients who had three and four dilations required surgery and nine of the 12 patients who underwent two dilations were operated on. There was no morbidity or mortality. The results were excellent or good in 11 (91%) cases. The mean LES pressure after pneumatic dilation(s) was 9.6 (SD 3.2) mmHg and after myotomy 8.2 (SD 2.4) mmHg, respectively. One patient in the dilation group and one in the myotomy group had pathological acid reflux after the treatment.

Discussion

Excellent or good results have been reported in about 67% of the patients after a single dilation with a hydrostatic or pneumatic bag.[13] Treatment with repeated dilations has produced excellent or good results in 77% of the patients. Only 7% were not improved.[15] The major disadvantage of this treatment is the 1–5% rate of perforation of the distal esophagus.[1,3,5,13] If, however, the perforation is detected early after the procedure, the situation can be safely dealt with. We prefer operative therapy in patients with esophageal perforation. After performing myotomy, the ruptured mucosa is sutured and covered with a fundic patch. Some authors, mainly gastroenterologists, believe that the perforation can be safely and effectively treated conservatively.[1,13]

The role of pneumatic dilation compared with surgical cardiomyotomy remains controversial.[1,3–6,13,14] The two treatments were compared in a prospective randomized trial in 38 patients. In this study, cardiomyotomy had significantly better long-term results.[6] In a retrospective study of 899 patients, Okike et al. found cardiomyotomy to have lower mortality and morbidity as well as better long-term results than forceful dilation.[5] The authors, however, stated that patients who have failed to benefit from forceful dilation respond to esophagomyotomy as well as if they had not had previous treatment. Csendes et al., on the other hand, found that the distal esophagus was firm and fibrous in three patients who had to be operated on due to failure of dilation. The authors had difficulty in separating the muscular layer from the mucosa. They had to open the mucosal layer to achieve complete muscular section.[6] The number of patients with pneumatic dilation as initial treatment in their study was 18. Seven had unsatisfactory results and three had to be operated on.[6]

It is our policy today to begin treatment with pneumatic dilation. If the first session does not relieve the symptoms or the relief is transient, we perform a modified Heller's myotomy with fundic patch operation (Thal fundoplasty) through the abdominal route. We have not had difficulties in performing myotomy after one or two pneumatic dilations. No mucosal ruptures occurred, and there was no morbidity or mortality. When comparing the patients with successful versus unsuccessful results with pneumatic dilations, we found that there were more patients under the age of 45 years in the latter group.

Whether an antireflux procedure should be added to cardiomyotomy is still debated.[4,7–9,15–17] The addition of an antireflux procedure to the myotomy was suggested by Belsey in 1966.[18] He found reflux esophagitis and fibrous stenosis in 11% of the 64 patients treated with myotomy without an antireflux procedure. After a modified antireflux repair was added to the cardiomyotomy, the development of esophagitis and fibrous stenosis was completely eliminated in the following 62 operations. The results related to dysphagia were comparable to those without an antireflux procedure.[18] On the other hand, Ellis and associates observed symptomatic postoperative reflux in only 3% of the patients after cardiomyotomy. The myotomy extended 4–5 cm over the distal esophagus and only a few millimeters onto the stomach. He did not perform an antireflux procedure. Complete relief of dysphagia was observed in 92% of patients.[4] In a collective review of 5002 patients with Heller's myotomy for achalasia, Andreollo and Earlam[9] reported roughly double the incidence (13.2%) of reflux with myotomy done through a laparotomy than through a thoracotomy (7.7%). When an antireflux procedure was added to the abdominal approach, the percentage was 7.4. The authors concluded that antireflux procedures are needed only to compensate for an incorrectly done myotomy and are unnecessary.[9] Some authors have recommended utilization of an antireflux procedure (even fundoplication) for selected patients. Hiatal hernia, extensive hiatal dissection on performing the myotomy, epiphrenic diverticulum, and mucosal perforation during the operation are conditions where those authors recommend performance of an antireflux procedure.[7,16]

We have added a fundic serosal patch (Thal procedure) in all patients after cardiomyotomy. The purpose of the procedure is three-fold. Suturing the muscular edges of the myotomy to the serosal surface of the stomach offsets the possibility of the future reapproximation of muscle fibers. If the mucosa has been opened, the procedure acts to prevent fistula development. The procedure also acts as an antireflux system.

Conclusion

Pneumatic dilation is a safe and effective method in the initial treatment of achalasia. If the first dilation fails to relieve symptoms, the great majority of cases will not benefit from further dilations. Modified Heller's myotomy with fundoplasty gives excellent or good results in these patients.

References

1. Vantrappen G, Hellemans J: Treatment of achalasia and related motor disorders. Gastroenterology 79:144–54, 1980.
2. Siewert JR, Früh E, Waldeck F, Schmidt H: Zur beeinflussbarkeit des unteren oesophagussphinktrers durch polypeptidhormone bei der achalasie. Z Gastroenterol 12:117–20, 1974.
3. Fellows IW, Olgive AL, Atkinson M: Pneumatic dilation in achalasia. Gut 24:1020–1023, 1983.
4. Ellis FH, Crozier RE, Watkins E: Operation for esophageal achalasia. Cardiovasc Surg 88;344–351, 1984.
5. Okike N, Payne WS, Neufeld DM, Bernatz PE, Pairolero PC, Sanderson DR: Esphagomytomy versus forceful dilation for achalasia of the esophagus: Results in 899 patients. Ann Thorac Surg 28:119–125, 1979.
6. Csendes A, Velasco N, Braghetto I. Henriquez A: A prospective randomized study comparing forceful dilation and esophagomyotomy in patients with achalasia or the esophagus. Gastroenterology 80:789–795, 1981.
7. Björck S, Dernevik L, Gatzinsky P, Sandberg N: Oesophagocardiomyotomy and antireflux procedures. Acta Chir Scand 148:525–529, 1982.
8. Duranceau A, LaFontaine ER, Vaillieres B: Effects of total fundoplication on function of the esophagus after myotomy for achalasia. Am J Surg 143:22–28, 1982.
9. Andreollo NA, Earlam RJ: Heller's myotomy for achalasia: Is an added antireflux procedure necessary? Br J Surg 74:765–769, 1987.
10. Heller E: Extramukose kardioplastik beim chronische cardiospasmus mit dilation der oesophagus. Mitt Grenzgeb Med Chir 27:141–149, 1913.
11. Zaaijer JH: Cardiospasm in the aged. Ann Surg 77:615–617, 1923.
12. Hatafuku T, Maki T, Thal AP: Fundic patch operation in the treatment

of advanced achalasia of the esophagus. Surg Gynecol Obstet 134:617–624, 1972.
13. Vantrappen G, Janssens J: To dilate or to operate? That is the question. Gut 24:1013–1019, 1983.
14. Schattenmann G, Lepsien G, Weiser HF, Siewert R: Endoscopischpneumatische Dilation (EPD) zur Behandlung der Achalasia. Z Gastroenterol 18:572–575, 1980.
15. Pai GP, Ellison RG, Rubin JW, Moore HV: Two decades of experience with modified Heller's myotomy for achalasia. Ann Thorac Surg 38:201–206, 1984.
16. Murray GF, Battoglini JW, Keagy BA, Starek PJK, Wilcox BR: Selective application of fundoplication in achalasia. Ann Thorac Surg 37:185–188, 1983.
17. Jara FM, Toledo-Pereyra LH, Lewis JW, Magilligan DJ: Long-term results of esophagomyotomy for achalasia of esophagus. Arch Surg 114:935–936, 1979.
18. Belsey R: Functional disease of the esophagus. J Thorac Cardiovasc Surg 52:164–168, 1966.

35

Comparison of Sleeve and Conventional Manometry Findings in the Assessment of Upper Esophageal Sphincter Disorders

André Duranceau, Edwin Lafontaine, C. Deschamps, E. Pellerin, Mannon Jadliwalla, Raymond Taillefer

Introduction

The upper esophageal sphincter (UES) is a high-pressure zone created by the cricopharyngeus muscle and the lower portion of the inferior pharyngeal constrictor.[1] The recording of upper esophageal sphincter function has shown that axial asymmetry exists, with higher pressures present in the anterior and posterior orientation, while lower pressures are observed in lateral positions.[2] This is caused by uneven pressure exerted on the lateral ports of the perfused recording catheter. Moreover, the upward excursion of the UES during deglutition makes it difficult to obtain an accurate and stable recording of the short high-pressure zone.

The aim of the present observation is to compare results of UES function when using two different manometric techniques: conventional side port perfused system and a sleeve perfused system.

Little AG, Ferguson MK, Skinner DB: Diseases of the Esophagus, Vol. II: Benign Diseases. Futura Publishing Company, Inc., Mount Kisco, NY, © 1990.

Materials and Methods

Patient Population

Twenty-four patients with oropharyngeal dysphagia were assessed. During an initial esophageal workup, conventional manometry was obtained, to be followed subsequently by sleeve manometry of the upper sphincter. Both studies were completed on the same day or in two different sessions. The 24 patients were classified in two separate categories of dysphagia. The first group of eight patients (mean age, 69.5 years) had oculopharyngeal muscular dystrophy, a primary striated muscle disorder transmitted genetically. The last 16 patients (mean age, 58.9 years) had oropharyngeal dysphagia of idiopathic origin. There were radiological functional abnormalities of the UES for eight patients and eight more had an associated hiatal hernia but without evident abnormality at the UES level.

Conventional Manometry Technique

A triple lumen esophageal motility tube (Renaldo Tube, U.S.C.I.) with side ports of 1.2 cm oriented radially at 180° from each other and with a distance of 5 cm between each port is passed in a nasoesophageal position. The proximal port, located in the pharynx, is water-filled and nonperfused. The middle port is held in a stationary position in the UES sphincter zone while the distal port records cervical esophageal function. The middle and distal ports are perfused by a syringe pump (Harvard) at a rate of 7.6 cc/minute. The maximal rise rate is 100 mmHg in 0.1 seconds. Ten voluntary swallows of a 2-cc water bolus are obtained while optimal sphincter readings are recorded.

Sleeve Manometry

The modified sleeve device (Dentsleeve, Adelaide, South Australia) is a silicone sleeve, 6 cm in length, flat in cross-section (3.2 × 7.2 mm), and records the highest pressure exerted over any point of its sensing membrane. It is passed through the nose, and the membrane is placed in a posterior position under direct vision, using an intubation laryngoscope. The motility tube is perfused with water at a rate of 1.3 ml/minute, using a pneumohydraulic infusion pump (Maui). The maximal rise rates is 100 mmHg in 0.2 seconds. Ten voluntary swallows are recorded with optimal UES recording in a stationary position.

Interpretation Criteria

The recording of the UES was stationary for both methods. Ten optimal readings of the pharyngoesophageal complex were obtained. Peak resting and contracting pressures was recorded. The ability of the UES to relax to resting intracervical pressure was interpreted as normal when the sphincter pressure fell to within 5 mmHg of the resting cervical pressure. Relaxation time was measured as the period between the fall in pressure in the sphincter to the point where the contracting slope of sphincter closure crosses back the level of the resting pressure prior to relaxation. The end-relaxation pressure gradient was calculated by subtracting intracervical pressure from the maximal relaxation pressure in the sphincter. The opening of the sphincter was said to be coordinated with pharyngeal contraction using two different methods of interpretation: *Method 1:* the coordination was normal if the nadir of the pharyngeal contraction met the nadir of UES relaxation at the same moment. *Method 2:* the coordination was normal if the opening time of UES relaxation encompassed totally the contraction period of the pharynx.

Statistical Analysis

Absolute pressures, percentages, and times resulting from both methods for both groups were compared. Student's *t*-tests for paired and unpaired values, when appropriate, were used as a measure of statistical significance with the 5% level being significant. Analysis of variance were used to compare groups and methods.

Results

The results of our recordings are summarized in the following tables.

Table I
UES Function in Dystrophy Patients (N = 8)

	Conventional	Sleeve	P Value
Resting pressure (mmHg)	27.0 ± 18	40.6 ± 20	0.08
Closing pressure (mmHg)	41.3 ± 22	46.9 ± 25	NS
Relaxation (%)	100	100	NS
End-Relaxation pressure	4.4 ± 4	8.8 ± 4	<0.01
Relaxation time (sec)	2.4 ± 3.1	1.9 ± 0.7	NS
Coordination 1 (%)	85.7 ± 37	77.1 ± 30	NS
Coordination 2 (%)	71.4 ± 40	77.0 ± 28	NS

Discussion

The upper esophageal sphincter is notoriously difficult to evaluate. Clinical symptoms and cine or videoradiology still remain the most reliable investigation means for analysis of dysfunctions of this area. Documentation of the true physiological abnormalities responsible for the numerous categories of oropharyngeal dysphagia remains elusive.

Dent and his colleagues[3,4] have provided us with a new instrument to assess UES function. Their reports, based on observations in healthy volunteers, show that sleeve recording of the UES results in pressure values that are lower with fewer variations than values ob-

Table II
UES Function in Idiopathic Patients (N = 16)

	Conventional	Sleeve	P Value
Resting pressure (mmHg)	47.6 ± 23	59.5 ± 22	.09
Closing pressure (mmHg)	94 ± 31	104.5 ± 31	NS
Relaxation (%)	100	100	NS
End-Relaxation pressure	4.6 ± 3.1	9.1 ± 4.3	<.003
Relaxation time (sec)	1.4 ± .55	1.4 ± .49	NS
Coordination 1 (%)	99.4 ± 17	97.5 ± 17	NS
Coordination 2 (%)	94.4 ± 14	92.5 ± 14	NS

tained with a motility system using perfused side ports. Sleeve pressures varied from 55 to 58 mmHg while side hole assemblies were in the range of 147 to 218 mmHg. Moreover, the maximal resting pressure of the UES high-pressure zone is more difficult to observe over a prolonged period when using a side hole system. The reason for this difficulty is the upward movement of the pharyngoesophageal junction during deglutition with consequent loss of recording of the very narrow UES for the perfused side port. The sleeve offers a more stable reading despite sphincter movement since it records the highest pressure exerted over any part of its length.

We looked at two populations of patients. The first group consisted of eight dystrophy patients, having an established muscle pathology with secondary oropharyngeal dysphagia. The second group consisted of 16 patients with oropharyngeal dysphagia who did not always offer an obvious etiology for their symptoms, although eight showed radiological evidence of UES dysfunction. In both groups of patients, sleeve recordings showed higher resting pressures than those seen with conventional manometry. There is a trend toward a significant difference between both methods for recording UES resting pressure. This difference between two groups of symptomatic oropharyngeal patients is not as impressive as in the reports by Kahrilas[3,4] based on values of normal asymptomatic volunteers. Our patients in the idiopathic group show pressures similar to those reported by those authors. Patients with muscular disease showed weaker resting pressures, probably resulting from their underlying condition. The differences between the two observations are possibly due to the single side port measurement that we used as opposed to the four and the eight lateral port assemblies used by these authors where anterior and posterior readings were compared with the sleeve recording.

Relaxation of the sphincter and maximal sphincter relaxation are measured accurately with the sleeve since it is a sensor that can record falling pressures in excess of 200 mmHg/second.[2,3] In patients with oropharyngeal symptoms, a significant difference in the pressure gradient that remained at the end of the sphincter relaxation was found when the sleeve was used. This gradient is twice as high when recorded with the sleeve as opposed to recordings with the side hole method. Whether this represents an incomplete relaxation with recording of a pressure gradient remaining with a partly opened sphincter is open to discussion. A careful comparison with values of a large control group should clarify this question. If this was confirmed, sleeve recording of UES function could prove useful in documenting incomplete relaxation of the sphincter in oropharyngeal dysphagia patients.

The evaluation of the relaxation, relaxation time, closing pressures, and coordination of the UES with pharyngeal contraction did not show major differences when comparing both recording methods.

In conclusion, it is known that sleeve recording of the UES in a normal population results in lower and less variable values of resting pressures. This observation is not reproduced in a population evaluated for symptoms of oropharyngeal dysfunction. The most significant finding when comparing sleeve and perfused side port manometry of the UES is a higher pressure gradient remaining at the end of sphincter relaxation. Sleeve manometry may represent a better tool to document incomplete UES relaxation.

References

1. Asoh R, Goyal RJ: Manometry and electromyography of the upper esophageal sphincter in the opossum. Gastroenterology 74:514–520, 1978.
2. Winans CS: The pharyngoesophageal closure mechanism: A manometric study. Gastroenterology 63:768–777, 1972.
3. Kahrilas PJ, Dent J, Dodds WJ, Hogan WJ, Arndorfer RC: A method for continuous monitoring of upper esophageal sphincter pressure. Dig Dis Sci 32:121–128, 1987.
4. Kahrilas PJ, Dodds WJ, Dent J, Haeberle B, Hogan WJ, Arndorfer RC: Effect of sleep, spontaneous gastroesophageal reflux and a meal on upper esophageal sphincter pressure in normal human volunteers. Gastroenterology 92:466–471, 1987.

36

Pharyngoesophageal Diverticulum (Zenker's): Clinical, Therapeutic and Morphological Aspects

Toni Lerut, D. Van Raemdonck, P. Guelinckx,
P. Van Clooster, Jacques A. Gruwez, R. Dom,
K. Geboes, J. Mebis

Introduction

The first description of a pharyngoesophageal pouch has been credited to Ludlow in 1769.[1] It was Zenker[2] who collected the first large series of 22 cases adding five from his own experience. The exact etiopathogenesis remains unclear although an incoordination of the cricopharyngeal muscle is frequently mentioned.[3] This uncertainty allowed the development of different therapeutic techniques of which diverticulectomy or diverticulopexy combined with an extramucosal myotomy of the cricopharyngeal muscle are the most commonly used surgical therapies[4,5] and the endoscopic myotomy according to Dohlman is the most commonly used nonsurgical therapy.[6]

In this chapter we present a series of 100 patients surgically treated between 1976 and June 1988, with special emphasis on the analysis of biopsy specimens taken at the time of operation compared to a control group.

Little AG, Ferguson MK, Skinner DB: Diseases of the Esophagus, Vol. II: Benign Diseases. Futura Publishing Company, Inc., Mount Kisco, NY, © 1990.

Table I
Zenker's Diverticulum: Associated Pathology

Cachexia	19
Pulmonary infection	37
Perforated diverticulum	1
Gastrointestinal	
hiatus hernia	36
reflux	30
diverticulum esophageal body	1
diffuse spasm*	4
nutcracker esophagus*	2
achalasia	1
gastro-duodenal ulcer	27
gastric polyp	1
duodenal diverticulum	2
internal herniation	1
cholecytolithiasis	11
hepatitis	1
colon carcinoma	1
volvulus	5
ulcer	1
Endocrine	9
Cardiac	10
Urologic	5
Neurologic	8

The braced group (hiatus hernia through gastro-duodenal ulcer) = 60 patients

* Manometric diagnosis

Symptomatology and Associated Pathology

This series consists of 57 men and 43 women with a mean age of 68 years (38 to 92 years). Fifty percent of the patients were older than 70 years and 22% were older than 80 years. All patients were symptomatic with a mean duration of 37.4 months. The cardinal symptom was dysphagia (85%), followed by regurgitation (76%) and hoarseness (8%). In addition to these symptoms, there was frequently associated pathology (Table I), the most important being cachexia (19%), chronic pulmonary infection (37%), and hiatal hernia and/or gastroesophageal reflux (GER) in 40%.

In 27 patients, a 24-hour pH study was performed and was found to be pathological in 13 (48%) patients, seven (26%) having combined reflux. Manometry of the esophageal body and lower esophageal

Table II
Zenker's Diverticulum

Postoperative Complications	
Fistula	1
Recurrent Nerve Paralysis	3
Temporary Phonetic Troubles	6
Infection-Abscess	4
Hematoma	2
Pneumonia	3
Respiratory Insufficiency	1
Thoracic Duct Leak	1
Other	3
Postoperative Mortality	0

sphincter (LES) was performed in 31 patients. Only eight (26%) patients had a normal recording. If GER as a possible cause was excluded, seven patients showed primary motility disorders: four times suggestive for diffuse spasm, two times for a nutcracker esophagus, and one patient confirming a long-standing history of achalasia. Overall, 60% of patients showed some form of synchronous or metachronous upper GI tract pathology. Preoperative manometry of the upper esophageal sphincter (UES) was possible in 13 patients. In eight (61.5%), a possible incoordination in the function of the cricopharyngeal muscle was suggested. The recorded pressures were normal in six, elevated in two, and abnormally low in five patients. These findings cannot be related to age, disturbances in the manometric recordings of the esophageal body, or to GER.

Postoperative Results (Table II)

The surgical treatment of choice was an extramucosal myotomy of the cricopharyngeal muscle with extension onto the cervical esophageal wall, combined with a diverticulopexy. This was done in 94 patients. In five patients, the diverticulum was judged too small to do a pexy, and in one patient, a resection was performed because of a suspicion of malignancy.

There was no postoperative mortality and only a minimum of morbidity. One small salivary fistula closed spontaneously after several days of parenteral feeding. The most frequently encountered

Table III
Zenker's Diverticulum: Follow-Up: Mean Duration: 4 Years (1 year–12 years)

Clinical
  Esophageal symptoms: 4
    1 insufficient myotomy ($>1°$ muscular disease ?) R/contralateral myotomy
    3 intermittent choking for liquids
  Tracheo-pulmonary symptoms: 6
    1 sensation of foreign body in throat
    3 bronchitis
    2 pneumonia ($>$CVA-Lungca)
X-Ray Cinematography
    1 insufficient diverticulopexy $>$asymptomatic
    1 aspiration contrast material (meningioma $>$N. glossopharyngeus paralysis)
Patient's Judgment
    Very good to excellent: 96%

problem (six patients) was a temporary change in phonation, most likely a consequence of postmanipulation edema. In three patients there was a temporary recurrent nerve paralysis. Wound infection was seen in four patients and in two patients a surgical drainage of a hematoma was required. There was no case of mediastinitis and no patient had a rise of temperature above 38.5°C, indicating a possible sepsis.

Oral feeding could usually be started on the first postoperative day. A nasogastric tube, which in our early experience remained 48 hours, is now removed immediately after the operation (64 patients). The mean duration of hospitalization is 7 days, but with increasing experience patients are now discharged earlier and 39 patients were able to leave the hospital within 5 days.

Long-Term Follow-Up Results (Table III)

All patients have been followed until the present or until death, either in clinic or through a detailed questionnaire. The mean follow-up is 4 years (6 months to 12 years). Clinically there are 90 patients who have had no symptoms whatsoever during the entire follow-up period. Four patients have residual esophageal symptoms: occasional choking while drinking in three and one patient required a second myotomy on the contralateral side. This patient showed on pathological examination strong evidence of a primary muscular disease. Six patients have tracheopulmonary symptoms: one patient complained of the sensation of a foreign body in the throat, three patients developed a single episode of bronchitis, and two others developed pneumonia (one an obstructive pneumonia behind a lung carcinoma and one a pneumonia as a sequella of a cerebrovascular accident).

No patient had any evidence for an aspiration pneumonia due to GER. Of the patients who had associated GER, two were treated surgically simultaneously (one Belsey procedure, one Toupet + HSV) and two received a Belsey procedure at a second operation. The remaining patients are all under control with a medical regime.

On X-ray examination, the typical finding is an additional trickle of contrast behind the esophagus at the level of the pexy. Only in one patient who had a very large diverticulum was an insufficient diverticulopexy seen and this patient was without any clinical symptoms 12 years after her operation. Finally, another patient showed aspiration of contrast material probably related to a glossopharyngeal nerve paralysis secondary to a meningioma of which she eventually died.

Ninety-six percent of the patients judged their results to be excellent (68%) or very good (28%).

Morphological, Enzymohistochemical, and Enzymoimmunological Examination

In 62 patients, a large biopsy specimen was taken intraoperatively at the level of the cricopharyngeal muscle. Pathological examination and enzymohistochemistry was performed on 41 biopsies and in 15 controls (HE staining, NADH, ATP pH: 4.3 pH: 6.45; pH: 9.4, Gomori PAS, PAS + Osmium). Acetylcholinesterase enzymohistochemistry and neurofilament immunohistochemistry was performed on 44 biopsies and on nine controls.

The obtained data demonstrate in patients a clear disturbance of all analyzed parameters (Table IV). Both atrophy and hypertrophy, size variation, necrosis, fibrosis, inflammation, and central nuclei were observed. Ragged red fibers (abnormal accumulation of mitochondria) were frequently seen and Nemaline bodies (abnormal densification of the Z-band) were occasionally noticed. All changes were

Table IV

Enzymohistochemical and Enzymoimmunological Findings in 19 Control Specimens and 62 Zenker's Patients

Dominant Fiber Type	Hyper-trophy	Atrophy	Necrosis	Size Variat.	Fibrosis	Central Nu-cleus	Inflam-mation	Nemaline Rods	Ragged Red Fibers	Acetyl-cholin-esterase	Neuro-filam.
				Controls							
I 9 II 3	1/15	1/15	0/15	2/15	2/15	1/15	0/15	0/15	2/15	0/9	0/9
				Zenker's Patients							
I 40	32/41	37/41	33/41	40/41	31/41	30/41	21/41	4/41	23/41	33/44	33/44

The denominator gives the number of patients in which a given parameter was examined.

important enough to be considered as pathological. In only two patients (5%) were all of the above-mentioned parameters normal. The fiber type distribution was predominantly fiber type I except in one patient, with a mean 70% type I versus 30% type II.

Acetylcholinesterase and neurofilament staining showed a heterogeneous and weak pattern compared to the controls in 75% of the 44 biopsies as more than 50% of the individual fibers didn't stain. In all but two biopsies, the plexus was normal. In nine patients, biopsies were also taken above the diverticulum at the level of the constrictor pharyngeous inferior muscle. Here type II is more represented (50–50%) and less frequent pathological changes can be seen.

In 10 other patients, a biopsy was taken just below the cricopharyngeal muscle at the level of the cervical esophageal muscle wall. In eight of them there was also a biopsy of the sternocleidomastoideus muscle together with a cricopharyngeal muscle biopsy. The sternocleidomastoid biopsies were all strictly normal. Fiber type II is clearly dominant (75–25%). The cervical esophageal muscle biopsies showed the same pathology as described for the cricopharyngeal muscle although it was somewhat less pronounced.

Discussion

Our results demonstrate Zenker's diverticulum as a typical geriatric condition. Its symptomatology is usually a longstanding one and in this respect it has to be stressed that symptoms are not only restricted to the esophagus but that many patients, 37% in our series, suffer from pulmonary infection due to chronic aspiration. This, together with old age and poor nutritional condition, may cause a life-threatening condition, unfortunately too often underestimated.

The most important form of associated pathology is the presence of a coexisting hiatal hernia and/or gastroesophageal reflux. This has already been stressed years ago by several authors.[5,7,8] In our series, 40% of the patients had a hiatal hernia and evidence for GER was found in 28% of the patients. Specifically, GER was present in 48% of those patients who underwent a 24-hour pH study.

In our study, it is remarkable that 60% of our patients were found to have some sort of associated upper GI tract disease. Moreover, the manometric studies were normal only in 8 out of 31 investigated patients. In seven patients with no evidence of GER, there was evidence strongly suggestive for diffuse spasm or nutcracker esophagus. These findings raise the question of a Zenker's diverticulum, one expression of a more complex pathology in which a disturbed vagal nerve function could be the common denominator. In this larger context, incoordination of the cricopharyngeal muscle could be considered as just one expression of a more complex functional disease rather than a disease on its own. This concept is supported by the clear pathological changes found in the muscle biopsies in our patients. Although some of them suggest myogenic degeneration, many are suggestive for neurogenic disease and this is not limited to the cricopharyngeal muscle but also affects the striated muscles of the cervical esophagus, resulting in weaker and slower contractility as we demonstrated in an earlier publication.[9] From this changed morphology and contractility as compared to the controls, it can be assumed that the so-called upper sphincter is more than just the cricopharyngeal muscle and that perhaps the whole of the striated esophageal wall acts as a sphincter of which the cricopharyngeal muscle is only a locally thickened and more pronounced part, an anatomical landmark. If so, it can easily be understood why, on manometry of the upper esophageal sphincter, there is not a well-defined sphincter but a high-pressure zone extending over the proximal esophagus.

In our series there were eight patients with so-called UES incoordination. This incoordination still remains a matter of controversy and findings differ from author to author, varying from a 100% incidence of incoordination to no disturbances at all,[10] probably related to different manometric techniques. In how far this incoordination causes increased intraluminal pressures and a blow-out phenomenon eventually causing a diverticulum is not clear since in our experience only two patients had increased pressures while five other patients had abnormally low pressures. This observation may find an explanation in the fact that laxity in the fixation of the laryngopharynx to the prevertebral fascia occurs with age. Based on our morphological studies we feel, however, that it is justified to extend the myotomy downward well into the high-pressure zone over a distance of at least 4 to 5 cm.

Regarding the treatment of the diverticulum itself, we prefer a diverticulopexy as it avoids the opening of the esophageal lumen and the consequent danger for leakage, which is observed after both a resection[4,11] and the Dohlman procedure.[12] Diverticulopexy allows immediate oral feeding from the first postoperative day resulting in an earlier hospital discharge now, usually within 5 days, and therefore has decreased morbidity within this geriatric group of patients. This is perhaps the reason why there was no mortality in our series.

The only criticism of a diverticulopexy consists of the risk of malignant degeneration.[13] Indeed, although rare, a carcinoma in the bottom of a Zenker's diverticulum has been reported. Its incidence is estimated around 4%. Therefore, a thorough preoperative endoscopic examination after a washout of the sac, together with a careful palpation intraoperatively are mandatory. Until now we have had no knowledge of a carcinoma in our series. The postoperative manometric studies confirm the persistence of a measurable pressure at the level of the UES which probably suffices to prevent aspiration of gastric juice in case of simultaneous reflux. Because of this risk, some authors have advocated an antireflux procedure in such cases.[14] We have experienced no instance of aspiration pneumonitis after myotomy and diverticulopexy in patients with coexisting GER. Of course, all patients are receiving medical treatment for their GER. In case of failure of this medical treatment, the indications for surgery are the same as for any form of refractory GER.

Regarding the long-term follow-up, we would like to stress not only the esophageal symptoms, but also the pulmonary aspects which require even more attention because of their life-threatening potential. In our series, 96% of the patients showed excellent to very good results as far as the esophageal symptoms are concerned, and for the whole scale of symptoms, this percentage was 90%, illustrating again the high quality of the results of diverticulopexy and extramucosal myotomy of the upper esophageal sphincter zone.

Summary

In a series of 100 surgically treated patients, Zenker's diverticulum appears as a typical geriatric pathology (50% over 70 years) in which not only esophageal but also pulmonary symptoms (37%) may lead to a life-threatening situation. In 60%, associated upper GI pathology was noticed, most frequently GER (30 patients). In 30% of the performed manometric studies of the esophageal body and LES, clearly pathological patterns were observed.

Morphological examination, enzymohistochemistry, and immunohistochemistry showed clear pathological changes not only at the level of the cricopharyngeal muscle but also at the level of the striated muscles of the cervical esophagus. These clinical, manometric, and morphological changes suggest that a pharyngoesophageal diverticulum is one expression of a more complex neurogenic disorder. They also justify the extramucosal myotomy of the cricopharyngeal wall as the cardinal step of the operation. This myotomy is combined with a diverticulopexy resulting in optimal results with no postoperative mortality and a minimum of morbidity. The mean long-term follow-up of 4 years in this series showed excellent or very good results in 96% of the patients for the esophageal symptoms and 92% for the full spectrum of symptomatology.

References

1. Ludlow A: A case of obstructed deglutition, from a preternatural dilation of, and bag formed in the pharynx. London Medical Observation and Inquiries 3:85, 1769.
2. Zenker FA, von Ziemssen H: Krankheiten des Oesophagus. In: Handbuch des Speciellen Pathologie und Therapie, Vol 7 (Suppl), von Ziemssen H (ed), Leipzig, FCW Vogel, 1877.
3. Ellis FH Jr, Crozier RE: Cervical oesophageal dysphagia. Ann Surg 198:279, 1984.
4. Payne WS, King RM: Pharyngo-esophageal (Zenker's) diverticulum. Surg Clin North Am 63:815, 1983,
5. Duranceau A, Jamieson G: Cricopharyngeal myotomy for pharyngoesophageal diverticula. Discussion. In: International Trends in General Thoracic Surgery, Vol 3, Benign Esophageal Disease, DeMeester TR, Matthews HR (eds), Philadelphia, CV Mosby, 1987, p 358.
6. Dohlman G: The endoscopic operation for hypopharyngeal diverticula. Arch Otolaryngol 71:744, 1960.
7. Belsey RHR: Disorders of function of the esophagus. In: Surgery of the Esophagus, Smith RA, Smith RE (eds), London, Butterworths, 1972, p 193.
8. Smiley TB: Pressure studies in the upper oesophagus in relation to hiatus hernia. In: Surgery of the Esophagus, Smith RA, Smith RE (eds), London, Butterworths, 1972, p 152.
9. Lerut T, Guelinckx P, Dom R, Geboes K, Gruwez J: Does the musculus cricopharyngeus play a role in the genesis of Zenker's diverticulum? Enzyme histochemical and contractility properties. In: Diseases of the Esophagus, Siewert JR, Hölscher AM (eds), New York, Springer Verlag, 1988, p 1018.
10. Knuff TE, Benjamin SB, Castell DO: Pharyngo-esophageal (Zenker's) diverticulum: A reappraisal. Gastroenterology 82:734, 1982.
11. Lerut T, Vandekerkhof J, Leman G, Guelinckx P, Dom R, Gruwez JA: Cricopharyngeal myotomy for pharyngoesophageal diverticula. In: International Trends in General Thoracic Surgery, Vol 3, Benign Esophageal Disease, DeMeester TR, Matthews HR (eds), CV Mosby, 1987, p 351.

12. Knegt PP, de Jong PC, van der Schans EJ: Endoscopic treatment of hypopharyngeal diverticulum with CO_2 laser. Endoscopy 17:205, 1985.
13. Huang B, Unni KK, Payne WS: Long-term survival following diverticulectomy for cancer in pharyngoesophageal (Zenker's) diverticulum. Ann Thorac Surg 38:207, 1984.
14. Hurwitz AL, Duranceau A, Haddad JK: Disorders of esophageal motility. Philadelphia, WB Saunders Co., 1979, p 67.

37

Manometric Patterns of Esophageal Diverticula

C. Iascone, M. Caporossi, R. Arca,
P. Addario Chieco, M. Picchio, C. Maffi,
Aldo Moraldi, Sergio Stipa

Introduction

Manometric studies have frequently documented the presence of functional disorders of the upper esophageal sphincter (UES). However, conflicting results have been published concerning their relationship to the development of pharyngoesophageal diverticula.[1–5] Little is known about manometric features of midthoracic[6,7] or epiphrenic diverticula.[8] As esophageal diverticula are frequently associated with primary motor disorders of the esophagus, manometric patterns of these diseases have been considered responsible for diverticular pouch formation. For this reason, we excluded patients with achalasia and diffuse esophageal spasms from this study and reviewed the manometric patterns of 47 patients with primary diverticular disease of the esophagus.

Patients and Methods

From 1972 to 1988, we studied 47 patients without previous upper GI operations with esophageal diverticula and primary motor dis-

Little AG, Ferguson MK, Skinner DB: Diseases of the Esophagus, Vol. II: Benign Diseases. Futura Publishing Company, Inc., Mount Kisco, NY, © 1990.

orders of the esophagus. There were 16 patients with Zenker's diverticula (34%), 18 with midthoracic esophageal diverticula (38.3%), and 13 patients with epiphrenic diverticula (27.6%). There were 31 males and 16 females with a mean age of 59.7 ± 9.9. All patients underwent clinical and radiological evaluation. Incidence and severity of heartburn, regurgitation, and dysphagia were similar in all groups of patients. Dysphagia was present in all subjects. Respiratory symptoms were more prominent in patients with Zenker's diverticula. Manometry[9] could be performed in 87% of subjects, endoscopy in 76%, 24-hour pH monitoring of the esophagus in 34%,[10] and esophageal scintegraphy in 51%.[11] The following manometric parameters were evaluated: upper and lower esophageal sphincter (LES) pressure, overall LES length and length of abdominal LES, relaxation and coordination of UES and LES activity, and overall motor activity of the body of the esophagus. A detailed analysis of manometric tracings was performed; from the lower end of the UES to the upper end of the LES, each tracing was divided into three parts of equal length. In each third, esophageal resting pressure, percent of peristaltic waves, mean wave amplitude (mmHg), and mean wave duration (sec) were determined. For the overall length of esophageal body, wave form, percent of peaks less than 30 mmHg in amplitude or higher than 70 mmHg were evaluated. These manometric findings were compared to those of 10 normal volunteers.

During the follow-up, a second manometry was performed in 12 subjects: three patients with Zenker's diverticula, two with midesophageal diverticula, and seven with epiphrenic diverticula. Results of this last group are reported in this study; three of these patients underwent surgery and follow-up manometry was performed after operative correction had been carried out.

Results

Uses

Complete relaxation of UES was found in 74.4% of swallowings in patients with Zenker's diverticula, in 90.4% in patients with midthoracic esophageal diverticula, in 94.7% of patients with epiphrenic diverticula, and in 100% of normal subjects (normals versus all others p < 0.05; Zenker versus epiphrenic diverticula p < 0.05). UES coordination with pharyngeal contraction on swallowings was 78.2%

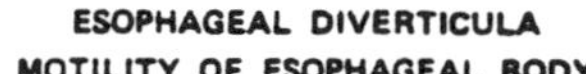

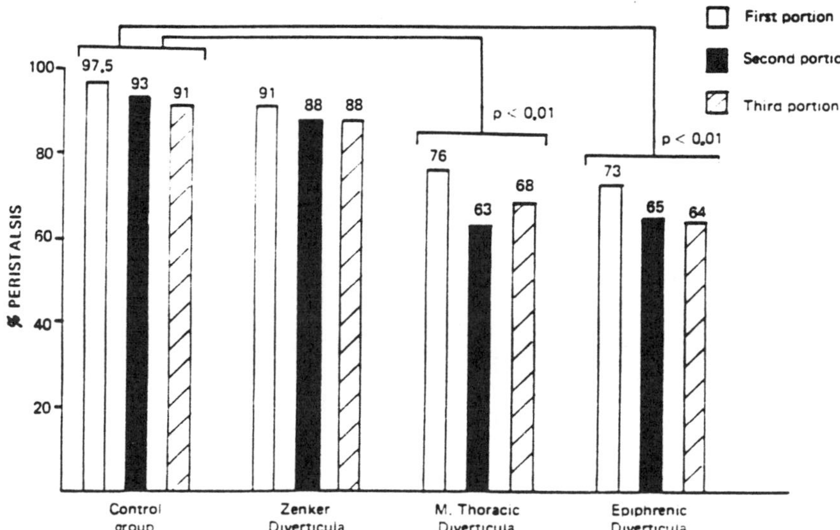

Figure 1: This graph shows the incidence of primary peristalsis which followed swallowings in each third of the esophageal body in normal subjects and in patients with esophageal diverticula. In patients with midthoracic and epiphrenic diverticula, peristaltic waves were registered significantly less frequently than in the control group.

in Zenker's diverticula, 90.3% in midthoracic esophageal diverticula, 91.4% in epiphrenic ones, and 100% in normal controls (Zenker's diverticula versus normals p < 0.001).

Esophageal Body

In patients with epiphrenic and midthoracic esophageal diverticula, primary peristalsis following swallowing was observed significantly less frequently than in normal subjects in each third of the esophagus (p < 0.01) (Fig. 1). For the overall body of the esophagus, the incidence of low amplitude waves (<30 mmHg) was 38.4% in Zenker's group, 41.2% in epiphrenic diverticula, 45% in midthoracic esophageal diverticula, and 14.1% in normal controls (normals versus all groups p < 0.01).

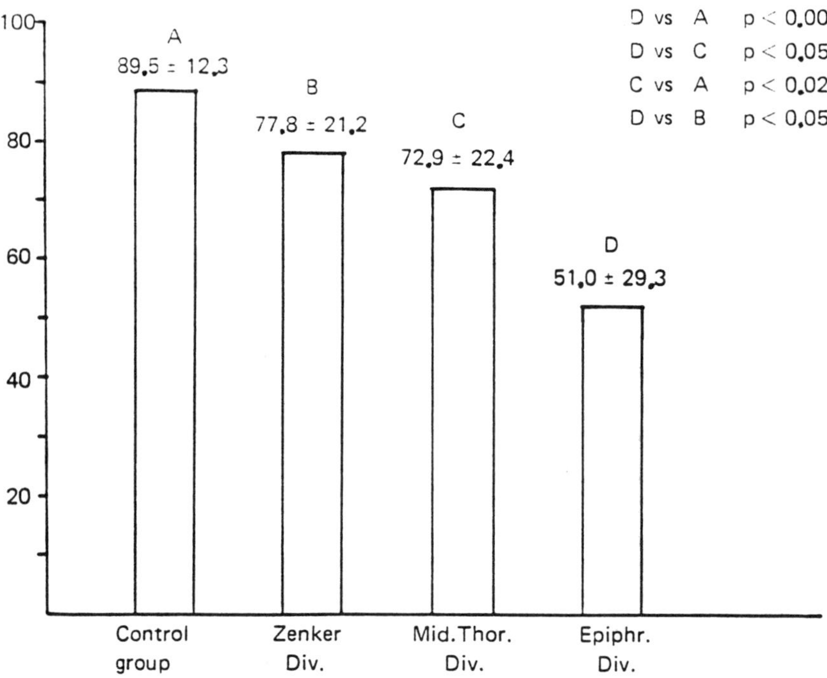

Figure 2: This graph shows LES coordination with peristaltic activity of the esophagus in normal subjects and in patients with esophageal diverticula. In patients with epiphrenic diverticula, LES coordination was significantly impaired compared to normals and to patients with pharyngoesophageal or midthoracic esophageal diverticula.

LES

A complete LES relaxation was detected in 69.5% of swallows in patients with epiphrenic diverticula, in 70.1% in patients with midthoracic esophageal diverticula, in 84% in Zenker's group, and 91.4% in normal controls (normals versus epiphrenic and midthoracic diverticula p < 0.01). LES coordination with the peristaltic waves in the esophagus was significantly poorer in epiphrenic diverticulum patients than in normals and in the remaining two groups of patients (Fig. 2).

Follow-up Results

Patients who were operated on (two diverticulectomies and one diverticulopexy plus myotomy), showed a postoperative decrease of wave amplitude of the lower third of the esophagus and an improvement of LES coordination (19.4% ± 9% preoperatively and 69.7% ± 16% postoperatively, $p < 0.01$). No substantial differences were observed in subjects who did not undergo surgery. However, an increase of esophageal body resting pressure was registered: -3 mmHg ± 0.07 versus 2.2 mmHg ± 2 ($p < 0.05$).

Comment

Factors leading to the development of esophageal diverticula are still unclear. Manometric findings in patients with pharyngoesophageal diverticula are frequently controversial; both increased UES resting pressure[12] or pressures lower than normals[1,4] have been reported. Similarly, normal UES function was found by some investigators[2,5] and UES achalasia or incoordination by others.[1,4] In this study about 25% of swallows in subjects with Zenker's diverticula showed abnormal relaxation or incoordination. This finding must be compared to the 100% normal swallowing coordination observed in the control group. In fact, only 2 out of 11 patients with pharyngoesophageal diverticula showed completely normal UES function in all swallows. A high incidence of similar abnormalities, such as sphincter achalasia and incoordination, was observed in the LES function of subjects with midthoracic or epiphrenic diverticula. It is not surprising to find that in these patients, hypertensive esophageal body activity and hypertensive LES were not observed, as we excluded subjects with achalasia and diffuse esophageal spasm from the study. The presence of low-amplitude and dysmorphic waves in the body of the esophagus in this selected group of patients suggests that midthoracic and epiphrenic diverticula do not have typical manometric patterns in the body of the esophagus and that LES dysfunctions, in terms of incoordination or abnormal relaxation, are the most relevant abnormalities.

These data support similar findings of previous investigators.[7,8] Common pathogenetic factors, i.e., abnormal relaxation and incoordination of esophageal sphincters, may be the basic derangement responsible for functional obstruction leading to the development of diverticular pouches in weak areas of the muscular wall of the esophagus.

These observations indicate that a myotomy of the LES and esophageal body, extended up to the diverticular neck, is the primary goal of surgery for treatment of all esophageal diverticula; this approach guarantees the correction of the underlying motor disorder and is followed by excellent long-term results.[1,4,8,13] Surgical approach to the treatment of the diverticular pouches is determined by the surgeon's preference and the size of the diverticulum, since either diverticulectomy or diverticulopexy achieve the same final long-term results, as long as the basic motor disorder is corrected.

In conclusion, our study shows that similar sphincter abnormalities are associated with diverticular pouch development in the esophagus. Areas of low amplitude and aperistaltic waves and malfunctioning LES, more than hypertensive esophageal body and/or LES activity, are the findings observed in midthoracic and lower esophageal diverticula. These results suggest that similar functional abnormalities are associated with each type of esophageal diverticulum; therefore, additional factors, such as areas of weakness in the muscular wall of the esophagus, are necessary to the final development of a diverticular pouch.

References

1. Ellis FH, Crozier RE: Cervical esophageal dysphagia: Indications for and results of cricopharyngeal myotomy. Ann Surg 194:279, 1980.
2. Pedersen SA, Hansen JB, Alstrup P: Pharyngo-oesophageal diverticula. Scand J Thorac Cardiovasc Surg 7:87, 1973.
3. Kodicek J, Creamer B: A study of pharyngeal pouches. J Laryngol Otol 75:406, 1961.
4. Duranceau A, Rheault MJ, Jamieson GG: Physiologic response to cricopharyngeal myotomy and diverticulum suspension. Surgery 94:655, 1983.
5. Knuff TE, Benjamin SB, Castell DO: Pharyngoesophageal (Zenker's) diverticulum: A reappraisal. Gastroenterology 82:734, 1982.
6. Kaye MD: Esophageal motor dysfunction in patients with diverticula of the midthoracic esophagus. Thorax 29:666, 1974.
7. Dodds WJ, Stef JJ, Hogan WJ, et al: Radial distribution of esophageal peristaltic pressure in normal subjects and patients with esophageal diverticulum. Gastroenterology 69:584, 1975.
8. Debas HT, Payne WS, Cameron AJ, et al: Physiopathology of lower esophageal diverticulum and its implications for treatment. Surg Gynecol Obstet 151:593, 1980.
9. Winans CS, Harris LD: Quantitation of lower esophageal sphincter competence. Gastroenterology 52:773, 1967.

10. Johnson LF, De Meester TR: 24-hour pH-monitoring of the distal esophagus: Quantitative measure of gastroesophageal reflux. Am J Gastroenterol 62:325, 1974.
11. Moraldi A, Iascone C, Zerilli M, et al: Patterns of radioisotopic esophageal transit in patients with symptoms of gastroesophageal reflux. In: Diseases of the Esophagus: Pathophysiology, Diagnosis, Conservative and Surgical Treatment. Siewert JR, Hoelsher AH (eds), Monaco, Springer-Verlag, 1988, p 827.
12. Hunt PS, Connell AM, Smiley TB: The cricopharyngeal sphincter in gastric reflux. Gut 11:303, 1970.
13. Belsey R: Functional disease of the esophagus. J Thorac Cardiovasc Surg 52:164, 1966.

38

Comparison Between Manometry and Radionuclide Esophageal Transit Study in Detection of Esophageal Motility Dysfunction

Raymond Taillefer, Mannon Jadliwalla, E. Pellerin, Edwin Lafontaine, André Duranceau

Introduction

Evaluation of esophageal function using radionuclide esophageal transit study (RETS) was initially proposed by Kazem[1] in 1972. Introduction of computer-based analysis and modifications in the acquisition parameters of the originally described procedure contributed to improve the diagnostic accuracy and subsequent clinical use of this new method.[2-8] RETS offers many advantages over the other standard clinical methods used in the investigation of esophageal disorders. It is a physiological, noninvasive test, simple to perform, well accepted by patients, and it provides quantitative measurement of esophageal emptying, a unique feature unavailable with other clinical procedures. However, some discrepancies in the results obtained with RETS have been reported and questions have been raised on

Little AG, Ferguson MK, Skinner DB: Diseases of the Esophagus, Vol. II: Benign Diseases. Futura Publishing Company, Inc., Mount Kisco, NY, © 1990.

the clinical usefulness of this test in the evaluation of different types of esophageal disorders.[9,10]

Since the primary purpose of RETS is to evaluate esophageal motility dysfunction, this study was undertaken to compare RETS to esophageal motility studies (EMS), used as a gold standard, in a patient population referred for the investigation of various esophageal diseases. The aim was to determine the sensitivity and specificity of this noninvasive test for the detection of esophageal motility disorders in a clinical context.

Materials and Methods

Patient Population

One hundred and nine consecutive patients without previous surgery of the esophagus were prospectively studied with both RETS and EMS within one month of each other. There were 57 males and 52 females with an age range of 21–81 (mean, 52) years. All patients were referred to the esophageal disorders clinic of our institution for esophageal symptoms or noncardiac chest pain. Their esophageal investigation also included radiological procedures, 24-hour pH-metry, and endoscopy. Final diagnosis was based on the global results of the esophageal investigation and divided into three categories: motor disorders, reflux disease, and noncardiac chest pain.

Esophageal Motility Studies

Technical aspects of EMS as performed at our institution have been described in detail elsewhere.[11] Briefly, EMS were performed in a supine position using a continuously perfused, triple-lumen motility catheter. The external pressure transducers (Hewlett-Packard 1290) were placed at the level of the table and pressures were recorded on a HP 7754 A recorder. The transducers were calibrated before and after each study, using a mercury-filled manometer and taking atmospheric pressure as the zero baseline. All measurements were made in mmHg.

The following parameters were determined: (1) upper esophageal sphincter: resting and closing pressures, relaxation, relaxation time, and coordination; (2) body of esophagus: proximal and distal resting pressure, peak contraction pressure, response to swallowing (primary and tertiary waves), and spontaneous activity; (3) lower esophageal sphincter resting and closing pressures, relaxation, relaxation time, and coordination.

Radionuclide Esophageal Transit Studies

RETS was carried out after a 6–8 hour fast. After a few practice swallows with water, the patient was placed in a supine position under a computer-interfaced, large-field-of-view scintillation camera fitted with a low-energy, all-purpose, parallel-hole collimator. The anterior projection was used and patients were positioned so that the mouth, hypopharynx, entire esophagus, and when possible, the proximal part of the gastric fundus were clearly visualized in the same field. The patient's head was placed in a slight anterior oblique rotation. A bolus of 0.5 to 1.0 mCi of ^{99m}Tc-sulfur colloid diluted in 15–20 ml of water was then taken into the mouth through a straw and the patient was asked to retain the bolus in the mouth. On completion of the radionuclide oral administration, a 2-minute analog and digital acquisition was started immediately. A few seconds after the beginning of acquisition, the patient was instructed to swallow the entire bolus in only one phase and not to move for 2 minutes. After 30 seconds, patients were instructed to have a dry swallow, and additional dry swallows were allowed at 15-second intervals for 2 minutes.

Analog images were obtained at 2-second intervals for 2 minutes. After data were recorded, time-activity curves were generated for seven regions of interest: oral cavity, hypopharynx, proximal, middle and distal esophageal segment, gastric fundus, and entire esophagus. Emptying time for each segment was determined and defined as the time for 90% or more of the maximal activity in each region of interest to be eliminated. Global esophageal emptying time corresponded to the time from entry of the bolus in the proximal esophagus to the clearance of more than 90% from the entire esophageal region of interest. Percentage of residual activity (defined as residual activity divided by maximal activity) was also determined.

Control Groups

EMS

Forty normal volunteers (23 men, 17 women), totally asymptomatic with a mean age of 27 years, were studied using the same EMS procedure described below.

RETS

Thirty normal volunteers (20 men, 10 women) with a mean age of 30 years, without digestive symptoms or systemic illness, were evaluated with RETS and were used as a control group.

Statistical Analysis

The values in the text are expressed as arithmetic mean ± 1 standard deviation. Statistical terms are defined as follows: *sensitivity:* TP/(TP + FN) $\times$ 100; *specificity:* TN/(TN + FP) $\times$ 100; *predictive value of a negative result:* TN/(TN + FN) $\times$ 100; *predictive value of a positive result:* TP/(TP + FP) $\times$ 100, where TP = true positive, TN = true negative, FP = false positive, FN = false negative.

Results

Patient Population

According to their final diagnosis, the 109 patients were divided into three diagnostic groups: *Group I:* 39 patients with esophageal motor disorder; *Group II:* 48 patients with gastroesophageal reflux disease; and *Group III:* 22 patients with noncardiac chest pain and/or dysphagia.

Patients with gastroesophageal reflux disease had a diagnosis that was confirmed by a 24-hour pH-metry and patients with noncardiac chest pain had a negative cardiac work-up before their esophageal investigation.

Control Groups

RETS

In the group of normal volunteers, the esophageal emptying time was 1.5 $\pm$ 0.5 seconds, 3.5 $\pm$ 1.0 seconds, and 6.0 $\pm$ 2.5 seconds for upper, middle, and distal esophageal segments, respectively. For the entire esophageal region of interest, the emptying time was 9.0 $\pm$ 2.5 seconds. Residual radioactivity at 2 minutes after the initial swallow was always less than 12% of the maximal activity recorded in a

Table I
Comparision Between Radionuclide Esophageal Transit Studies (RETS) and Esophageal Motility Studies (EMS) in Patients with Motor Dysfunction of the Esophagus (Group I)

		RETS	
		Positive	*Negative*
EMS	Positive	36	1
	Negative	2	0

n = 39
sensitivity: 97.3%

given region of interest.[12] The upper limit of normality included 2 standard deviations.

EMS

Data obtained form the 40 normal volunteers were described in detail in a previous article.[11] Criteria of interpretation were rigorous. Any deviation from these criteria were considered to be abnormal.

Group I: Esophageal Motor Disorders

Thirty-nine patients had a final diagnosis of esophageal motor disorder. Distribution was as follows: achalasia (n = 7), diffuse esophageal spasm (n = 5), scleroderma (n = 4), Zenker's diverticulum (n = 5), oculopharyngeal muscular dystrophy (n = 9), and oropharyngeal dysphagia (n = 9). Table I shows the correlation between RETS and EMS in this group of patients. Sensitivity of RETS was 97.3% and predictive value of a positive test was 94.7%. The number of normal cases was too low to determine the specificity. In one case, RETS was normal in a patient with oropharyngeal dysphagia while EMS demonstrated 80% primary waves in response to swallowing in the proximal esophagus. Endoscopy and pH-metry were normal. EMS was normal in two cases while RETS showed esophageal motility dys-

Table II
Comparision Between Radionuclide
Esophageal Transit Studies (RETS)
and Esophageal Motility Studies
(EMS) in Patients with Reflux Disease
(Group II)

		RETS	
		Positive	*Negative*
EMS	Positive	24	2
	Negative	2	20

n = 48
sensitivity: 92.3% specificity: 90.9%

function. One patient had a Zenker's diverticulum and the other suffered from oropharyngeal dysphagia of central origin.

Group II: Gastroesophageal Reflux Disease

Forty-eight patients had gastroesophageal reflux disease demonstrated by 24-hour pH-metry. Table II shows the results of both RETS and EMS in detection of esophageal motility disorders related to gastroesophageal reflux disease. Sensitivity and specificity of RETS were 92.3% and 90.9%, respectively. Predictive value of a negative test was 90.9% and 92.3% for a positive test. There were two false negatives: one patient had a hypotensive LES and abnormal contractions in the proximal esophagus and one patient had abnormal contractions in the esophageal body. The two false positive cases on RETS showed hiatal hernia and reflux disease on pH-metry.

Group III: Noncardiac Chest Pain

Twenty-two patients had a final diagnosis of noncardiac chest pain. Table III shows results of both procedures in this group of patients. Sensitivity and specificity of RETS were 76.9% and 100%, respectively. The predictive value of a negative test was 75% and 100% for a positive test. In this group, RETS was normal in three patients in whom EMS detected slight nonspecific abnormalities: one patient

Table III
Comparision Between Radionuclide
Esophageal Transit Studies (RETS)
and Esophageal Motility Studies
(EMS) in Patients with Noncardiac
Chest Pain (Group III)

		RETS	
		Positive	Negative
EMS	Positive	10	3
	Negative	0	9

n = 22
sensitivity: 76.9% specificity: 100%

had a hypertensive lower esophageal sphincter, one had a hypotensive lower esophageal sphincter, and another had 60% primary waves in response to swallowing in the proximal esophagus. RETS did not show false positive cases in this group of patients.

Global Results

Table IV summarizes the global results obtained in 109 patients. When compared to EMS, RETS had a sensitivity of 92.1% and a spec-

Table IV
Comparision Between Radionuclide
Esophageal Transit Time (RETS) and
Esophageal Motility Studies (EMS):
Global Results (Groups I, II, and III)

		RETS	
		Positive	Negative
EMS	Positive	70	6
	Negative	4	29

n = 109
sensitivity: 92.1% specificity: 87.9%

ificity of 87.9% in detection of esophageal motor dysfunction. The predictive value of a positive test is 94.6% and 82.9% for a negative test. There were six false negatives (5.5%) and 4 false positives (3.7%).

Discussion

Although several articles have been published on RETS in the investigation of esophageal disorders, there is no consensus on its role in clinical practice.[9] This may be partially explained by the large number of different procedures that were used to perform this test. Many technical variants were reported, including the radiopharmaceutical, amount of ingested activity, patient positioning, single versus multiple swallows, duration of acquisition, type of computer analysis, and interpretation criteria. This led to confusing reports and results obtained with RETS are quite variable.

Furthermore, RETS has been compared to other tests commonly used in clinical esophagology such as endoscopy, radiological studies, and pH-metry. RETS does not have the anatomic resolution of endoscopy or radiological studies and it is not designed to detect gastroesophageal reflux like pH-metry. Rather, RETS has been developed to assess the motor function of the esophagus and the end result of its emptying capacity. In this study, RETS was compared to EMS used as a gold standard in the assessment of motor function. The sensitivity and specificity of RETS in detection of esophageal motility disorders were 92.1% and 87.9%, respectively. It should be emphasized that these results were obtained using rigorous EMS criteria. All six (5.5%) false negative cases on RETS has only minor "nonspecific" abnormalities on EMS. Thus, no significant lesions were missed by RETS. Furthermore, the four (3.9%) false positives on RETS had esophageal disorders demonstrated by endoscopy, pH-metry, or radiological procedures.

RETS with computer data processing offers advantages over other standard clinical methods used in the investigation of esophageal motility disorders. It fulfills the major criteria of evaluating esophageal emptying function: it is safe, noninvasive, very well accepted by patients, easy to perform, readily available to an average nuclear medicine laboratory, and has a low radiation dosimetry. Most importantly, it uses physiological markers and provides quantitative data on esophageal emptying function. RETS is a complementary procedure evaluating different parameters that would be unavailable by other means. While EMS measures the duration, velocity, and pressure of the esophagus and sphincters, RETS evaluates the combined effects of these factors on the segmental and global esophageal emptying.

Conclusion

RETS is a useful noninvasive test for the screening of patients with symptoms thought to be of esophageal origin and it can quantitate esophageal emptying abnormalities in patients with motor disorders, reflux disease, or other conditions affecting esophageal function.

References

1. Kazem I: A new scintigraphic technique for the study of the esophagus. Am J Roentgenol Radiol Ther Nucl Med 115:681, 1972.
2. Tolin RD, Malmud LS, Reilley J, et al: Esophageal scintigraphy to quantitate transit. Gastroenterology 76:1402, 1979.
3. Russell COH, Hill LD, Holmes ER, et al: Radionuclide transit: A sensitive screening test for esophageal dysfunction. Gastroenterology 80:887, 1981.
4. Gross R, Johnson LP, Kaminski DJ: Esophageal emptying in achalasia quantitated by a radioisotope technique. Dig Dis Sci 24:945, 1979.
5. Kjellen G, Svedberg JB, Tibbling L: Solid bolus transit by esophageal scintigraphy in patients with dysphagia and normal manometry and radiography. Dig Dis Sci 29:1, 1984.
6. Taillefer R, Beauchamp G: Radionuclide esophagogram. Clin Nucl Med 9:465, 1984.
7. Taillefer R, Beauchamp G, Duranceau A, et al: Nuclear medicine and esophageal surgery. Clin Nucl Med 11:445, 1986.
8. Taillefer R, Duranceau A: Manometric and radionuclide assessment of pharyngeal emptying before and after cricopharyngeal myotomy in patients with oculopharyngeal muscular dystrophy. J Thorac Cardiovasc Surg 95:868, 1988.
9. Gilchrist AM, Laird JD, Rodney Ferguson W: What is the significance of the abnormal esophageal scintigram? Clin Radiol 38:509, 1987.
10. Richter JE, Wu WC, Ott DJ: Nutcracker esophagus: Diagnosis with radionulide esophageal scintigraphy versus manometry. Radiology 164:877, 1987.
11. Duranceau A, Devroede G, LaFontaine E, et al: Esophageal motility in asymptomatic volunteer. In: The Surgical Clinics of North America, Duranceau A (ed), WB Saunders Company, p. 377.
12. Taillefer R, Beauchamp G, Duranceau A: Radionuclide esophageal transit studies. In: Atlas of Nuclear Medicine, Van Nostrand D, Baum S (ed), Philadelphia, J.B. Lippincott Company, 1988, p 1.

39

The Hypercontracting-Hypertensive Lower Esophageal Sphincter as a Cause of Dysphagia and Chest Pain

Ernst P. Eypasch, Hubert J. Stein,
Tom R. DeMeester, K. H. Vestweber,
Antony P. Barlow, Harry Jenkins

Introduction

In 1960 Code et al. first described the hypertensive lower esophageal sphincter as a separate esophageal motor disorder in patients with dysphagia and/or chest pain.[1] The disorder was characterized by the presence of an elevated resting pressure of the lower esophageal sphincter (LES) with normal relaxation following deglutition in the absence of other structural esophageal abnormalities. Subsequent studies showed that a considerable proportion of these patients have associated motility disorders of the esophageal body which could account for their symptoms. What remains unclear is why patients with normal esophageal peristalsis and the isolated finding of a high resting pressure in a lower esophageal sphincter, which relaxes normally on deglutition, should experience dysphagia and chest pain. Re-

Little AG, Ferguson MK, Skinner DB: Diseases of the Esophagus, Vol. II: Benign Diseases. Futura Publishing Company, Inc., Mount Kisco, NY, © 1990.

cently, it has been suggested that the cause is a hypercontraction of the sphincter following its relaxation.[1–6]

In the present study, the incidence of patients who met the criteria for the hypertensive LES was determined in a series of symptomatic patients undergoing esophageal manometry. The patients were separated into those with and those without manometric abnormality of the esophageal body. The manometric lower esophageal sphincter characteristics in the two patient groups were compared to findings in normal asymptomatic volunteers with elevated LES pressures.

Materials and Methods

Study Population and Design

The study population consisted of a series of 250 consecutive patients and 50 normal healthy volunteers undergoing esophageal manometry. The patients were referred to the senior author (TRD) or the Swallowing Center at Creighton University for evaluation of foregut symptoms. In all patients, symptoms were recorded on a standardized questionnaire. All patients had an endoscopy or a roentgenographic barium contrast study of the upper gastrointestinal tract or both to exclude or document the presence of a structural abnormality in the esophagus. A particular effort was made to exclude patients with the classic findings of achalasia or structural abnormalities of the esophagus from the study.

Patients who met the manometric criteria of the hypertensive LES, i.e., elevated sphincter resting pressure with complete relaxation on deglutition, were divided into those with and those without associated manometric abnormalities of the esophageal body. The manometric characteristics of LES relaxation and postrelaxation contraction in both patient groups were compared to findings in normal asymptomatic volunteers who had a lower esophageal sphincter pressure above the 90th percentile of normals.[5]

Esophageal Manometry

Esophageal manometry was performed according to a standard protocol using a 5-lumen water-perfused catheter connected to a low

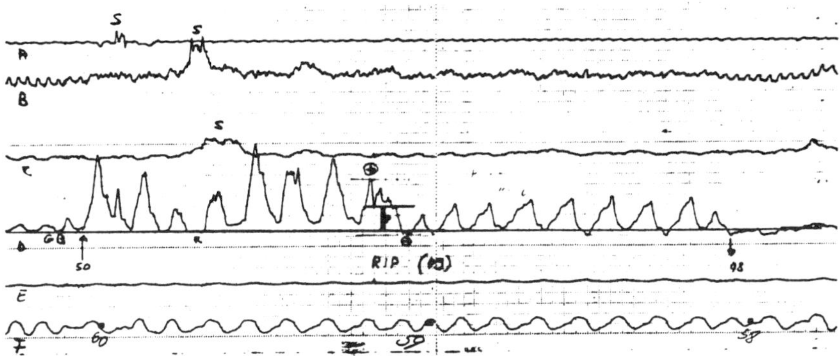

Figure 1: Station pull-through manometry profile of a normal lower esophageal sphincter. The sphincter pressure is measured at the RIP taking the mean of the two closest positive (+) and negative (−) respiratory deflections. (A) microphone attached to the neck; (B–D) pressure channels in the esophageal lumen (5 cm apart); (E) gastric pressure; (F) pneumograph recording (belt around the lower chest). S = swallow; R = relaxation. Arrows indicate lower and upper border of the high pressure zone.

compliance pneumohydraulic capillary infusion system. The side hole openings of the catheter were placed at 5-cm intervals from the tip and oriented radially at 72° from each other. The LES was evaluated with a station pull-through technique.[6] LES pressure was measured at the respiratory inversion point with each of the five radially oriented side holes and an average pressure was calculated (Fig. 1). A mean LES pressure which exceeded the 90th percentile of the average LES pressure in the 50 normal healthy volunteers, i.e., a mean LES pressure greater than 25 mmHg, was considered a hypertensive sphincter. The overall length and abdominal length of the LES were calculated as described previously.

For the evaluation of the relaxation and postrelaxation contraction of the LES, one side hole of the catheter was positioned within the sphincter with a distal side hole located within the stomach and the proximal side holes within the esophageal body. Sphincter relaxation was assessed by a series of five dry and five wet (5 cc water) swallows. Normal relaxation of the LES was defined as a drop of the LES pressure to the fundic baseline pressure following wet swallows. The maximum amplitude, duration, and the up and down slopes of the sphincter contraction following the relaxation (postrelaxation sphincter contraction) were measured for all swallows. Up and down

Table I
Clinical Data in Patients with the Manometric Findings of a Hypertensive Lower Esophageal Sphincter

	Group 1	Group 2
Incidence	5/250 (2.0%)	3/250 (1.2%)
Symptoms		
Heartburn	1/5	2/3
Regurgitation	2/5	1/3
Dysphagia	4/5	3/3
Chest pain	4/5	2/3
Associated Esophageal Body	NCE: 3	–
Motility Disorders:	DES: 2	

Group 1: Patients with hypertensive sphincter and associated motor abnormalities of the esophageal body.
Group 2: Patients with hypertensive sphincter without motor abnormalities of the esophageal body.
NCE = Nutcracker esophagus
DES = Diffuse esophageal spasm

slopes of the postrelaxation sphincter contraction were calculated as the rise or drop of sphincter pressure per second over resting sphincter pressure.

The function of the esophageal body was assessed with the most proximal side hole of the catheter located 1 cm below the lower border of the cricopharyngeal sphincter and the distal orifices trailing at 5-cm intervals over the whole length of the esophageal body. Ten dry and 10 wet swallows were performed. The presence of diffuse esophageal spasm, nutcracker esophagus, and nonspecific esophageal motor disorders was diagnosed according to standard criteria.[7]

Results

An elevated LES pressure with normal relaxation on deglutition was present in 12/250 (4.8%) consecutive patients with foregut symptoms. Four of these patients had structural foregut disorders accounting for their symptoms. These patients were excluded from the subsequent analysis. Five of the remaining eight patients with the manometric characteristics of hypertensive LES had an associated abnormality of the esophageal body, two patients had diffuse esophageal spasm, and three patients had the so-called nutcracker esoph-

Table II
Manometric Data in Normal Subjects and Patients with a Mean Lower Esophageal Sphincter (LES) Pressure Greater than 25 mmHg

	Normal Subjects	Group I	Group II
LES Pressure (mean, SD; mmHg)	26.7 (1.9)	35.0 (3.5)	32.8 (7.3)
Length of the LES			
abdominal	1.7 (0.8)	2.8 (1.0)	1.7 (1.8)
total	3.9 (0.8)	4.0 (0.8)	3.0 (1.4)
(mean, SD; cm)			
Duration of Postrelaxation Contraction (mean, SD; s)	5.3 (4.5)	4.9 (4.3)	13.6 (4.5)*
Maximum Amplitude of Postrelaxation Contraction (mean, SD; mmHg)	77 (33)	120 (43)	105 (37)
Slope of Postrelaxation Contraction (mmHg/sec)			
up	69.2 (35)	27 (10)**	17.4 (2)**
down	59.6 (42)	25 (8)	15.0 (6)

* $p < 0.05$ compared to normals and patients
** $p < 0.05$ compared to normals
Group 1: Patients with hypertensive sphincter and associated motor abnormalities of the esophageal body.
Group 2: Patients with hypertensive sphincter without motor abnormalities of the esophageal body.

agus. In the remaining three patients, the hypertensive LES occurred as an isolated abnormality.

The clinical presentation of the patients with a hypertensive LES is summarized in Table I. Dysphagia and chest pain were the main complaints in patients who had a hypertensive LES as an isolated abnormality and in patients who had an associated esophageal motor disorder. Due to the small number of patients, statistical differences in the symptoms between the two groups could not be described.

Table II compares the manometric lower esophageal sphincter characteristics in the two patient groups to findings in normal healthy volunteers with elevated lower esophageal sphincter pressures. Mean LES pressure, overall length, and abdominal length of the sphincter were not different in the groups. The postrelaxation contraction of

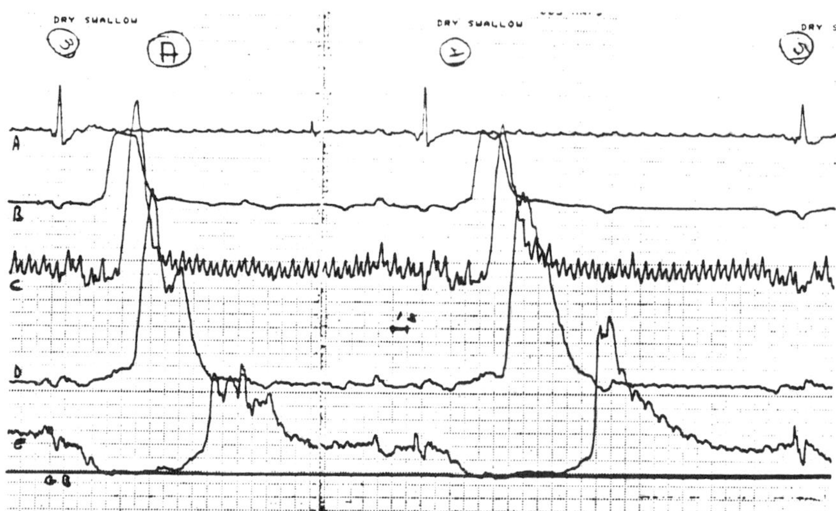

Figure 2: Peristaltic wave and postrelaxation contraction profile of the lower esophageal sphincter in a healthy volunteer with a mean pressure greater than 25 mmHg. (A) microphone attached to the neck; (B–D) pressure channels in the esophageal lumen; (E) sphincter channel; GB = gastric baseline.

the LES in patients who had an isolated hypertensive esophageal sphincter was significantly prolonged compared to asymptomatic volunteers or patients with an associated esophageal motor disorder ($p < 0.05$). In both patient groups, the rise in pressure of the postrelaxation sphincter contraction was significantly slower than in the asymptomatic volunteers ($p < 0.05$).

The typical patterns of postrelaxation sphincter contraction in asymptomatic volunteers with elevated LES pressure and a patient with an isolated hypertensive LES are shown in Figures 2 and 3. Figure 4 demonstrates that sphincter relaxation is not impaired in patients with an isolated hypertensive LES.

Discussion

The improvements in the technology of esophageal manometry and its increased use in the evaluation of patients with foregut disorders has led to the description of a variety of esophageal function abnormalities. The finding of a lower esophageal sphincter with ele-

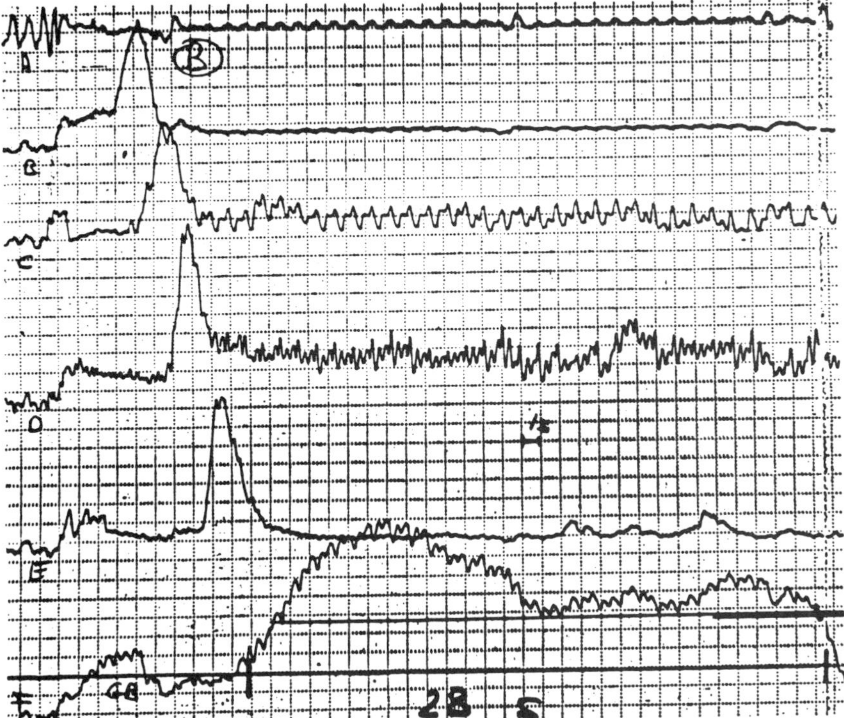

Figure 3: Peristaltic wave and postrelaxation contraction profile of the lower esophageal sphincter in a patient with hypercontracting sphincter. Note the long duration and the slow onset of the contraction. (A) microphone; (B–E) pressure channels in the esophageal lumen; (F) sphincter channel. GB = gastric baseline.

vated resting pressure but normal relaxation on deglutition has been repeatedly reported in patients with dysphagia and/or chest pain of noncardiac origin and has been termed hypertensive lower esophageal sphincter.[1–4,8–11] In the present study we showed that the incidence of a hypertensive LES in a population of symptomatic patients is not higher than in normal asymptomatic volunteers. A hypertensive lower esophageal sphincter, defined by a sphincter pressure exceeding the 90th percentile of normal volunteers in the absence of structural foregut abnormalities, occurred in only 8/250 (3.2%) consecutive symptomatic patients undergoing esophageal manometry.

As in previous reports, dysphagia was the primary symptom in these patients. It is difficult to comprehend how a sphincter that

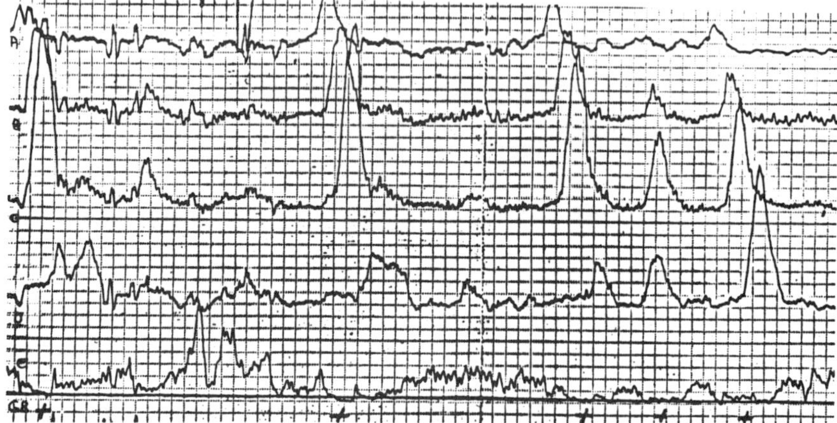

Figure 4: A series of repetitive swallows in short intervals in the same patient as Figure 3 demonstrates no impairment of sphincter relaxation. (A–E) pressure channels in th eesophagus. GB = gastric baseline; (+) indicates full relaxation.

Table III
Associated Esophageal Body Motor Abnormalities in Patients with a Hypertensive Lower Esophageal Sphincter

Author/Ref.	Year	Associated Motor Disease (% of Patients)	Sphincter Hypercontraction (% of Patients)
Code[1]	1960	diffuse spasm 60%	25%
Garrett[2]	1969	diffuse spasm 20%	100%
Pederson[3]	1972	diffuse spasm 25%	54%
Kaye[8]	1973	—	20%
Graham[4]	1978	diffuse spasm 30%	30%
Present study	1989	diffuse spasm 16% hypertensive contractions 25%*	25%

* So-called nutcracker esophagus

Table IV
Characteristics of the Lower Esophageal Sphincter
Postrelaxation Contraction in Patients with a Hypertensive
Lower Esophageal Sphincter

Author	Year	Duration of Postrelaxation Contraction	Slope of Contraction
Code[1]	1960	"vigorous contractions"	—
Garrett[2]	1969	11.3 seconds	—
Pederson[3]	1972	12 seconds	—
Kaye[8]	1973	up to 45 seconds	—
Graham[4]	1978	15 to 30 seconds	reduced
Present study	1989	13.6 seconds	reduced

shows normal relaxation on deglutition can cause dysphagia. In the majority of our patients with the hypertensive LES, the disorder was associated with a primary motor disorder of the esophageal body known to cause dysphagia and chest pain. This finding is consistent with reports by other authors (Table III), suggesting that the associated motor disorder of the esophageal body accounts for the symptoms of dysphagia in most of their patients.[1-4,8-11]

In our study hypertensive LES occurred as an isolated abnormality in only 3/250 (1.2%) patients undergoing manometry. All three patients complained of severe dysphagia (Table II). Each of these patients showed a markedly prolonged duration of the postrelaxation contraction of the LES compared to asymptomatic volunteers or patients with an associated motor disorder of the esophageal body. In-

Table V
Diagnostic Criteria for Hypercontracting Lower Esophageal
Sphincter

1. Dysphagia and chest pain as the predominant symptoms.
2. Lower esophageal mean resting pressure greater than 25 mmHg.
3. Mean duration of postrelaxation contraction greater than 14 seconds.
4. Mean slope of contraction pressure rise under 25 mmHg/second.
5. No other primary esophageal motor disorder.
6. No endoscopic or radiological evidence of organic causes of symptoms.

creased duration of the postrelaxation sphincter contraction in patients with the hypertensive LES has been observed previously (Table IV) and has been termed hypercontracting sphincter. Our data suggest that in the absence of an associated motor abnormality of the esophageal body, the prolonged duration of postrelaxation sphincter contraction (a hypercontracting-hypertensive sphincter) may account for the dysphagia occurring in these patients. The finding of a hypertensive sphincter without postrelaxation hypercontraction or associated motor abnormality of the esophageal body may not constitute an abnormal finding as it also occurs in normal asymptomatic volunteers.

In summary, a hypertensive sphincter occurs only in a minority of patients undergoing esophageal manometry for the evaluation of foregut symptoms. Dysphagia in these patients appears to be frequently due to an associated motility disorder of the esophageal body. A prolonged contraction of the LES following relaxation (the hypercontracting-hypertensive sphincter) may be responsible for the dysphagia in patients without associated esophageal body disorders. The diagnostic criteria for the hypercontracting-hypertensive sphincter are summarized in Table V. Appropriate medical or surgical treatment should be guided by the symptoms.

References

1. Code DF, Schlegel JF, Kelley ML, et al: Hypertensive gastroesophageal sphincter. Proc Mayo Clinic 35:391, 1960.
2. Garrett JM, Godwin DH: Gastroesophageal hypercontracting sphincter. JAMA 208:992, 1969.
3. Pederson A, Alstrup P: The hypertensive gastroesophageal sphincter. Scand J Gastroent 7:531, 1972.
4. Graham DY: Hypertensive lower esophageal sphincter: A reappraisal. South Med J 71:31, 1978.
5. Zaninotto G, DeMeester TR, Schwizer W, et al: The lower esophageal sphincter in health and disease. Am J Surg 155:104, 1988.
6. Winans CS, Harris LD: Quantitation of lower esophageal sphincter competence. Gastroenterology 65:1235, 1967.
7. Castell DO, Richter JE, Dalton CB: Esophageal Motility Testing. New York, Elsevier Science Publishing Co, 1987, p 138.
8. Kaye MD: Dysfunction of the lower esophageal sphincter in disorders other than achalasia. Am J Dig Dis 18:734, 1973.
9. Ellis FH, Code CF, Olsen AM: Long esophagomyotomy for diffuse spasm of the esophagus and hypertensive gastroesophageal sphincter. Surgery 48:155, 1960.

10. Jamieson GG, Maddern GJ: Long esophageal myotomy through the diaphragmatic hiatus in the treatment of hypertensive lower esophagus associated with gastroesophageal reflux. In: Diseases of the Esophagus, Siewert JR, Hölscher AH (eds), New York, Springer Heidelberg, 1988, p 918.
11. Samuelson SL, Nyhus LM: Hypertensive lower oesophageal sphincter. In: Surgery of the Esophagus, Jamieson GG (ed), Churchill Livingstone, 1988.

VII.

Esophageal Varices:
Editors' Overview

Chapter 40 documents the efficacy of vasopressin in controlling bleeding from esophageal varices as bleeding stopped in 28 of the 31 patients receiving this drug. Unfrotunately, there was no comparison group receiving an alternative acute therapy. These results do, however, support the author's contention that use of vasopressin is effective and can be used until endoscopic sclerosis becomes available for the patient.

Chapter 41 documents the high rate of success when endoscopic sclerotherapy is performed. Using the approach outlined in their chapter, definitive control of hemorrhage was accomplished in 94% of acute bleeders. They make the important point that, if experienced endoscopists are available, sclerotherapy can be performed in an emergency setting, but if such experience is not available around the clock, then acute control of bleeding should be obtained by other means and sclerotherapy reserved until the appropriate endoscopist becomes available. From the same group, Chapter 42 reports results utilizing the Sugiura operation in patients with portal vein thrombosis. This chapter shows that utilization of this devascularization procedure can be carried out with acceptable mortality and morbidity figures and with good long-term results. They recommend this approach for patients in whom a shunt operation is not possible and long-term endoscopic injection sclerotherapy is not successful.

40

Glypressin (Triglycyl-Lysine Vasopressin) in the Control of Bleeding from Esophageal Varices:
A Placebo-Controlled Double-Blind Clinical Trial

C. Söderlund, U. Seligsson, S. Törngren, and Lars Lundell

Introduction

Balloon-tamponade, vasopressin infusion, and endoscopic sclerotherapy either as monotherapy or in combination, are widely used for the acute treatment of bleeding esophageal varices. All these modalities have, however, disadvantages; balloon-tamponade is complicated to use for the physician, unpleasant, and potentially dangerous for the patient.[1] Vasopressin infusion has few serious side effects if given as a low dose and as a continuous intravenous infusion,[2] but its hemostatic effect has not been established in controlled randomized trials.[3,4] Emergency sclerotherapy is a widely used technique preferred by many,[5,6] but this endoscopic technique requires time for a resuscitation of the patient and is difficult to carry through

Little AG, Ferguson MK, Skinner DB: Diseases of the Esophagus, Vol. II: Benign Diseases. Futura Publishing Company, Inc., Mount Kisco, NY, © 1990.

during ongoing bleeding. Sclerotherapy is preferably carried out during the daytime by a highly trained endoscopist.

In order to avoid protein load to the liver from blood absorbed from the gut, bleeding must be stopped without delay in patients with liver cirrhosis. Continued bleeding may precipitate renal and multi-organ failure and worsen an already disturbed coagulation profile. Triglycyl-lysine vasopressin (Glypressin[R], GLY) in itself biologically inactive, is activated through cleavage of the triglycin residue and which releases the active lysine vasopressin. Consequently, the pharmacological activity of lysine vasopressin lasts 6–10 hours after a single dose of GLY as opposed to 20–40 minutes after an equipotent dose of lysine vasopressin. The potential advantages of GLY are: administration simplicity, and improved hemostatic effect due to a longer duration of action and a greater biological availability. We have in a prospective, randomized trial evaluated the hemostatic effect of GLY in patients with acute hemorrhage from esophageal varices. In view of the lack of clinical effect of lysine vasopressin per se, we have chosen to administer a placebo to the control group.

Materials and Methods

Included in the study were patients who presented with extensive upper gastrointestinal bleeding within 24 hours prior to the endoscopy and who also had clinically suspected liver cirrhosis. Diagnostic endoscopy was performed within 12 hours of hospital admission. The course of bleeding was considered to be from esophageal varices when at endoscopy current bleeding was actually seen from varices or when varices of at least size 3[6] were identified along with fresh blood in the stomach and when no other lesions were observed. Extensive bleeding was defined as that requiring a blood transfusion, within 24 hours, of at least 2 units of blood (900 ml) or an equal amount in packed red blood cells. Pregnant women and patients with a body weight below 55 kg were excluded from the study.

After randomization, a placebo (mannitol) or 2 mg of GLY was administered intravenously as a bolus and then repeated every fourth hour until control endoscopy with sclerotherapy was performed after 24 to 36 hours. Failure was defined as a need for active intervention (balloon-tamponade and/or sclerotherapy) to stop hemorrhaging during the treatment period. Each patient was observed and treated at the intensive care unit. Blood pressure, pulse rate (continuous ECG monitoring), and hemoglobin were assessed, laboratory screening was performed, and a nasogastric tube was inserted after endoscopy to monitor continuous or recurrent bleeding.

The control endoscopy was carried out with dual aims: to evaluate the presence or absence of active variceal hemorrhage and to carry out sclerotherapy. The clinical course was then followed for another 24 hours, during which time period the transfusion requirements were recorded in addition to the clinical course.

The therapy was evaluated both as an overall assessment of success or failure and also as to the efficacy and safety of the test medication. Efficacy was defined as no blood mixing in two consecutive gastric rinses carried out through the nasogastric tube, 4 hours apart in a hemodynamically stable patient and with no ongoing bleeding or fresh blood at control endoscopy.

Statistics and Ethics

Comparisons between proportions were made by application of Fisher's exact test. Analyses of variance were applied to evaluate differences in blood pressure, pulse rate, and hemoglobin levels. The study protocol was approved by the local ethical committees and informed consent was obtained from each patient.

Results

Sixty consecutive patients entered the study. The two study groups were quite similar regarding all relevant, clinical demographic data (Table I). About 80% of the patients had liver cirrhosis secondary to alcohol abuse and 1/3 patients had poor hepatic function (classified as Child-C).[7] The treatment was judged as successful in 17 patients (59%) among those given placebo compared to 29 (90%) among those given GLY (p < 0.01) (Fig. 1). Active intervention because of continuous bleeding was necessary in 12 placebo-treated patients whereas only three patients given active substance required endoscopic sclerotherapy (Fig. 1) during the test period.

There was no difference between the study groups in the pre-entry amounts of blood transfused. During the treatment period, however, significantly more blood was transfused into patients ran-

Table I
Demographic Data

	Placebo (n = 29)	Glypressin (n = 31)
Male/female	21/8	20/11
Age (years)	60 ± 13	57 ± 11
Weight (kg)	74 ± 14	73 ± 15
Alcoholic cirrhosis	24	25
Pugh score A + B	20	20
Bilirubin (mmol/L)	34.3 ± 23.7	51.4 ± 58.7
Albumin (g/L)	28.4 ± 5.7	28.9 ± 5.2
PP (% of normal)	46.6 ± 14.0	55.8 ± 26.1

Mean ± SD are given.

domized to placebo treatment ($p < 0.05$) (Fig. 2). Including also the 24-hour posttreatment observation period in the analysis, the total need for transfusions was still larger in patients receiving placebo ($p < 0.05$).

Side effects, usually of a mild nature, were more often experienced in patients given GLY. One patient allocated to GLY had to be withdrawn from the study due to severe bradycardia.

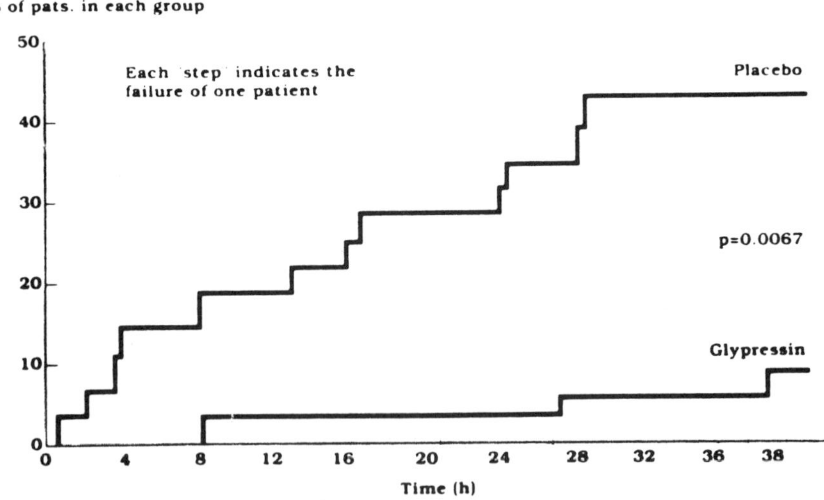

Figure 1: Cumulative failure rate in patients randomized to Glypressin or placebo administration.

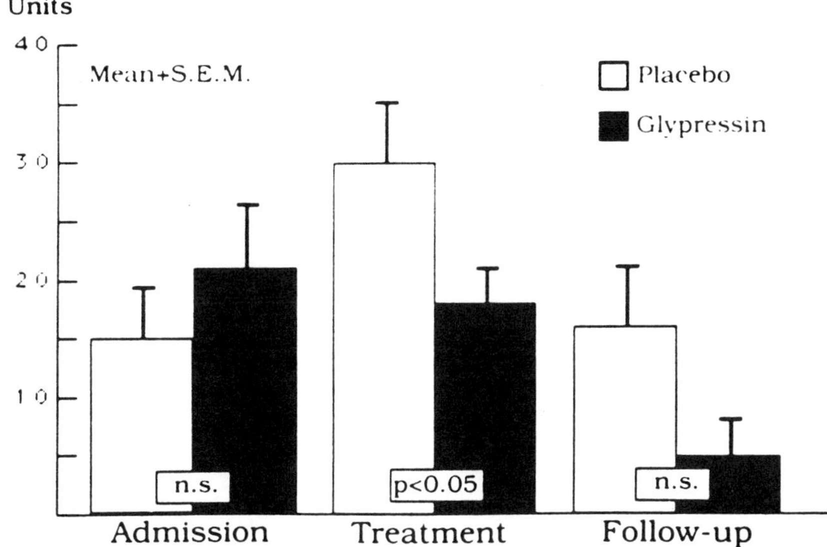

Figure 2: Blood transfusion requirements (units of blood) in patients randomized to placebo or Glypressin treatment.

Discussion

During the last 20 years vasopressin has been used to control bleeding from esophageal varices despite the lack of clinical efficacy.[3,4] There are a number of pitfalls when carrying out clinical studies in patients with bleeding esophageal varices such as the need for monitoring continuing or recurrent bleeding, stratification for the severity of liver dysfunction, the need for repeated endoscopy, and definition of clinically relevant end-points. We, like others, have taken steps in the design of the clinical trial to circumvent many of these difficulties. In addition, other mechanisms may also contribute to explain the lack of clinical effect of vasopressin. This hormone has been reported to exert a stimulating effect on the fibrinolytic system.[8] The cardiotoxic effects of vasopressin also limit its clinical usefulness and adequate local concentrations are not reached to exert a hemostatic effect in the splanchnic area. So far, no serious cardiac side effects or alterations in hemostasis have been observed after GLY administration.[9]

Triglycyl-lysine vasopressin was in an initial study found clinically useful and also to possess prolonged vasoconstrictive properties.[10] Clinical studies also suggested that this drug might be effective in arresting variceal hemorrhage,[11] and in fact a controlled trial suggested GLY to be superior to a vasopressin infusion both regarding its simplicity to administer and its ability to stop bleeding from esophageal varices.[12] However, when GLY was tested against placebo in a double-blind, randomized trial, Freeman and co-workers[13] were unable to demonstrate a significant, acute hemostatic effect although rebleeding during a 5-day follow-up period seemed to be more common among those who were given placebo. The present study, into which considerably more patients were entered, for the first time demonstrates a significant beneficial hemostatic effect of vasoconstrictive therapy in patients with bleeding esophageal varices.

Vasoconstrictor therapy can never replace sclerotherapy in the long-term management of patients with bleeding from esophageal varices. There is, however, a great clinical demand for a drug that is safe and causes prompt arrest of hemorrhage, particularly in patients with severe liver dysfunction, enabling time for resuscitation to prepare the patients for more definite therapy.[14] The efficacy and safety of GLY, as reported in the present study, suggests that this substance can make an important contribution in the immediate clinical treatment of variceal bleeding.

References

1. Conn HO, Simpson JA: Excessive mortality associated with balloon-tamponade bleeding varices: A critical appraisal. JAMA 202:587, 1967.
2. Shojker M, Groszmann RJ, Atterbury CE, et al: A controlled comparison of continuous intra-arterial and intervenous infusions of vasopressin in hemorrhage from esophageal varices. Gastroenterology 77:540, 1979.
3. Fogel MR, Knauer CM, Andres L, et al: Continuous intervenous vasopressin in active upper gastrointestinal bleeding. Ann Intern Med 96:565, 1982.
4. Dahl CR, Mallory A, Hansen R, et al: Continuous intravenous (IV) vasopressin (VP) for upper gastrointestinal hemorrhage. Gastroenterology 84:1132, 1983.
5. Söderlund C: Endoscopic sclerotherapy of esophageal varices: A clinical study. Acta Chir Scand (suppl) 524, 1985.
6. Dagradia Stempins Owens K: Bleeding esophagogastric varices. Surgery 92:944, 1966.
7. Pugh RNH, Murray-Lyon IM, Dawson JL, et al: Transection of the oesophagus for bleeding esophageal varices. Br J Surg 60:646, 1973.
8. Douglas JC, Forrest JAH, Prowse CW, et al: Effects of lysin vasopressin and Glypressin on the fibrinolytic system in cirrhosis. Gut 20:565, 1979.

9. Walker S, Stiehl A, Raedsch R, Kommerell B: Terlipressin in bleeding esophageal varices: A placebo controlled double-blind study. Hepatology 6:112, 1986.
10. Cort CJH, Albrecht I, Novakova J, et al: Regional and systemic hemodynamic effects of some vasopressins: Structural features of the hormone which prolongs activity. Eur J Clin Investigation 5:165, 1975.
11. Vosmik J, Jedlicka K, Mudler IL, Cort JH: Action of the triglycyl hormonogen form of vasopressin (Glypressin) in patients. Gastroenterology 72:605, 1977.
12. Freeman JG, Cobden I, Lishman AH, Record CO: Controlled trial of terlipressin (Glypressin) and vasopressin in the early treatment of esophageal varices. Lancet 1:66, 1982.
13. Freeman JG, Cobden I, Lishman AH, Record CO: Placebo controlled trial of terlipressin (Glypressin) in the management of acute variceal bleeding. J Clin Gastroenterol 11:58, 1989.
14. Westaby D, Hayes PC, Gimson AES, Polson RJ, Williams R: Controlled clinical trial of injection sclerotherapy for active variceal bleeding. Hepatology 9:274, 1989.

Immediate Endoscopic Sclerosis of Bleeding Esophageal Varices: A Propsective Evaluation Over Five Years

K.-J. Paquet, P. Koussouris, J.-F. Kalk, W. Rambach

Introduction

In most sclerotherapy reports, initial management of the variceal bleeding consists of vasopressin, vasopressin and nitroglycerin, glypressin, and/or balloon-tamponade for control of active bleeding, followed by late sclerotherapy once the bleeding stops. This allows the endoscopist to perform sclerotherapy in a clear field of vision, presumably in order to inject the sclerosant more accurately.

Balloon tamponade has been associated with a high complication rate of 8% to 38%,[2,21] usually from faulty techniques in inserting and monitoring the tubes. Fleig et al.[5] and Lewis et al.[7] reported the use of emergency endoscopic injection sclerosis for control of active variceal bleeding not controlled by balloon tamponade.

There is only one report comparing the efficacy of emergency sclerotherapy versus late sclerotherapy for the control of active bleeding.[17] On the other hand, we have demonstrated in a prospective controlled randomized trial that immediate endoscopic sclerosis dur-

Little AG, Ferguson MK, Skinner DB: Diseases of the Esophagus, Vol. II: Benign Diseases. Futura Publishing Company, Inc., Mount Kisco, NY, © 1990.

Table I
Child-Pugh-Classification[2,18] (Noncirrhotic
Patients are Classified as Child-Pugh A)

Classification	Number	Percent
Child-Pugh A	53	23
Child-Pugh B	70	30
Child-Pugh C	109	47
	232	100

ing emergency endoscopy is highly superior to Sengstaken balloon tamponade in stopping hemorrhage, (p < 0.01), reducing the episodes of rebleeding and improving clinic mortality and survival after 6 (p < 0.01) and 36 months (p < 0.001).[14] Similarly, emergency endoscopic sclerotherapy using a flexible endoscope and absolute alcohol was recently recommended by Sarin et al.[19] because of an initial successful control rate of variceal bleeding of 92% and an overall success rate of 87%.

As a consequence, since January 1, 1982 we have performed in every patient admitted to our hospital with active variceal hemorrhage acute endoscopic sclerotherapy (AES) during emergency endoscopy.

Patients and Methods

Between January 1982 to January 1987, a prospective nonrandomized sclerotherapy study was conducted at the Heinz-Kalk Hospital in Bad Kissingen with 232 consecutive patients receiving AES for variceal bleeding during emergency endoscopy. One hundred forty-four (62%) patients belong to the category Forrest I (active bleeding) and 88 (38%) to Forrest II (clot on a varix). No patients were excluded from this study. All patients were classified according to the Child-Pugh criteria[2,18] (Table I); 53 (23%) were classified as Child-Pugh A, 70 (30%) as B and 109 (47%) as Child C. The underlying disease of all patients is summarized in Table II; more than 93% had liver cirrhosis based on biopsy and nearly 60% had alcoholic liver disease. Sixteen (7%) noncirrhotic patients are included in the study and were classified as Child-Pugh A, but only nine (3.9%) of them had a prehepatic block.

All patients underwent emergency fiberoptic endoscopy and en-

Table II
Causes of Portal Hypertension in 232 Consecutive Patients

Underlying Disease	Number	Percent
alcoholic cirrhosis	138	59.5
posthepatitic cirrhosis	47	20.3
cirrhosis of unknown etiology	17	7.3
primary biliary cirrhosis	11	4.7
extrahepatic bile duct atresia	2	0.9
secundary biliary cirrhosis	1	0.4
liver cirrhosis	216	93.1
prehepatic block	9	3.9
liver fibrosis	5	2.2
schistosomiasis	1	0.4
mucoviscidosis	1	0.4
non-cirrhotic patients	16	6.9

doscopic sclerotherapy using an Olympus-GIF$_1$-T, K, or a Fujinon UGR$_{P2}$ or -F$_4$ endoscope. Five to 40 1-ml portions of 0.5% Polidocanol were injected with a flexible self-constructed injection needle. Clear identification of the esophageal bleeding point was a primary endoscopic goal. The second goal was to stop hemorrhage by the paravariceal "free-hand" injection technique. If this was not successful, an intravariceal approach was used. After the initial bleeding site was controlled, no further injection was performed and the fiberscope was withdrawn. Cessation of bleeding was defined as no bleeding for 24 consecutive hours as determined by gastric aspiration and stability of hematocrit and vital signs. If bleeding could not be stopped after a period of 15 minutes, the endoscope was withdrawn and a Linton-Nachlas tube inserted for 6–12 hours. Thereafter, the tube was deflated but remained in position another 24 hours to ensure the definitive cessation of bleeding.

All patients received blood transfusion, gastric lavage, cathartics (60 mg MgSO$_4$) and neomycin (2 g), cleansing sodium acetate enemas, and antacids. Hypertonic glucose (40%) was administered intravenously, and electrolyte abnormalities were corrected.

If bleeding recurred, the localization and origin of hemorrhage was again determined endoscopically for a second acute endoscopic injection sclerotherapy. If this was not successful, a gastroesophageal disconnection according to Hassab-Paquet[6,12] (Fig. 1), sometimes

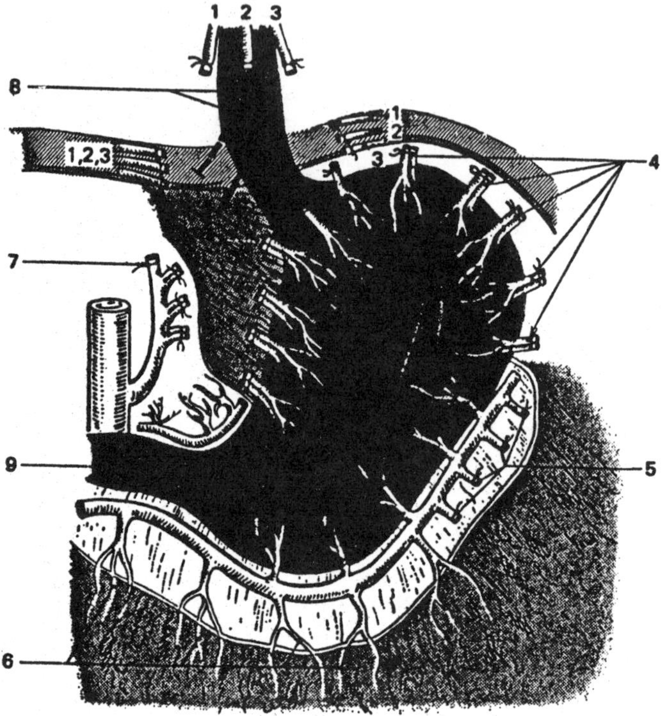

Figure 1: Gastroesophageal disconnection according to Hassab-Paquet with selective proximal vagotomy and sometimes pyloroplasty: 1, 2, 3 = devascularization of abdominal esophagus; 4, 5 = ligated left gastroepiploic vessels; 6 = retained right gastroepiploic vessels; 7 = ligated left gastric artery and vein; 8, 9 = vagotomy and pyloroplasty.

combined with a fundoplication and, if technically necessary, splenectomy was performed as an urgent procedure. In Child-Pugh A and B patients, our selection criteria[13,15] including liver volume, total liver blood flow, and portal perfusion were determined by noninvasive investigations. With positive results (liver volume between 1000 and 2500 ml and portal perfusion more than 10%), they were completed by laparoscopy with liver biopsy in order to exclude active hepatitis and an indirect lieno-, mesenterico-, hepatico-, and portography. Angiography was used to exclude stenosis of the hepatic artery and to visualize the suitability of the splenic or mesenteric vein. If all these criteria were positive, an elective shunt was recommended. In case of recurrent variceal hemorrhage in Child-Pugh C patients, a

Table III
Surgical Procedures Following Failed Immediate Endoscopic
Injection Sclerotherapy (n = 56/232 = 24%)

	Number of Patients and Time of Operation		
Procedures	*Elective*	*Emergent*	*Total*
Gastroesophageal disconnection according to Hassab-Paquet, often with fundoplication, sometimes with splenectomy	11	8	19
Semiselective or selective shunt operation	35	2	37
Meso-caval	18	2	20
Proximal spleno-renal	1		1
Distal spleno-renal	16		16

gastroesophageal disconnection was performed. Number, type and time of intervention of surgical procedures are listed in Table III.

In case of successful cessation of bleeding by AES, it was repeated at two to five sessions at 6- or 7-day intervals. An average of four sessions were necessary in this initial phase of therapy. Four months later, endoscopy was repeated, and if varices were seen, the second phase of sclerotherapy was performed. Thereafter, controls every 6, 9, or 12 months were sufficient. Statistical analysis was performed using Fischer's exact probability tests and paired Student's *t*-test.

Results

Bleeding was controlled in 214 of 232 patients (92%) with AES and in 225 of 232 (97%) with the combination of sclerotherapy and the Linton-Nachlas tube. Thus, seven patients exsanguinated. Recurrence of hemorrhage occurred in 49 of 225 patients (22%). Rebleeding was again controlled in 43 of 49 patients (88%). Thus, definitive control of hemorrhage was accomplished in 219 of 232 patients (94%) (Table IV).

Complications of AES, in 18 cases in combination with the Linton-Nachlas tube, consisted of esophageal ulceration in 21 patients (9%), three cases of aspiration pneumonia, three cases of a stricture of the

Table IV
Results

Primary control of hemorrhage by AES	214 (92%)
Primary control of hemorrhage by AES and Linton-Nachlas tube	225 (97%)
Recurrence of hemorrhage	49 (22%)
Control of recurrent hemorrhage	43 (88%)
Definitive control of hemorrhage	219 (94%)

esophagus that required dilatation, and three cases of pleural effusion that required drainage (3.9%). There was no case of esophageal wall necrosis with mediastinatis or pleural empyema.

Thirty-five patients died during the first 30 days after admission (15.1%). Main causes of death were liver failure and variceal hemorrhage or a combination of both (Table V). Eleven of them died after surgical procedures (Table VI): two after elective and four after urgent or emergent gastroesophageal disconnection (32%) and five following an elective semiselective or selective elective shunt operation (14%).

Only two patients were lost to follow-up. The main causes of 69 late deaths (29.8%) were liver failure, hepatocellular cancer, and hemorrhage (Table VII). A cumulative survival curve calculated using the method of Kaplan and Meier[8,12] is shown in Figure 2. The 5-year life expectancy rate is about 45%.

Table V
Causes of Early Death (In-Hospital Mortality During the First 30 Days After Admission)

Causes	*Number*	*Percent of Total*
Liver failure and hemorrhage	10	28.6
Variceal bleeding	10	28.6
Liver failure	9	25.6
Hepatocellular cancer	2	5.7
Hepatorenal syndrome	2	5.7
Pancreatitis	1	2.9
Bronchopneumonia	1	2.9
	35	100.0

Table VI
Early and Late Mortality of Surgical Procedures Following AES
(n = 56/232 = 24%)

Procedures	Mortality		
	Elective	*Emergent*	*Total*
Gastroesophageal disconnection according to Hassab-Paquet, often with fundoplication, sometimes with splenectomy	2/11 (18%)	4/8 (36%)	6/19 (35%)
Semiselective or selective shunt operation	5/35 (14%)		5/35 (14%)
	7	4	11/56 (19.5%)

Table VII
Causes of Late Death

Causes	Number	Percent	
		(death)	*(patient)*
Liver failure	22	31.9	9.5
Hepatocellular cancer	12	17.4	5.2
Liver failure and hemorrhage	8	11.6	3.4
Variceal bleeding	6	8.7	2.6
Hepatorenal syndrome	5	7.2	2.2
Heart failure	3	4.3	1.3
Bronchopneumonia	3	4.3	1.3
Peritonitis	2	2.9	0.9
Colon cancer	2	2.9	0.9
Unknown	2	2.9	0.9
Lung infarct	1	1.5	0.4
Sepsis	1	1.5	0.4
Stroke	1	1.5	0.4
Accident	1	1.4	0.4
	69	100.0	29.8

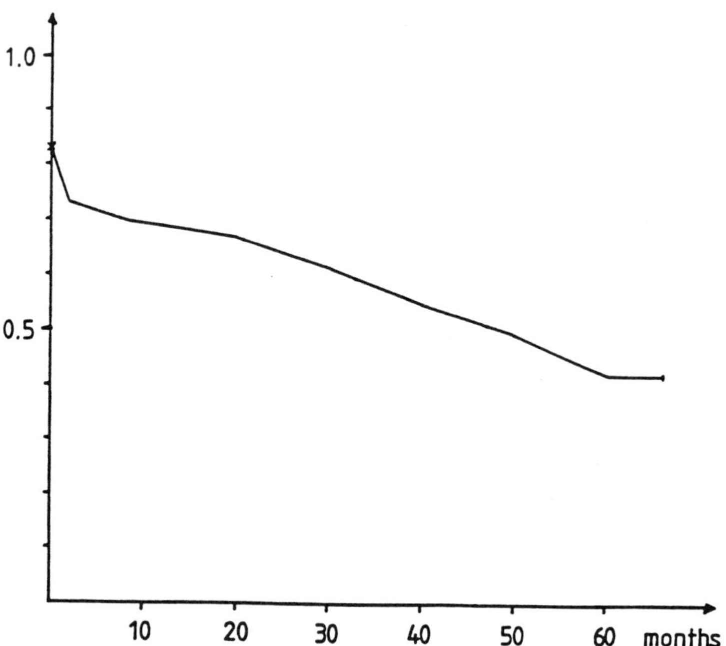

Figure 2: Survival after immediate endoscopic injection sclerosis (AES) of bleeding esophageal varices according to Kaplan-Meier.

Discussion

During the past 10 years, endoscopic injection sclerotherapy has become a widely accepted method of treating bleeding varices. Two randomized controlled trials of AES have been published. One was by Barsoum et al.,[1] which was performed primarily in patients with schistosomiasis. In that study, AES was shown to be superior to Sengstaken-Blakemore tamponade. The second study was performed by our group.[10] In this study, AES was also superior to Sengstaken-Blakemore tamponade as a sole form of therapy in stopping actively bleeding esophageal varices.

Other controlled trials of endoscopic sclerosis have dealt with elective sclerotherapy, i.e., in patients in whom the active bleeding was controlled prior to endoscopic sclerosis.[4,9,10,21,22,24] In each of these investigations, endoscopic sclerosis decreased the rate of recurrent bleeding and showed improved survival.[10,24]

Only one recently published study has compared immediate[16] versus delayed endoscopic injection sclerosis of bleeding esophageal varices.[17] Immediate control of active bleeding was achieved in all patients whose varices were injected (100%), whereas in the delayed sclerotherapy group, initial control of bleeding was 79%. Control at 48 hours was 89% versus 64%. Both values are statistically superior in favor of immediate endoscopic injection sclerosis. Furthermore, rebleeding rate, complications, and death from examination were greater in the delayed group, whereas survival was similar in both groups. The authors therefore conclude that immediate sclerotherapy effectively controls acutely bleeding esophageal varices with a lower complication rate than sclerotherapy performed after conventional or medical therapy with vasopressin and Sengstaken-Blakemore tamponade. These results are confirmed by our prospective evaluation of the value of immediate endoscopic injection sclerosis in bleeding esophageal varices during emergency endoscopy.

In comparison with Prindiville and Trudeau,[17] our primary control of hemorrhage was 92% by AES and 97% by the combination of AES and the Linton-Nachlas tube (225 of 232 patients). In 219 patients (94%), hemorrhage was definitely controlled. Ten emergency operations were performed, eight gastroesophageal disconnections, and two emergency mesocaval shunts. In three patients, neither the repeated sclerotherapy nor the surgical procedure was successful. In-hospital mortality within 30 days following admission was only 15% and total mortality during the whole observation time of 5 years was 45%; only two patients were lost to follow-up. Thus the 5-year life expectancy rate was nearly 50%.

The results of our prospective study are better concerning the frequency of rebleeding and identical concerning the survival time in comparison to the prospective randomized trial of the Kings College group of elective sclerotherapy.[10,24] This group has published the best results of all prospective randomized studies using elective sclerotherapy; patients were choosen for inclusion into the trial days and weeks after the active variceal hemorrhage had been stopped by conservative treatment or endoscopic sclerotherapy. However, it has been demonstrated by Smith and Graham[20] that the later patients are included into a prospective randomized trial (Fig. 3), the better the results will be. If our results concerning life expectancy seem similar

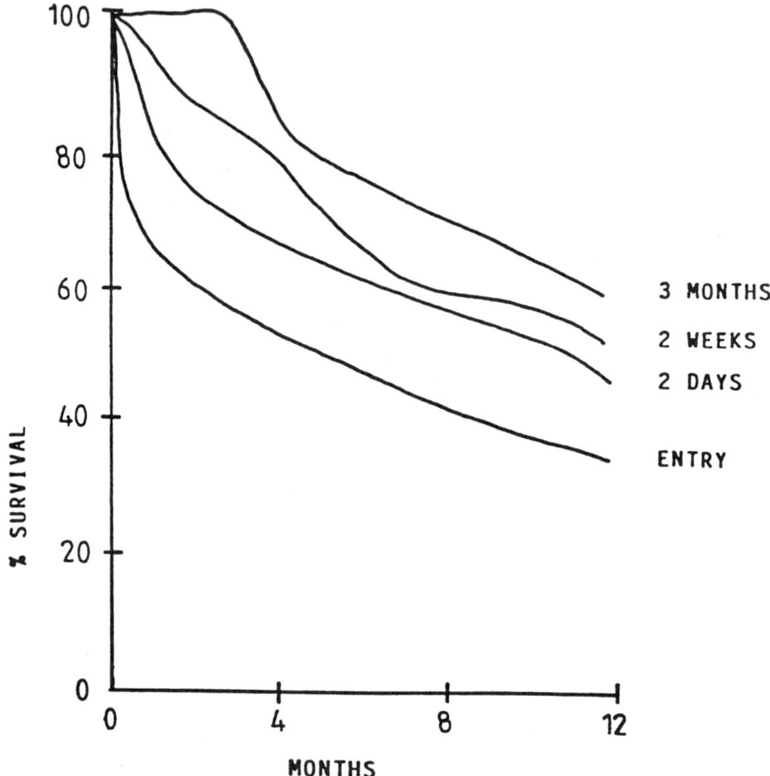

Figure 3: The calculated life-table analysis survival curve for 85 consecutive patients with variceal bleeding and predominantly Child C-grade cirrhosis of the liver (entry-curve). In addition, the effect of varying "zero" time for calculating survival from entry to 2 days, 2 weeks and 3 months is clearly shown. (From Graham and Lacey Smith (1981), with permission of the authors and the editor of Gastroenterology).

to the prospective controlled randomized trial of the Kings College Hospital group, they must actually be better, because in our prospective evaluation all actively bleeding patients are included.

Thus, acute injection sclerotherapy during emergency endoscopy is established as a primary therapeutic mode to successfully control hemorrhage from bleeding esophageal varices which can be done with a high degree of patient and operator tolerance. With sclerotherapy performed at the time of the diagnostic emergency endoscopy, prior stabilization with a Blakemore tube and/or vasopressin is not necessary. Rebleeding can also successfully be controlled by immediate sclerotherapy and in very rare cases by emergency operations. On the other hand, we recommend this strategy for experienced endoscopists who are available day and night and have an experienced endoscopy team with at least two additional persons at hand.

References

1. Barsoum MS, Boulus FI, ElRobby AA, Moore HWE: Tamponade and injection sclerotherapy in the management of bleeding esophageal varices. Br J Surg 69:76–78, 1982.
2. Child CG: The liver in portal hypertension. In: Major Problems in Clinical Surgery. Philadelphia, WB Saunders, 1974.
3. Conn HO, Simson JA: Excessive mortality associated with balloon tamponade of bleeding varices: A critical apraisal. JAMA 202:587–592, 1967.
4. The Copenhagen Esophageal Varices Sclerotherapy Project: Sclerotherapy after first variceal hemorrhage in cirrhosis: A randomized multicenter trial. New Engl J Med 311:1594–1600, 1984.
5. Fleig WE, Stange ET, Rüttenauer K, Ditschuneit H: Emergency endoscopic sclerotherapy for bleeding esophageal varices: A prospective study in patients not responding to balloon tamponade. Gastrointest Endosc 29:8–14, 1983.
6. Hassab MA: Gastroesophageal decongestion and splenectomy: A new method of preventing bleeding from esophageal varices. J Int Coll Surg 41:232–239, 1964.
7. Lewis JW: Survival and rebleed after acute and chronic injection sclerotherapy. In: Endoscopic Sclerotherapy of Esophageal Varices, Sivak MV Jr (ed), New York, Praeger, 1984, pp 89–97.
8. Kaplan EL, Meier P: Nonparametric estimation from incomplete observation. J Am Stat Assoc 53:457–481, 1958.
9. Korula J, Balart LA, Radvan G, Zweiban BE, Larson AW, Kao HW, Mamda S: A prospective randomized controlled trial of chronic esophageal variceal sclerotherapy. Hepatology 4:584–589, 1985.
10. McDougall BRD, Theodossi A, Westaby D, Dawson JL, Williams R: Increased long-term survival in variceal hemorrhage using injection sclerotherapy. Lancet 1:124–127, 1982.
11. Peto R, Pike MC, Armitage P, Breslow NE, Cox DR, Howard SV, Mantel N, McPherson K, Peto J, Smith PC: Design and analysis of randomized clinical trials requiring prolonged observation of each patient. Br J Cancer 35:1–40, 1977.
12. Paquet K-J, Oberhammer E: Sclerotherapy of bleeding esophageal varices by means of endoscopy. Endoscopy 10:7–12, 1978.
13. Paquet K-J, Thelen M, Koischwitz G, Biersack H-J: Ein neues therapeutisches Konzept für die Auswahl von Leberzirrhotikern mit rezidivierender Ösophagusvarizenblutung für den elektiven Shunt. Chirurg 50:313–317, 1979.

14. Paquet K-J, Feussner H: Endoscopic sclerosis and esophageal balloon tamponade in acute hemorrhage from esophagogastric varices: A prospective controlled randomized trial. Hepatology 5:580–583, 1985.
15. Paquet K-J, Koussouris P, Kalk J-Fr, Janson R, Biersack H-J: Spätergebnisse nach semiselektivem und selektivem splenorenalen und mesokavalem Shunt bei Leberzirrhotikern über einen Zeitraum von 2-16 Jahren-Zum Wert verschiedener Selektionskriterien. Acta Chir 21:252–256, 1986.
16. Paquet K-J, Kalk J-F, Koussouris P: Immediate endoscopic sclerosis of bleeding esophageal varices. Surg Endosc 2:18–23, 1988.
17. Prindiville E, Trudeau W: A comparison of immediate versus delayed endoscopic injection sclerosis of bleeding esophageal varices. Gastrointest Endosc 32:385–388, 1986.
18. Pugh RM, Dawson J, Prétroni MC, Williams R: Transection of the esophagus for bleeding esophageal varices. Br J Surg 60:646–649, 1973.
19. Sarin SK, Nanda DMR, Kummer N, Vij JC, Amand BS: Repeated endoscopy sclerotherapy for active bleeding. Ann Surg 202:708–711, 1986.
20. Smith JL, Graham DY: Variceal hemorrhage: A critival evaluation of survival analysis. Gastroenterology 82:968–973, 1982.
21. Söderlund C: Endoscopic sclerotherapy of esophageal varices: A clinical study. Acta Chir Scand (Suppl) 151:1–23, 1985.
22. Terblanche J, Bornmann PC, Kahn D, Jonker MA, Campell JAH, Weight J, Kirsch R: Failure of repeated injection sclerotherapy to improve long-term survival after esophageal variceal bleeding: A five-year prospective controlled clinical trial. Lancet 2:1328–1334, 1983.
23. Terés J, Caecilia A, Bordas JM, et al: Esophageal tamponade for bleeding varices. Gastroenterology 75:566–569, 1979.
24. Westaby D, McDougall BRD, Williams R: Improved survival following injection sclerotherapy for esophageal varices: Final analysis of a controlled trial. Hepatology 5:627–631, 1985.

42

Sugiura Operation for Recurrent Variceal Hemorrhage in Patients with Portal Vein Thrombosis After Long-Term Injection Sclerotherapy

K.-J. Paquet, M. A. Mercado, P. Koussouris,
F. Cuan-Orozco, F. Siemens

Introduction

Two basic approaches are currently used in the surgical management of bleeding esophageal varices. One is the decrease of portal pressure by diminishing resistance to the outflow of blood from the portal system, that is, porta-systemic shunting. The other is the interruption of the flow to the bleeding sites by porta-azygos disconnection, esophageal transection, ligation of varices or their combination. Porta-systemic shunt, though effective in controlling variceal hemorrhage, has an accompanying high incidence of encephalopathy, particularly in older patients. In patients with severely impaired hepatic function, the shunting procedure increases the likelihood of worsening hepatic function and causes an even higher incidence of

Little AG, Ferguson MK, Skinner DB: Diseases of the Esophagus, Vol. II: Benign Diseases. Futura Publishing Company, Inc., Mount Kisco, NY, © 1990.

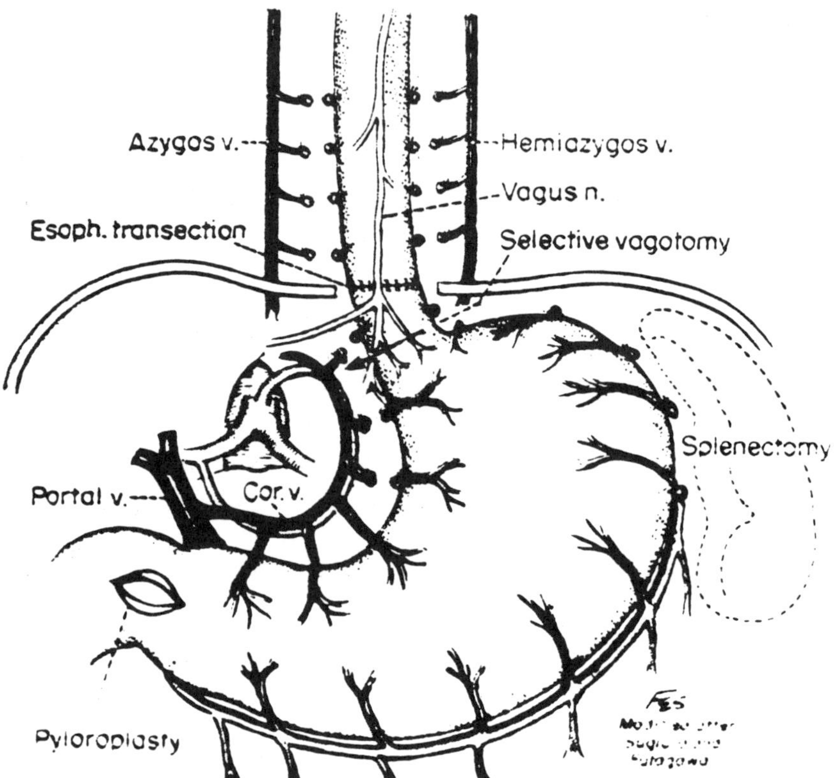

Figure 1: Esophageal transection with paraesophagogastric devascularization and splenectomy in selected cases (modified Sugiura procedure).

encephalopathy, thus leading to an appreciable increase in mortality. In addition to these complications, a shunting procedure may be technically impossible in some patients. No vein in the portal circulation may be suitable to anastomose to a systemic vein, as in patients who have had previous shunting procedures or thrombosis of major branches of the portal system or prior splenectomy. This is particularly true in patients with congenital or acquired portal vein thrombosis and no liver disease. In the majority of them, splenectomy and shunt procedures were performed during childhood, often with the late result of recurrence of hemorrhage and thrombosed shunts. However, the introduction of endoscopic injection sclerotherapy has changed the indication for shunting procedures.[11]

In 1973, Sugiura and Futagawa[13] described an operation designed to eliminate proximal gastric and esophageal varices but maintain the extraesophageal acquired porta-systemic shunts that developed in the upper abdomen and lower thorax in response to portal hypertension. The original procedure includes esophageal transection and reanastomosis, proximal gastric and distal esophageal devascularization and splenectomy (Fig. 1). Separate abdominal and thoracic approaches were utilized in one operation or in two separately staged operations. A selective vagotomy was performed, thereby necessitating a gastric drainage procedure. In 1987, Sugiura[14] described the results of 780 cases. In 687 (88%) liver cirrhosis was the underlying disease and operative mortality was 4.5%; there was no postoperative death in 44 cases (5.6%) of extrahepatic portal vein thrombosis. The frequency of rebleeding during the following 10 years in both groups was 5% and the 5-year survival rate was 60% in patients with liver cirrhosis and 95% in patients with portal vein thrombosis. Outside of Japan, the Sugiura procedure is less popular because the Japanese results have not been confirmed in Europe and the United States. Only a group in Mexico City[6] has described acceptable results in patients with liver cirrhosis applying the Sugiura procedure.

This was the reason why our group, treating regularly more than 100 patients with portal hypertension and bleeding esophageal varices per year, has limited the indication for this operation to a very small selected group with a good prognosis. These are primarily patients with congenital portal vein thrombosis not responding to long-term injection sclerotherapy and without a suitable vein for a porta-systemic shunt operation.

Methods and Materials

Operative Technique

We have modified the Sugiura operation but not the concept. The operation was usually performed in two separately staged operations with an interval from 3 to 6 months. The main trunk vagus nerves were preserved, and only a highly selective vagotomy performed, thus obviating the need for a gastric drainage procedure. If technically possible, the spleen was preserved.

Table I
Age and Cause of Portal Hypertension in 10
Consecutive Patients Treated by Long-Term
Paravariceal Sclerotherapy and Sugiura Operation

No. of Patients	Age (years)	Cause of Portal Hypertension
7	18–35 (23)	congenital portal vein thrombosis
3	35–53 (41)	acquired portal vein thrombosis (chronic pancreatitis)

Patient Selection

The indication for operation was first based on the results of long-term injection sclerotherapy. If at least four phases of endoscopic sclerotherapy—each phase included two to five sessions with 20 to 40 1-ml injections of 0.5% or 1.0% Polidocanol,[8,10,12]—had been performed and were not able to prevent recurrent variceal hemorrhage or to reduce the varices in size, patients were considered for the Sugiura operation. Furthermore, angiography had to exclude a suitable vein for a porta-systemic anastomosis.

From March 1, 1982 to March 1, 1989, 721 patients with bleeding esophageal varices were admitted to the Heinz-Kalk Hospital. Ten of them were selected using the above-mentioned criteria for a Sugiura operation. The patients' ages and causes of portal hypertension are listed in Table I. Seven patients had a congenital and three an acquired portal vein thrombosis. In three of them, no previous operation had been performed to stop variceal hemorrhage; in the remaining seven patients, one or more unsuccessful operations had been performed (Table II). Furthermore, the majority of patients had multiple episodes of variceal hemorrhage in spite of both shunt and nonshunting procedures and endoscopic sclerotherapy; the latter was performed at least in two phases in every patient and in the majority of patients four to eight times (Table III).

In seven patients, the operation was performed in two steps with 3 to 5 months' interruption; one patient was operated on in one step. In the remaining two patients, a transabdominal approach was not

Table II
Number of Operations Performed Before the Sugiura Procedure (n = 10) to Stop Variceal Hemorrhage

Number of Patients	Number of Operations
3	0
1	1
2	2
3	3
—	4
—	5
1	6 and more
10	23

necessary because a partial Sugiura procedure had been performed at another hospital (Table IV).

Early and Late Results

We assessed the early and long-term results of the modified Sugiura procedure with regard to mortality, early and late morbidity, early and late rebleeding, and encephalopathy.

Table III
Number of Esophageal Variceal Bleeding Episodes and Phases of Sclerotherapy Performed Before the Sugiura Procedure

Number of Variceal Hemorrhages	Number of Patients	Number of Phases of Endoscopic Paravariceal Sclerotherapy	Number of Patients
2	1	2	1
3	2	3	0
4	0	4	4
5	0	5	0
6–10	5	6 or more	5
11 or more	2		

Table IV
Type of Sugiura Operation

Transthroacic	Transabdominal	Combined*
2	0	8

* In seven patients the operation was performed in two steps with 3–6 months' interruption; one patient was operated on in one step.

No patient was lost to follow-up. Each patient came once every postoperative year for a short outpatient or an in-hospital control follow-up. No patient died up to July 1, 1989. We observed one severe postoperative complication: a leakage at the esophageal anastomosis, detected fluoroscopically by gastrografin swallow investigation, usually performed in every patient at the fifth postoperative day; up to this time, the patients were fed parenterally. In this case, there was no connection to the mediastinum and no signs of mediastinitis; the parenteral nutrition was continued for another 5 days; thereafter the leakage healed spontaneously (Table V). No stricture was observed and no major esophageal or gastric necrosis has occurred because of the devascularization. No early or late episodes of encephalopathy could be observed after the procedure. All patients are eating normal diets.

There have been no episodes of rebleeding from esophageal or gastric varices. The variceal grading according to our classification (Fig. 2)[9] is described in Table VI. In two patients, no varices could be seen endoscopically during follow-up; in six patients varices degree

Table V
Results of Sugiura Operations

Postoperative Complications	Mortality up to July 1, 1989	Recurrence of Hemorrhage under Regular Endoscopic Control (once per year)
one leakage without mediastinitis	0	0

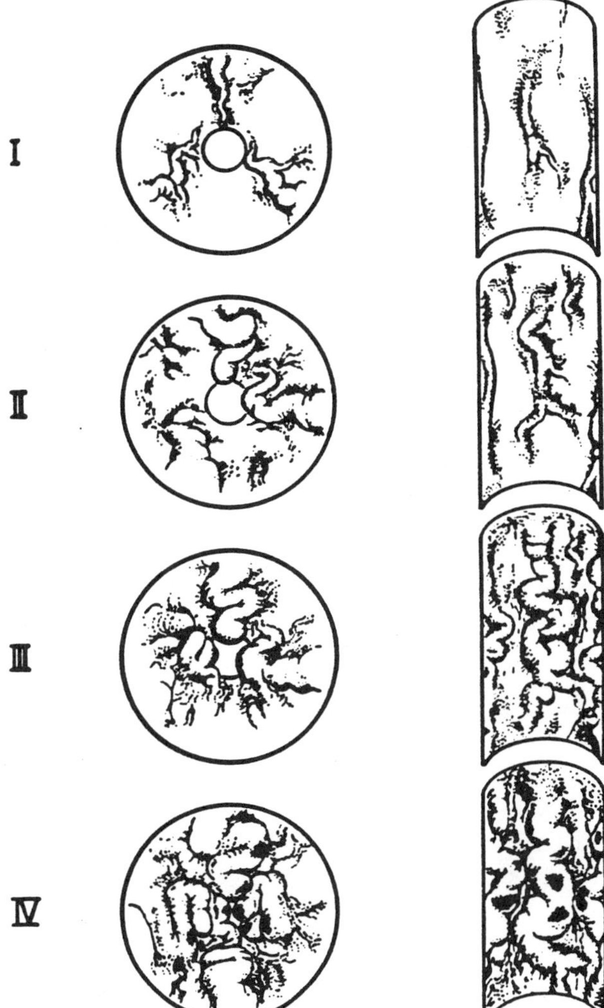

Figure 2: Classification of varices according to our group (Paquet 1978): I = Dilated vein or veniectasias, fluoroscopically negative; II = Varices detectable fluoroscopically and obstructing half of the lumen of the esophagus during endoscopy; III = Varices obstructing two-thirds of the lumen of the esophagus endoscopically and sometimes accompanied by telangiectasias (varices on a varix); and IV = Varices obstructing the total lumen of the esophagus endoscopically; in the majority, telangiectasias (varices on a varix) can be found on the top of the varices.

Table VI
Variceal Grading According to Paquet (Fig. 2) in Postoperative Endoscopic Investigations of 10 Consecutive Patients Following Long-Term Paravariceal Sclerotherapy and Sugiura Procedure

	Classification of Varices				
	0	*I*	*II*	*III*	*IV*
Number of patients	2	6	2	0	0

I and in two patients varices degree II developed during the late follow-up period.

Gastroesophageal Reflux

Gastroesophageal reflux was investigated in all patients 12 months postoperatively by endoscopy, manometry, and pH-metry. Figure 3 demonstrates the lower esophageal sphincter pressure (LES) in normal patients (a), in patients with liver cirrhosis and portal hypertension (b), in patients with portal hypertension and prehepatic block, bleeding from esophagal varices and managed by paravariceal endoscopic sclerotherapy (c), and in patients with prehepatic block, treated by long-term endoscopic sclerotherapy and Sugiura procedure (d). No significant differences could be detected.

Thus, manometrically and endoscopically in no patient was an incompetent LES or reflux esophagitis seen. By pH-metry in all patients the total reflux time in 24 hours was normal (Table VII).

Discussion

The surgical treatment of portal hypertension complicated by bleeding esophageal varices may be classified in two major categories: porta-systemic shunting operations and nonshunting procedures. If the cause of portal hypertension is extrahepatic portal obstruction, treatment is often unsatisfactory. A portal systemic anastomosis, usually splenorenal, is the operation of choice to decompress the portal trunk, but is only successful if a stoma more than 10 mm in diameter can be constructed and if splenectomy has not been performed before.

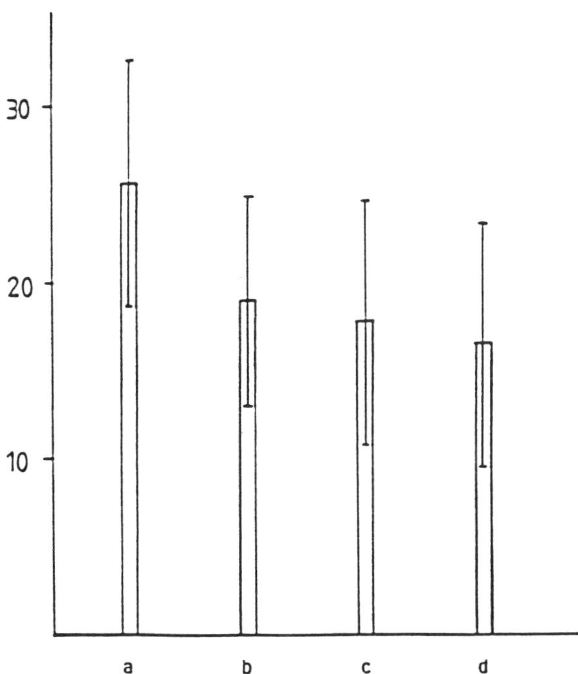

Figure 3: LES pressure in normal patients (a), patients with liver cirrhosis and portal hypertension without endoscopic treatment (b), patients with prehepatic block and portal hypertension after long-term endoscopic and paravariceal sclerotherapy (2–10 phases) (c), and after long-term endoscopic paravariceal sclerotherapy and modified Sugiura operation I + II (I + II: n = 8, II: n = 2) (d). No significant reduction in sphincter pressure could be demonstrated from b to c and d.

The thrombosis rate is 36% overall in children and 16.5% in adults.[11] The results with mesocaval or cavomesenteric anastomosis are not more satisfactory. Frequently no suitable vein of the portal system is available for anastomosis, or an anastomosis may subsequently thrombose. Such patients present a major surgical challenge when they continue to have repeated hemorrhages. Recently there has been a surge of interest in endoscopic sclerotherapy; however, these techniques are frequently complicated by esophageal ulcer, stricture, the

Table VII
Total Reflux Time (pH <4) and Frequency of Reflux Episodes in 10 Consecutive Patients Following Long-Term Paravariceal Sclerotherapy in 10 Consecutive Patients

	Number	*Total Reflux Time*	*Frequency of Reflux*
Group I	7	26 s/24 hr 6 s	5 peaks/24 hr
Group II	1	61 s/24 hr 12 s	9 peaks/24 hr
Group III	1	116 s/24 hr 16 s	13 peaks/24 hr
Group IV	1	167 s/24 hr 19 s	18 peaks/24 hr

need for recurrent injections, and are accompanied by recurrence of hemorrhage despite regular resclerosis, and make further operative intervention in this area extremely complicated.[1,4,15]

Because of dissatisfaction with the shunt procedures currently in vogue for preventing rebleeding from esophagogastric varices, we began a noncontrolled trial of a modified Sugiura procedure in a limited group of patients, seven with congenital and three with acquired portal vein thrombosis, in whom a shunt operation was either not possible because of the lack of suitable veins or had been previously performed without lasting success. This technique has the unique advantages of preserving porta-systemic shunts, including those in the periesophageal plexus. It has other advantages as well. Sugiura and Futagawa[13,14] reported an extremely low (about 5%) operative mortality in patients with liver cirrhosis and no mortality in patients with extrahepatic portal obstruction and virtually no rebleeding following elective procedures. No groups have reported any instance of postoperative encephalopathy.[4–7,16] Last but not least, our selected group had been treated with many phases of endoscopic sclerotherapy without being able to prevent recurrence of hemorrhage on a long-term basis. As mentioned above,[1,4,15] further operative intervention in the sclerosed area can be extremely complicated, if not impossible.

This is the first group of patients in whom a modified Sugiura operation was performed after long-term injection sclerotherapy with a very low morbidity (one fluoroscopically detected leak without clinical signs) and neither early nor long-term mortality. Finally, during a follow-up time up to 7 years, no recurrence of hemorrhage was observed.

Thus, the modified Sugiura procedure in recurrent variceal hemorrhage of patients with portal vein thrombosis after long-term injection sclerotherapy has proven to be very successful and is fully justified.

Conclusion

Among the nonshunt operations, the Sugiura operation guarantees the best early and long-term results in treating recurrent variceal hemorrhage in patients with portal hypertension. This includes an operative mortality and a frequency of rebleeding during the following 10 years under 5% and a 5-year survival in patients with portal vein thrombosis of 95% and in patients with liver cirrhosis of 60%. Unfortunately, this operation has only gained popularity in Japan, where Sugiura and his group have performed more than 750 operations. There are few promoters of this type of operation in Europe and in the United States. Furthermore Sugiura recommends performing this operation only in patients without prior sclerotherapy. Since 1982, our group has gained experience with this modified type of operation in 10 patients with portal vein thrombosis who had received at least four phases of endoscopic injection sclerotherapy and rebled.

Additionally, with three exceptions, all patients had been operated on at least two (up to seven) times before without permanent success. Seven men and three women with a mediam age of 32 (18–53 years) were operated on electively. There was no postoperative death. In one case, on the fifth postoperative day a leak with a blind fistula was detected which healed spontaneously. All patients were followed up to July 1, 1989 and are living. There were no instances of recurrent bleeding. Thus, the Sugiura procedure can be performed without great technical difficulty in patients who have received more than one phase of endoscopic sclerotherapy. It seems to be the operation of choice in patients with prehepatic block, in whom a shunt operation is not possible, and in whom endoscopic long-term injection sclerotherapy has not been successful.

References

1. Ayers SJ, Goff JS, Warren GH: Endoscopic sclerotherapy for bleeding esophageal varices: Effects and complications. Ann Int Med 98:900–903, 1983.
2. DeMeester TR, Wang C-I, Wernly JA, et al: Technique, indications and

clinical use of 24-hour esophagal pH-monitoring. J Thorac Cardiovasc Surg 79:656–670, 1980.

3. Ginsberg RJ, Waters PF, Zeldin RA, Spratt EH, Shandling W, Stone RM, Strasberg S: A modified Sugiura procedure. Ann Thorac Surg 34:258–264, 1982.

4. McDougall BRD, Theodossi A, Westaby D, Dawson JL, Williams R: Increased long-term survival in variceal hemorrhage using injection sclerotherapy. Lancet 1:124–127, 1982.

5. Matory WE, Sedgwick CE, Rossi RL: Nonshunting procedures in management of bleeding esophageal varices. Surg Clin North Am 60:281–95, 1980.

6. Orozco H, Guevara L, Mercado MA: Comparative study of the distal splenorenal shunt (Warren) vs Sugiura procedure in the treatment of the hemorrhagic portal hypertension syndromes (abstr). Dig Dis Sci 39:535, 1986.

7. Peracchia A, Ancona E, Battaglia G: A new technique for the treatment of esophageal bleeding in portal hypertension. Int Surg 65:401–404, 1980.

8. Paquet K-J, Oberhammer E: Sclerotherapy of bleeding esophageal varices by means of endoscopy. Endoscopy 10:7, 1978.

9. Paquet K-J: Prophylactic endoscopic sclerosing treatment of the esophageal varices: A prospective controlled randomized trial. Endoscopy 14:4, 1982.

10. Paquet K-J: Endoscopic paravariceal injection sclerotherapy of the esophagus—indications, technique, complications: Results of a period of 14 years. Gastrointest Endoscopy 29:310–315, 1983.

11. Paquet K-J: Ten years experience with paravariceal injection sclerotherapy of esophageal varices in children. J Pediatr Surg 20:109–112, 1985.

12. Paquet K-J: Indication and early and long-term results of paravariceal immediate, elective and prophylactic injection sclerotherapy. In: Treatment of Esophageal Varices, Idezuki Y (ed), Amsterdam/New York/Oxford, Excerpta Medica, 1988 (p 1–22).

13. Sugiura M, Futagawa S: A technique for treating esophageal varices. J Thorac Cardiovasc Surg 66:677–685, 1973.

14. Sugiura M, Watanabe I: Stellenwert der Sugiura operation zur Verhütung von rezidivierenden Ösophagusvarizenblutungen bei Leberzirrhotikern: Indikation und Langzeitresultate. Chir Gastroenterol 3:77–88, 1987.

15. Terblanche J, Yakoob HI, Bornman PC, Stiegmann EV, Barne R, Jonker M, Wright J, Kirsch R: Acute bleeding varices: A five-year prospective evaluation of tamponade and sclerotherapy. Ann Surg 194:521–530, 1981.

16. Weese JL, Starling JR, Yale CE: Control of bleeding esophageal varices by transabdominal esophageal transection, gastric devascularization, and splenectomy. Surg Gastroenterol 3:31–36, 1984.

VIII.

Operative Treatment of Complex Benign Disease:
Editors' Overview

After emphasizing that the operations discussed are only for very selected and complex patients, the two chapters in this section describe alternative operations for patients requiring esophagectomy and/or partial gastrectomy for complex, benign esophageal disease. The operation described in Chapter 43 combines antrectomy and a Roux-en-Y gastrojejunostomy for complete diversion of duodenal contents and maximum suppression of acid production. This is a major operation but it is clearly demonstrated to be an effective one for selected patients. Chapter 44 reports experience with esophagectomy and colon interposition and, although it must be read to appreciate fully the author's contentions, their conclusion is that although the operation can be done with acceptable morbidity and short segments of colon provide very good long-term functional results, construction of a long segment colon interposition does not seem to be better, either functionally or clinically, than gastric interposition.

43

Acid Suppression and Alkaline Diversion:
A Safe and Effective Operation for Patients with Complex Benign Esophageal Disease Requiring Reoperation

F. Henry Ellis, Jr., S. Peter Gibb

Introduction

The proper operative approach for the patient with complex benign esophageal disease is controversial. A number of alternatives have been proposed, including resection with jejunal interposition[1] or colon interposition[2] and transhiatal esophagogastrectomy.[3] In a recent review of our surgical experience with the management of these difficult cases,[4] the results after the acid-suppression alkaline-diversion procedure far surpassed those of other techniques. This chapter reviews this operation in more detail, emphasizing its origins, its results as reported in the literature, and our own clinical experience.

Origin and Reported Results

More than 30 years ago, dissatisfaction with the available methods of surgical management of the complications of reflux esophagitis

Little AG, Ferguson MK, Skinner DB: Diseases of the Esophagus, Vol. II: Benign Diseases. Futura Publishing Company, Inc., Mount Kisco, NY, © 1990.

Table I
Acid-Suppression and Alkaline-Diversion Results of Operation

Author/Ref.	Year	Patients	Resection	Result (%)	
				Improved	Poor
Wells & Johnson[11]	1955	12	0	100	0
Holt & Large[12]	1961	11			
Weaver et al.[13*]	1970	10	6	100	0
Payne[10]	1970	15	6	73	27
Roysten et al.[14]	1975	8	0	88	12
Herrington & Mody[15]	1976	6	0	100	0
Payne[16]	1984	13	3	85	15
Matikainen[17]	1984	6	0	83	17
deMiguel[18]	1985	7	0	100	0
Washer et al.[19]	1986	57	0	86	14
Present study	1989	23	18	86	14
Total		157	33	90	10

* Late follow-up of cases originally reported by Holt and Large.[12]

led the senior author to seek a solution in the experimental laboratory. An operation was devised consisting of cardiectomy, bilateral vagotomy, and antrectomy with restoration of gastrointestinal continuity by gastroduodenostomy and esophagogastrostomy.[5] The technique of the operation as applied to man was described in some detail in a later publication,[6] and its early results in nine patients were favorably reported the same year.[7] Further favorable experience with its clinical use was reported 2 years later.[8] However, longer follow-up revealed the need to divert the alkaline secretions by employing a Roux-en-Y gastrojejunostomy instead of a gastroduodenostomy.[4,9,10]

A number of reports have discussed the clinical application of these principles to the patient with complications of reflux esophagitis (Table I). Wells and Johnston[11] were the first to report the clinical results of vagotomy, gastrectomy, and Roux-en-Y gastrojejunostomy without esophageal resection. Twelve patients with hiatus hernia and reflux esophagitis treated this way experienced good results although the follow-up was short. Holt and Large[12] were the first in the United States to employ the approach and reported its use in 11 patients in 1961. A report on 10 of these patients,[13] six of whom required resection of the strictured area, 8 to 12 years after operation described successful results in all patients. Subsequently, there have been other similar reports,[14–19] usually on small numbers of patients, most of whom did not require resection. The largest experience with the acid-suppression alkaline-diversion procedure is that of Washer and associates,[19] who reported an 86% success rate after a median follow-up of 6 years in 57 patients, none of whom required cardiectomy.

Operative Technique

The surgical approach for the acid-suppression alkaline-diversion procedure depends on whether resection of the distal esophagus and cardia is required because of an "undilatable" stricture or severe ulcerative esophagitis with hemorrhage. When a localized resection of the involved area (cardiectomy) must be performed, a thoracic approach is required (Fig. 1). A left posterolateral thoracotomy entering the chest through the bed of the nonresected seventh or eighth rib is the preferred approach (Fig. 1A).

After the mediastinal pleura is opened and the distal esophagus is mobilized, the hiatal attachments are divided so as to permit freeing of the proximal stomach by division of some of the short gastric and posterior gastric vessels (Fig. 1B). Use of a stapling device applied to the stomach just distal to the cardia permits division of the gastrointestinal tract at an appropriate level. Continuity is restored after resecting the esophagus proximal to the diseased area by advancing part of the gastric greater curvature after freeing its vascular connections and performing an end-to-side esophagogastrostomy (Fig. 1C). An open anastomosis with an inner layer of running catgut and an outer layer of interrupted silk sutures is preferred. A nasogastric tube is passed transnasally across the anastomosis into the intrathoracic stomach for decompression.

Although the thoracic incision may be extended as a thoracoabdominal incision permitting performance of the intra-abdominal portion of the procedure without repositioning the patient, we currently prefer a separate abdominal incision in order to avoid some of the potential complications of transecting the costal arch as well as to avoid the necessity of partial denervation of the diaphragm by such an approach. Accordingly, the thoracotomy is closed with intercostal drainage in the usual fashion, and the patient is repositioned in a supine position for an upper midline incision to provide adequate exposure of the upper abdomen (Fig. 2A). When cardiectomy is not

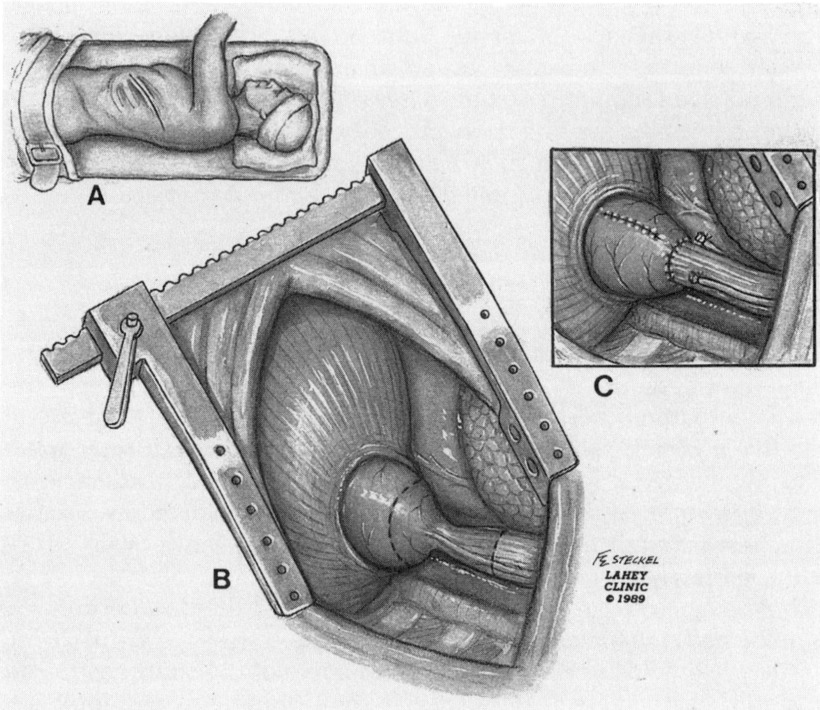

Figure 1: Operative technique of cardiectomy. (A) Location of incision. (B) Operative exposure indicating area to be resected. (C) Completed anastomosis. (Used with permission of Lahey Clinic.)

needed, the entire operative procedure is performed through an upper midline incision.

Exposure of the upper stomach and hiatus is provided by mobilization of the left lobe of the liver (Fig. 2B). If a cardiectomy has not been performed, both vagus nerves are isolated and divided, and the operation continues as an antrectomy with partial division of the stomach beginning at the greater curvature and extending cephalad. A stapler is used on the lesser curvature to provide a small gastric opening for the anastomosis. The stapled lesser curvature portion of the stomach is oversewn with interrupted silk sutures, and the antrectomy is completed by ligation of the right gastroepiploic and right gastric arteries. The duodenum is closed with a stapler and oversewn with interrupted silk sutures. It is important that the left gastric artery remain intact as this artery will constitute the major gastric blood

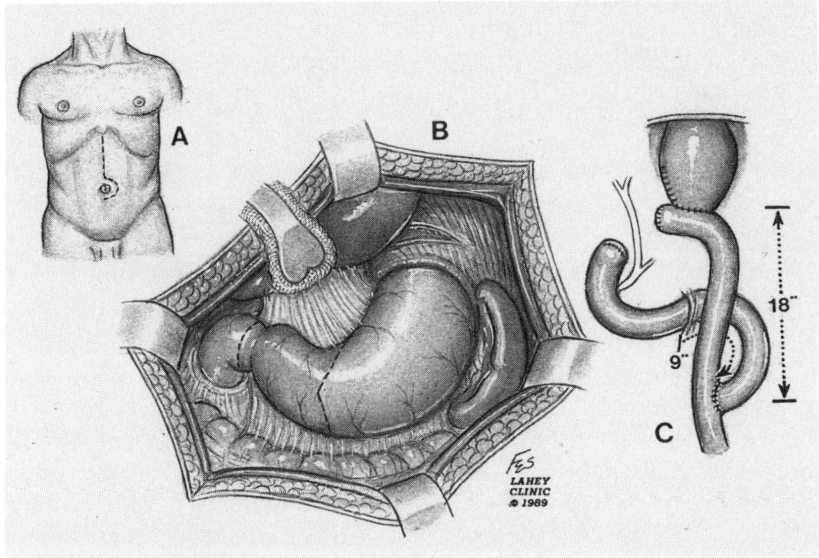

Figure 2: Operative technique of antrectomy and Roux-en-Y gastrojejunostomy. (A) Location of incision. (B) Operative exposure indicating area to be resected. (C) Completed anastomosis. (Used with permission of Lahey Clinic.)

supply when the fundus has been mobilized by division of the short gastric vessels when cardiectomy is required.

The colon is then elevated, the ligament of Treitz identified, and a point on the jejunum 9 inches from the ligament selected for division of the jejunum using the GIA stapler (US Surgical Corp., Norwalk, CT). A retrocolic gastrojejunostomy is then performed to the distal divided jejunum in an end-to-side fashion, the previously stapled jejunal end being oversewn with interrupted silk sutures (Fig. 2C). The gastrojejunostomy is performed using a running inner layer of catgut and an outer layer of interrupted silk sutures. The proximal divided jejunum is then implanted in a side-to-side fashion, after closing its stapled end with interrupted silk sutures, to the jejunum at a point 18 inches beyond the gastrojejunostomy using an anastomotic technique similar to that described for the gastrojejunostomy (Fig. 2C). The area is peritonealized to prevent development of an internal hernia, and the abdomen is closed in the usual fashion after placement of Penrose drains through a separate stab wound to the duodenal stump.

The anastomotic integrity of the esophagogastrostomy is determined radiographically 4 to 5 days postoperatively, and oral feedings are gradually resumed. Hospital discharge is anticipated 7 to 10 days after operation.

Clinical Experience

Patients

From January 1970 until July 1989, 23 patients underwent the acid-suppression alkaline-diversion procedure as described. Eighteen of these patients required a limited esophagogastrectomy and esophagogastrostomy. Two patients with stricture underwent cardioplasty to relieve the obstruction, whereas for three other patients, no operative procedure on the cardia was required. The procedure was performed in two stages in only four patients; two other patients had previously undergone resection of the cardia elsewhere, one on two occasions; and another patient had previously required a subtotal gastrectomy with Roux-en-Y gastrojejunostomy.

The patients' ages ranged from 26 to 75 years, with a median of 60 years. Eleven patients were men and 12 were women. Pertinent associated disorders were achalasia in 13 patients and scleroderma in two patients, one of whom also had Barrett's esophagus. There was one case each of gastric ulcer and esophageal ulcer. The indication for a reconstructive esophageal operation was severe gastroesophageal reflux disease (GERD) in all patients; 20 patients also had a stricture.

Twenty-one of these patients had undergone a total of 40 previous operative procedures on the distal esophagus and stomach (Table II). Only two patients had not undergone previous surgery, and they had scleroderma with "undilatable" strictures at the esophagogastric junction. Fundoplication was the most common procedure, usually of the Nissen variety. Esophagomyotomy was the next most common previous operation, usually of the modified Heller type. Two patients had a long myotomy for suspected but unproved diffuse esophageal spasm.

Results

No hospital deaths were recorded. The three postoperative complications (13%) included respiratory complications as a result of re-

Table II
Acid-Suppression and Alkaline-Diversion
Previous Operations

Operation	No. of Patients
Fundoplication	16
Nissen	7
Collis-Nissen	3
Belsey	2
Collis-Belsey	1
Hill	1
Thal-Nissen	1
Angelchik	1
Esophagomyotomy	14
Esophageal exploration and/or repair	4
Cardiectomy	3
Miscellaneous	3
Total	40

tained secretions in one patient, development of a duodenal stump leak in another patient, and an empyema requiring open drainage in a third patient.

Clinical evaluation after hospital discharge was available in all patients but was too early after operation to be meaningful in two patients. Results were classified as excellent if the patient was virtually asymptomatic, good if there were occasional symptoms, and fair if symptoms persisted but were less intense than before operation. If the patient's condition remained unchanged or was worsened by operation, the results were classified as poor. The follow-up interval ranged from 6 months to $16\frac{1}{4}$ years, with a median of $3\frac{3}{4}$ years. Eighteen (86%) of the patients were considered to have improved (Table III). Of the three patients classified as having poor results, two had recurrent dysphagia, and the third had troublesome nausea and vomiting with inability to maintain normal weight. Dumping, diarrhea, and nocturnal aspiration were not seen in any of our patients.

Comment

In a review of patients requiring esophageal reconstruction for complex benign esophageal disease,[4] severe GERD and esophageal

Table III
Acid-Suppression and Alkaline-Diversion
Results of Operation*

Result	No. of Patients	%
Improved	18	86
Excellent	6	
Good	8	
Fair	4	
Poor	3	14
Total	21	100

* Follow-up of ½ to 16¼ years (median, 3¾ years).

perforation were the major indications. Based on that study, we now restrict the use of colon interposition to patients with esophageal perforation and mediastinitis who require esophageal defunctioning and subsequent reconstruction. Colon interposition is also used for some patients with carcinoma of the esophagus. However, we have encountered some anastomotic problems with this technique, and others[2] have reported a high incidence of graft necrosis, aspects of the technique that have dampened our enthusiasm for its use in patients with GERD.

All of the patients who underwent the acid-suppression alkaline-diversion procedure had severe GERD as the indication for operation, 20 of whom had an esophageal stricture. This operation is suitable for such patients after failure of previous operative procedures regardless of the cause of reflux, whether associated with operative procedures on the cardia, scleroderma, or a sliding diaphragmatic hiatus hernia. Many of the patients being reported on also had esophageal achalasia, and although resection of normal stomach and retention of proximal diseased esophagus may offend the sensibilities of some surgeons, the excellence of the result speaks for itself. Although total esophagectomy by the transhiatal route with cervical esophagogastrostomy is a satisfactory alternative surgical approach, we believe our approach is simpler and subject to fewer complications.

Our success with the operation as described in these extraordinarily difficult reoperative cases has encouraged us to continue its use and to employ it earlier in the course of the disease than heretofore. We now recommend its use after one or at most two previous conservative operations for the complications of GERD. It should be used only rarely as a primary operation, as was true for two patients with sclerodermatous strictures in this series.

Summary

From January 1970 to July 1989, 23 patients with severe GERD who had undergone 40 previous conservative operations had reconstruction using the acid-suppression alkaline-diversion procedure. Eighteen of these patients also required cardiectomy and two required cardioplasty. There were no hospital deaths and three (13%) postoperative complications. Eighteen (86%) of the 21 patients available for follow-up were improved over a median follow-up of 3¾ years. We currently prefer this reconstructive procedure to other available procedures for complex benign esophageal disease requiring reoperation.

References

1. Wright C, Cuschieri A: Jejunal interposition for benign esophageal disease. Technical considerations and long-term results. Ann Surg 205:54, 1987.
2. DeMeester TR, Johansson KE, Franze I, et al: Indications, surgical technique, and long-term functional results of colon interposition or bypass. Ann Surg 208:460, 1988.
3. Orringer MB, Stirling MC: Cervical esophagogastric anastomosis for benign disease: Functional results. J Thorac Cardiovasc Surg 96:887, 1988.
4. Ellis FH Jr, Gibb SP: Esophageal reconstruction for complex benign esophageal disease. J Thorac Cardiovasc Surg (in press).
5. Ellis FH Jr: Experimental aspects of surgical treatment of reflux esophagitis and esophageal stricture. Ann Surg 143:465, 1956.
6. Ellis FH Jr: Physiologic operation for ulceration and stricture of terminal esophagus. Mayo Clin Proc 31:615, 1956.
7. Ellis FH Jr, Andersen HA, Clagett OT: Surgical management of complications of reflux esophagitis. Arch Surg 73:578, 1956.
8. Ellis FH Jr, Andersen HA, Clagett OT: Treatment of short esophagus with stricture by esophagogastrectomy and antral excision. Ann Surg 148:526, 1958.
9. Payne WS, Andersen HA, Ellis FH Jr: Reappraisal of esophagogastrectomy and antral excision in the treatment of short esophagus. Surgery 55:344, 1964.
10. Payne WS: Surgical treatment of reflux esophagitis and stricture associ-

ated with permanent incompetence of the cardia. Mayo Clin Proc 45:553, 1970.

11. Wells C, Johnston JH: Hiatus hernia: Surgical relief of reflux esophagitis. Lancet 1:937, 1955.
12. Holt CJ, Large AM: Surgical management of reflux esophagitis. Ann Surg 153:555, 1961.
13. Weaver AW, Large AM, Walt AJ: Surgical management of severe reflux esophagitis: Eight to seventeen year follow-up study. Am J Surg 119:15, 1970.
14. Roysten CMS, Dowling BL, Spencer J: Antrectomy with Roux-en-Y anastomosis in the treatment of peptic esophagitis with stricture. Br J Surg 62:605, 1975.
15. Herrington JL Jr, Mody B: Total duodenal diversion for treatment of reflux esophagitis uncontrolled by repeated antireflux procedures. Ann Surg 183:636, 1976.
16. Payne WS: Surgical management of reflux-induced oesophageal stenoses: Results in 101 patients. Br J Surg 71:971, 1984.
17. Matikainen M: Antrectomy: Roux-en-Y reconstruction and vagotomy for recurrent reflux oesophagitis. Acta Chir Scand 150:643, 1984.
18. deMiguel J: Tratamiento de ciertas estrecheces pépticas del esófago mediante vagotomía, gastrectomía parcial y anastomosis gastroyeyunal en "Y" de Roux. Rev Esp Enferm Apar Dig 67:511, 1985. (Eng abst)
19. Washer GF, Gear MW, Dowling BL, et al: Duodenal diversion with vagotomy and antrectomy for severe or recurrent reflux oesophagitis and stricture: An alternative to operation at the hiatus. Ann R Coll Surg Engl 68:222, 1986.

44

Colon Interposition for Esophageal Disease: A Good Procedure for Selected Patients?

Brice Gayet, O. Farges, G. Etienne, Françoise Fékété

Introduction

After esophagectomy or esophageal bypass, the choice of organ for esophageal substitution is still debated.[1-6] None of the several techniques proposed has given satisfactory morbidity and mortality rates even despite having been reduced during the last years.[7,8] The stomach has a high rate of immediate complications such as postoperative aspiration pneumonia or fistula. The two main reasons for using colonic interposition are an unpredictable capacity of the stomach to raise the neck in Western countries[9,10] and a disadvantage in gastric long-term results compared to the colon.[1-3] However, construction of a long-segment colon substitution can be difficult and any technical error can have disastrous consequences for its viability.[2,11] Some publications on long-term function of a colon graft report less than satisfactory results.[12-14] The present report analyzes our experience in colonic interposition with special evaluation of clinical long-term results.

Little AG, Ferguson MK, Skinner DB: Diseases of the Esophagus, Vol. II: Benign Diseases. Futura Publishing Company, Inc., Mount Kisco, NY, © 1990.

Table I
Indication for Surgery in 81 Patients
Undergoing Colon Interposition

Indication	Number of Patients
Malignant disease	
Esophagus or cardia	34
Mediastinum	1
Total	35
Benign disease	
Caustic injury	32
Peptic stricture	8
Traumatic injury	4
Benign tumor	1*
Vesicular epidermolysis	1
Total	46

* Patient undergoing two colon interpositions.

Patients

Chart analysis of 81 consecutive patients undergoing 82 colon interpositions at the Beaujon Department of Surgery between 1979 and 1988 was undertaken. During the same period of time, 751 other patients had esophageal disease treated by another type of esophagoplasty, including gastroplasty (502 patients) and jejunoplasty (167 patients).

The mean age ± SD of the patients was 45.3 ± 14 years (range, 7–70); 64 were men and 17 were women. The underlying diseases warranting operation are summarized in Table I. Thirty five patients had malignant disease(s) involving the esophagus and 46 patients had a variety of benign diseases of which caustic injury was the predominant cause. The colon was chosen as the esophageal substitute for a number of reasons. (1) Most patients underwent prior to or at the time of coloplasty a surgical procedure on the stomach precluding its use as an esophageal substitute. These were mainly gastrectomies (34 patients) but also gastroenterostomies or gastrostomies, in particular as part of esophageal exclusion procedure or as a nutritional support in patients with caustic injuries. Another reason for not using the stomach was the presence of an associated disease such as Menetrier disease or gastric caustic burn. (2) The second main reason was the use of the graft to bypass the esophagus as part of a two-stage resection procedure when resection of the esophagus was anticipated to be associated per se with a high risk as was the case in 10 patients with late strictures from caustic injury, in five patients with malignant tumors that were either large, complicated, or developed on Barrett's esophagus, and in one patient with a post-traumatic esophageal fistula. (3) Five patients with unresectable esophageal carcinomas and one patient with a mediastinal carcinosis from bronchial neoplasia were selected for a palliative bypass. These patients were young, aphagic, or insertion of an endoprosthesis had failed or could not be performed. (4) The colon was chosen as the substitute of choice in eight patients with gastroesophageal reflux (Belsey procedure) (seven with acquired short esophagus, one with suspicion of associated carcinoma) and in three patients aged less than 35 years with caustic injuries of the esophagus in an attempt to preserve the gastric reservoir.

Current follow-up was obtained by mailed questionnaires and telephone interviews when recent (within 6 months) information was not available in the patient record. The long-term result in patients with a malignancy was classified as good if they were able to resume oral eating without significant dysphagia or reflux and was classified as poor in the other patients. In the latter, it proved sometimes difficult to differentiate between symptoms related to a dysfunction of the plasty itself or to the persistence or recurrence of the tumor, the investigations being limited for ethical reasons. Therefore, unless obviously related to end-stage malignancy, these symptoms were included irrespective of their mechanism. Two patients were lost to follow-up.

In patients operated on for a benign disease, the criteria for dysfunction included dysphagia precluding the ability to eat a normal meal, frequent episodes of reflux, poor progression of the bolus in the plasty or its mechanical obstruction, or persistent weight loss in the postoperative period. These patients were evaluated by upper gastrointestinal barium study, endoscopy with biopsies, and in recent years manometry or pH monitoring. Patients experiencing persistent dysphagia were either reoperated (anastomotic plasty) or treated by endoscopic dilatation. Three patients were lost for follow-up 6–12 months after the operation. During the same interval, two patients died from associated neoplasia or intestinal obstruction. Mean follow-up in the others was 5.1 years.

Table II
Main Pre- Peri-, and Postoperative Features in Six Patients Dying After Esophageal Colosplasty

Patient	Sex	Age (years)	Indication for Surgery	Type of Surgery	Cause of Death
1	M	57	aphagia from carcinoma	retrosternal bypass	pneumopathy, previous pneumonectomy
2	M	49	aphagia from carcinoma	retrosternal bypass	pneumopathy, hemomediastinum (erosion of vessel by tumor)
3	M	70	aphagia from carcinoma	retrosternal bypass	pneumopathy, malignant tracheoesophageal fistula
4*	M	62	aphagia from carcinoma	retrosternal bypass	pneumopathy, malignant tracheoesophageal fistula
5	M	56	carcinoma	esophagogastrectomy	liver failure (hepatic artery thrombosis)
6	M	51	carcinoma	esophagogastrectomy	pulmonary embolism (clotting of central catheter)

* Patient 4 died 2 weeks after discharge from hospital.

Methods

Most of these operations were performed during the past 7 years. The coloplasty was performed according to a standard procedure. Briefly, the left, right, and transverse colon were mobilized. The vessels of the transverse colon including the ascending branch of the left colic artery, the middle colic artery when present, and the right superior colic artery were dissected free as close as possible to the superior and inferior mesenteric arteries respectively. The diameter of these arteries and their connections were determined. They were thereafter successively clamped to assess on which would be based the vascularization of the transverse colon used as the esophageal substitute. In 67 procedures, the superior branch of the left colonic artery provided sufficient blood supply and the veins provided sufficient blood drainage to use the transverse colon as an isoperistaltic graft. In 12 patients, however, these vessels, especially the veins, were too small (two patients), absent (two patients), or although large provided insufficient blood supply (eight patients); in these patients the transverse colon was used as an antiperistaltic graft based on the middle colic artery and (or) the right superior colic artery. In the remaining three patients, the transverse colon could not be used because of previous transverse coloplasty (two patients) or perioperative ischemia of a transverse coloplasty (one patient); hence, an isoperistaltic ileocolic graft was constructed.

The colon segment was passed through a retrosternal tunnel in 55 patients and was placed in the mediastinum in 27 patients. The esophagocolic anastomosis was created under the aortic arch in 10 patients, above the aortic arch in five patients, and at the cervical level in 67 patients. It was either sewn using interrupted resorbable sutures (38 patients) or completed with an EEA (19 patients), or ILS stapler (35 patients). An upper digestive tract follow-through radiological examination with water-soluble contrast was routinely performed on the seventh postoperative day. If normal, nasogastric suction was discontinued and the patient allowed progressive realimentation. Clinical fistulas were classified as severe if they warranted reoperation or transcutaneous drainage for the thoracic ones and as benign in the other patients.

Results

Early Postoperative Mortality

In-hospital mortality was nil in patients with benign esophageal disease as compared to 14.3% (5/35) in patients with esophageal malignancies (p < 0.01). Moreover, one other patient with an esophageal malignancy died 2 weeks after discharge from the hospital. Indication for surgery, type of surgery, and main cause of death in these six patients are summarized in Table II. Four patients had undergone a palliative procedure; death in these patients was primarily related to a complication from the unresected tumor. Two patients had undergone a curative resection; death in these patients was related to iatrogenic complications (extensive dissection of the hepatic artery, prolonged parenteral nutrition). The esophageal substitute per se was in no patient the main cause of death.

Table III
Major Postoperative Complication as a Function of Underlying Esophageal Disease

Complications	Benign Esophageal Disease (46 pts.)	Esophageal Carcinoma (29 pts. surviving over 2 months)
Complications of the graft requiring reoperation	4	1
Upper anastomotic leak	2	0
Mechanical perforation[a]	2	0
Graft necrosis	0	1
Other complications requiring reoperation[b]	1	3
Pulmonary complications[c]	3	11
Bilateral recurrent nerve injury	0	2

[a] one acute distension of the plasty resulting in rupture of upper anastomosis, one erosion of the plasty by a drain.
[b] evisceration, subphrenic abscess, postoperative bleeding, leak of the ileocolic anastomosis: one each.
[c] are included pneumonia and severe hypoxia.
pts = patients.

Postoperative Complications

Twenty two other patients developed 25 major complications in the postoperative period. These complications are listed in Table III as a function of the underlying esophageal disease. The incidence of major postoperative complications was higher in patients operated for malignant esophageal tumor (14/29, 48.3%) than in patients operated for benign esophageal disease (8/46, 17.4%) (p < 0.01).

Pulmonary complications, mainly pneumonia, were the predominant complications that developed in 40% of the patients with neoplasia. A clinical anastomotic leak of the esophageal anastomosis developed in 15 patients, related in one to an acute distension and in another to graft necrosis. Four of these were severe, requiring reoperation, seven resulted in sepsis of the cervical wound, and four were cutaneous fistulas without significant clinical consequences. The development of a fistula was not associated to the etiology of the esophageal disease (benign: 9/47, 19%; malignant: 6/35, 17%), the time of operation during the past 7 years, or to the site of the upper anastomosis (cervical: 12/66, 18.2%; other: 3/15, 20%), but was significantly influenced by the type of anastomosis (manual: 13/38, 34%; mechanical: 2/44, 4.5%; $p < 0.05$). Four other patients had a small blind radiological fistula without any clinical manifestation. One patient had a mechanical ulceration of the plasty by a drain that resulted in its rupture. Two other patients (benign disease, 1; malignant disease, 1) developed small bowel obstruction from postoperative adhesions, one of whom died.

Length and Quality of Survival in Patients with Malignant Disease

Five patients experienced persistent dysphagia. Three patients had stenosis of the upper anastomosis and underwent repeated endoscopic dilatation. Two patients with retrosternal coloplasty had long stenosis of the graft related to extrinsic compression in one and chronic ischemia in the other. One patient had major gastrocolic reflux which required a total duodenal diversion.

Functional Results in Patients with Benign Disease

The functional result of the coloplasty after discharge from the hospital was unsatisfactory in 20 patients. Dysphagia was the predominant complaint, related in most patients to stenosis of the esophagocolic anastomosis. These patients had experienced an anastomotic leakage postoperatively (five patients) and/or had had their anastomosis performed manually (11 patients) or mechanically but with a small-sized cartridge (two patients). A surgical plasty or endoscopic dilatations of the anastomosis relieved this symptom in all patients. In one other patient experiencing early postoperative dysphagia, reoperation documented an ischemic colitis that warranted a Gavriliu procedure. The final functional results in this patient were good. In two other patients, dysphagia was not related to a stenosis but to kinking of the coloplasty or to its obstruction by a bezoar. These patients were not reoperated.

Biliary or gastric reflux within the graft was not infrequent (60%) in the early postoperative period. The reflux was incapacitating in six patients and three with alkaline reflux through a jejunocolic anastomosis required a reoperation (total duodenal diversion, 9; lower colic anastomosis on a Roux-en-Y jejunal loop, 1). Reflux occurred irrespective of whether the graft was isoperistaltic or whether an antireflux procedure had been associated, although the number of patients is too small for reliable comparision.

Finally, one patient experienced a perforation of the colon probably from a medical tablet retained within a redundant portion of the graft. Most patients experienced an increase in weight postoperatively although most did not reach their basal level.

Discussion

This series allows some conclusions. The interposition can be done in most cases with an isoperistaltic segment of transverse colon vascularized by the left colic artery. The proximal dissection and ligation of the right or midcolic vessels seemed absolutely necessary. The operative mortality is low when the patient's condition is fair.

The fistula rate might be reduced by the use of staplers but it doesn't seem possible in Western countries to reach the results of Asia. We do not use preoperative arteriography, advocated by others,[15,16] because the assessment of arteries after clamping and the venous drainage are, in our opinion, much more important than the vessel size.

For benign disease, we had many immediate complications which occurred in most cases in patients for whom a thoracotomy was performed in order to remove the esophagus. According to the patients' assertions, late results were acceptable. Actually, our long-term results are quite similar with gastric esophagoplasty.[6] Some complications as redundancy, are specific to colon interposition but might be diminished by some technical modifications.[2] Finally, these patients had great difficulty swallowing before the operation; therefore, the subjective postoperative course may be biased. In this series, biliary (pain, colitis) or acid (ulceration) reflux in the colon was sometimes a significant complaint. We advocate, with a colon graft, performing a vagotomy, an antireflux procedure, and, if the stomach is removed, an anastomosis to a Roux-en-Y jejunal loop.[14]

We believe, as others do, that for carcinoma, the usual poor prognosis does not justify a procedure responsible for a longer in-hospital stay. Our pulmonary complication rate (43%) in this group of patients was incompatible with a safe outcome.

These results suggest that after colon interposition: (1) mortality and morbidity are very high in patients with malignant disease, especially in case of bypass; (2) the operative risk is low in patients with benign disease, and is mainly related to the associated resection of the esophagus; (3) long-term functional results are perfect in 59% of the patients with benign disease of the esophagus; and (4) reflux into the coloplasty can become incapacitating. According to our experience, a long segment interposition of colon does not fare better, functionally or clinically, than gastric interposition.

References

1. Solauri J: Colonic interposition for benign esophageal disease. Am J Surg 155:498, 1988.
2. DeMeester TR, Johansson KE, Franze I, et al: Indications, surgical technique, and long-erm functional results of colon interposition or bypass. Ann Surg 208:460, 1988.
3. Skinner DB: Esophageal reconstruction. Am J Surg 139:810, 1980.
4. Akiyama H, Hiyama M: A simple esophageal bypass operation by the high gastric division. Surgery 75:674, 1974.
5. Ellis F: Esophagogastrectomy for carcinoma: Technical consideration based on anatomic location of lesion. Surg Clin North Am 60:265, 1980.
6. Fekete F, Gayet B, Favas A, et al: Indications et résultats du traitement chirurgical du cancer de l'oesophage thoracique. Ann Chir 3:185, 1988.
7. Akiyama H, Tsurumaru M, Watanabe G, et al: Development of surgery for carcinoma of the esophagus. Am J Surg 147:9, 1984.
8. Lorentz T, Fok M, Wong J: Anastomotic leakage after resection and bypass for esophageal cancer: Lessons learned from the past. World J Surg 13:472, 1989.
9. Goldsmith HS, Akiyama H: A comparative study of Japanese and American gastric dimensions. Ann Surg 190:690, 1979.
10. Koskas F, Gayet B: Anatomical study of 70 retrosternal gastric esophagoplasties. Anat Clin 7:237, 1985.
11. Postlethwait RW: Colonic interposition for esophageal substitution. Surg Gynecol Obstet 156:377, 1983.
12. Belsey RW: Reconstruction of the esophagus. Ann Royal Col Surg Engl 65:360, 1983.
13. Glasgow JC, Cannon JP, Elkins RC: Colon interposition for benign esophageal disease. Am J Surg 137:175, 1979.
14. Fekete F, Hugentobler JP, Breil P: Ulcères anastomotiques des esophagoplasties coliques. Ann Chir 36:334, 1982.

15. Wilkins EW Jr: Long-segment colon substitution for the esophagus. Ann Surg 192:722, 1980.
16. Ventemiglia R, Khalil KG, Frazier OH, et al: The role of preoperative mesenteric arteriography in colon interposition. J Thorac Cardiovasc Surg 74:98, 1977.

Index